THE LUNG BLOCK

HISTORY OF THE URBAN ENVIRONMENT

MARTIN V. MELOSI AND JOEL A. TARR, EDITORS

THE
LUNG BLOCK

PLAGUES, PARKS, AND POWER
IN PROGRESSIVE ERA NEW YORK

ADRIENNE D. DeNOYELLES

UNIVERSITY OF PITTSBURGH PRESS

Published by the University of Pittsburgh Press, Pittsburgh, Pa., 15260
Copyright © 2024, University of Pittsburgh Press
Manufactured in the United States of America
Printed on acid-free paper
10 9 8 7 6 5 4 3 2 1

Cataloging-in-Publication data is available from the Library of Congress

ISBN 13: 978-0-8229-4786-8
ISBN 10: 0-8229-4786-2

Cover art: 4044-1 Cherry St. looking west from Market St., New York City.
Fred F. French Companies Record, Manuscripts and Archives Division, New
York Public Library. Disease map from the Tenement House Exhibition
showing the block bounded by Cherry, Catherine, Hamilton, and Market
streets. Collection of the New-York Historical Society.

Cover design: Melissa Dias-Mandoly

In memory of Leon Hernandez, my great-grandfather, an immigrant New Yorker who died of tuberculosis in a tenement at the age of twenty-five. To him, to so many others who met the same cruel and untimely end generations ago, and to the 1.5 million still dying of tuberculosis every year all over the world, this book is sincerely dedicated.

CONTENTS

ACKNOWLEDGMENTS

Just as it takes a village to raise a child, so the conventional wisdom goes, the same can be said for this book. This analogy is especially apt, given that the timeline for producing said book wound up paralleling my daughter's journey to adulthood almost exactly. Throughout this prolonged, messy, and ultimately rewarding creative process, encouragement at key moments proved absolutely critical for channeling my curiosity about the Lung Block story into book form. To my deep and lasting regret, I cannot recall the name of the public librarian in Alachua County, Florida, who processed my first of many interlibrary loan requests, but my gratitude for the way her enthusiasm sustained me through the project's vulnerable early stages will stay with me always. I'm likewise grateful to architectural historian and consummate New Yorker Andrew Alpern for his valuable time, perspective, and materials from his extensive holdings, but most of all for taking my interest in New York City history seriously before I had any institutions or credentials to vouch for me.

Working with a dynamic and multitalented group of scholars at the University of Florida, my Lung Block study blossomed. Here I am indebted to Jeffrey Adler, Joseph Spillane, Mitchell Hart, Jack Davis, Pamela Gilbert, and Judith Walzer Leavitt, for their valuable clarity and contributions; and Sheryl Kroen and Nina Caputo, for their keen interest and confidence in my abilities. My debts extend beyond this immediate circle to a wider community of scholars, Alan Kraut, Howard Markel, Edward O'Donnell, Emily Abel, and Bonnie Yochelson figuring prominently among them. Josh Shanholtzer and the editorial and production staff at the University of Pittsburgh Press deftly guided my project through its final stages into the book you are reading now.

As my research angles gained definition, a small-but-mighty archival army emerged to supply me with steady streams of boxes, folders, digital copies, and inspiration. Here, I wish to thank Tal Nadan, from the New York Public Library; Sydney Van Nort and Jane Madembo, from the City College of

ACKNOWLEDGMENTS

New York Archives; Tom McCutcheon, Tara Craig, and Thai Jones, from the Columbia University Rare Book and Manuscript Library; Jeanne Abrams and Thyria Wilson, from the Jewish Consumptive Relief Society Archives at the University of Denver; Kate Feighery, from the Archives of the Archdiocese of the City of New York; Kenneth Cobb and Dwight Johnson, from the New York City Municipal Archives; Mariam Touba, from the New-York Historical Society; and Paul Mercer, from the New York State Archives. These research expeditions were funded through grants awarded by the University of Florida's Department of History, Graduate School, College of Liberal Arts and Sciences, and Center for Humanities and the Public Sphere.

Crowded as this book's village is getting, it would not be complete without the good cheer and forbearance of people outside the academy who helped me navigate all of this project's seemingly interminable stages. First among these is Edward Klein, who listened patiently for hours and years as I mulled over possibilities, fumed over dead ends, puzzled over what to do next, and agonized over whether or not the project would ever reach a favorable conclusion. If I can be said to have "birthed" this book, his was the face closest to mine in the delivery room, his hand always nearby to squeeze as the contractions intensified. Next comes Magdala Klein, for her grace in tolerating an exceedingly demanding and obnoxious brain-sibling for most of her conscious life. Just outside this tight familial core stretches a network of rock-solid friends who grounded me in coffee chats and park playdates, dispelled my writing-induced fogs with memorable road trips, hoisted cocktails regularly with me over Zoom, and encouraged me to laugh at myself when I needed it, which was often. To Jennifer Spillane, Michael Joseph, Elizabeth Richey, Jennifer Dunn, Louise Hamlin, and Jill Nilles, I offer heartfelt thanks for the light and oxygen they pumped into the stale air and dark rooms that engulfed me mentally while I was researching and writing this book. Whether or not the final product made all these villagers' efforts worth it, I will let them—and you—be the judge.

THE LUNG BLOCK

INTRODUCTION

On October 10, 1933, camera bulbs flashed and thousands of New Yorkers cheered as former governor Al Smith wielded a sledgehammer in front of 164 Cherry Street. The first in a block of aging Lower East Side tenements slated for demolition, it would soon make way for clean, modern apartment buildings that offered middle-class tenants a shorter commute to their office jobs downtown. Smith, a onetime Lower East Sider himself, was standing just a short walk from his childhood home on South Street when he hailed "a new chapter in the movement to provide modern housing to replace slum buildings."[1]

While demolition was a common enough sight in Manhattan, the slum facing the wrecking ball that day was no ordinary slum. This was the "Lung Block," a working-class immigrant neighborhood notorious for its high tuberculosis mortality. Two blocks inland from the East River, bounded by Cherry, Catherine, Hamilton, and Market Streets, it had persisted in the public eye as an unsavory intersection of poverty, dissipation, and disease. When Smith's sledgehammer came down on the old, ramshackle tenement, it struck a blow against the overcrowded squalor and misery that for decades had defined the immigrant experience for New York and other large American cities.

In actuality, the "new chapter" that Smith ushered forth had been decades in the writing. In 1903 a Progressive Era coalition launched its own campaign to replace the neighborhood bounded by Cherry, Catherine, Hamilton, and Market Streets with a park. Despite the activists' collective expertise, arsenal of facts, and widespread support from newspapers and well-known public figures, the park failed to materialize—a reform setback absent from most American urban histories.[2] Likewise, standard survey-course textbooks tend to highlight social activism's successes from this period: "watchdog" federal agencies, public parks, labor and housing legislation, and social work organizations. Against these prevalent patterns, the failed park campaign of 1903 reveals a more richly nuanced picture of Progressive Era social activists in moments of conflict and resistance. How did these individuals and groups react to challenges exposing their limitations, or respond to public critiques of their motives and methods? How accurately do these responses-under-fire reflect the image of humanitarian, right-thinking, and determined civic crusaders that filled their own memoirs and subsequent histories?

To answer these questions, I trace the park campaign's rise and fall through the diverse, yet interconnected perspectives of people and interests shaping it. Hermann Biggs, chief bacteriologist for New York City's Department of Health, represented the intersection of germ theory and expanding government oversight that enabled this neighborhood to emerge as a public menace. Biggs's disease maps provided powerful ammunition for housing reformer Lawrence Veiller and his allies in the Charity Organization Society of the City of New York (COSCNY), who pursued tighter housing regulations and the speedy removal of "infected" buildings through slum-clearance projects. Biggs's maps also supplied Jacob Riis and other park advocates with a rationale for replacing slums with green spaces that provided "lungs" for the city's social body. Working together through the COSCNY's Committee on the Prevention of Tuberculosis (CPT), these public health, housing, and parks activists wielded information to galvanize support for rearranging working-class spaces. They appealed to New Yorkers' sensibilities through the tables and analysis of CPT statistician Lilian Brandt, which outlined the demographic risk categories for tuberculosis with seemingly impartial professionalism. They also appealed to New Yorkers' fears through the vivid imagery of muckraker Ernest Poole, which cemented the association of the the "Lung Block" neighborhood with irredeemable physical and moral contamination. As the campaign picked up momentum, Father James Curry, a local Catholic priest, rejected park supporters as professional do-gooders who placed their aesthetic preferences above his parishioners' desperate need for housing. His outspoken opposition promoted an alternate view of Progressive Era social activism as intrusive, predatory, and detrimental to New York working-class immigrant communities.

Taken together, these perspectives form a story of contested space that illuminates significant class and cultural tensions between reform-minded park supporters and the marginalized populations they aimed to help. Park supporters' preoccupation with germs, mapping, and statistics yielded abstracted and pathological views of the neighborhood that did not reflect the experiences of the people living there. Firmly focused on long-term urban-planning objectives, these supporters remained indifferent toward the immediate humanitarian crisis that their project would unleash on a thousand displaced families. Their refusal to consider less drastic alternatives rendered the park campaign vulnerable to criticism from local political and religious figures, who promoted an unflattering counterimage of reformers as cold, impractical elitists. Following city leaders' tabling of the project, park supporters bypassed opportunities for self-reflection to lash out bitterly against their opponents: one more example of the narrow, uncompromising approach that undermined not only their own park campaign but arguably the broader New York City reform movement.

While historians have long been aware of the class and cultural tensions that accompanied Progressive Era activism, they have discussed and explored them to varying degrees.[3] Public health historians have made significant headway over the past thirty years by showing how changing demographics, combined with changing conceptualizations of disease, brought out these tensions in specific times and places.[4] Spatialization has emerged as a strong theme in some of these works, particularly with respect to how changing demographics combined with changing conceptualizations of disease to influence the production of space.[5] In establishing space as the common denominator between reform-minded proponents and ethnically based opponents of the park project, this study enables us to examine more closely the gulf between their perspectives as they envisioned the same piece of land very differently.[6]

Maintaining a tight focus on one conflict from start to finish, as I do in this study, affords an opportunity to dig beyond commonplace observations about Progressive Era social policing by showing exactly how the process unfolded. I show how the effort to claim and transform this tenement neighborhood began in abstracts: pathologizing tenement buildings and people with disease maps; using powerful but unsubstantiated terms such as "infected houses," "city wildernesses," "Lung Block" to frame the problem, and "breathing spaces" to promote solutions. I then show how these abstracted methods laid the groundwork for contesting the space in three-dimensional reality, arming activists with the scientific knowledge they needed to advocate replacing the neighborhood with a park. Likewise, maintaining a tight focus on one campaign from start to finish enables us to see how activists' strategies affected a specific community: what happened when new and sinister meanings became imposed upon the space that working-class immigrants occupied and moved through every day, and the threats that reform activity posed to political and religious leaders.

What emerges from these clashing perspectives is not just a story of tuberculosis and contested spaces but a story of how tuberculosis provided the driving catalyst and the medium for contesting citizenship, which linked directly to power. Who determines a space's character and purpose: those who occupy it, those who own it, those who regulate it, or those who study it from an (ostensibly) objective distance? At what point must the individual's or community's right to forge their own identity, assess their own needs, and solve their own problems yield to a greater public good, and who determines that point? If space figures prominently in the production of knowledge—if the literal spaces we occupy convey meanings about our relative power in society, as poststructural theorists have long argued—how do contested spaces like the Lung Block present opportunities to examine the intentions of well-heeled, Progressive Era urban reformers toward the working-class immigrant populations they aimed to influence?[7] Likewise, how do these contested spaces present opportunities to examine how these reformers and their intentions were received in the tenement districts?

The conflicts in the Lung Block park campaign of 1903 went beyond tuberculosis or diseased houses to illuminate competing visions of what American cities—and city dwellers—should look and act like. As such, they provide a portal into the concerns driving early twentieth-century experts in immigration, public health, social reform, and urban planning—topics that rarely occupy the same frame in American histories. A forerunner of urban renewal, this campaign highlights the need for balancing the broad vision of community improvement projects with working-class priorities and cultural identities. This is a timely message for twenty-first-century America, where gentrification of working-class urban neighborhoods, and growing social discontentment expressed through the Occupy and Black Lives Matter movements, demonstrate how space functions as a sociocultural battleground. As a deadly pandemic once again compels Americans to reassess how they occupy and navigate space, the *Lung Block* offers a reminder to conduct such reassessments as inclusively as possible. The term *social distancing* did not exist in the 1900s, yet it resembles closely what urban reformers sought to enforce in crowded tenement neighborhoods through tightened housing codes and outdoor "breathing spaces." Then as now, socially conscious elites asserted their educational and moral qualifications for directing other people's spatial movements; then as now, reactionary critics interpreted such directives as veiled acts of class aggression. In modern-day America, where contested meanings of "progressive" and "reform" complicate our efforts to improve public health and welfare, the *Lung Block* highlights the need for solutions to our social problems that transcend our divisions, rather than reinforce them.

A NOTE ON TERMINOLOGY

While including now-problematic terms like "infected houses," "city wildernesses," and "breathing spaces" is necessary for discussing the mindsets and methods behind the Lung Block campaign, I have attempted to maintain a degree of detachment from them in the text, often through the use of quotation marks. This reflects my conviction that to do otherwise risks neutralizing the class and cultural biases of the park advocates who framed urban problems in these powerfully loaded metaphors more than a century ago. What one faction of New Yorkers reviled as "city wildernesses," another experienced as working-class immigrant homes and neighborhoods. Similarly, where park proponents saw untapped potential for "breathing spaces," park opponents saw wholesale evictions and communities ripped apart. Relying too heavily and uncritically on these phrases, therefore, risks obscuring the wholesale disruption that urban reformers' visions exacted on the human beings and communities inhabiting these "city wildernesses."

The term "Lung Block" is especially challenging in this regard in that it embodies too many different meanings in different contexts for punctuation to fully capture. In stark contrast to longstanding, popular New York City–area nicknames like Mulberry Bend or Hell's Kitchen, the "Lung Block" would have been neither recognized nor accepted by the residents of Cherry, Catherine, Hamilton and Market Streets. The Lung Block was an idea, or cluster of ideas, projected by urban reformers onto a physical space in order to claim it for their own purposes. When using this term as a geographic reference, or to invoke broader metaphors for urban contamination, as contemporary outsiders often did during and after the park campaign, I do not lose sight of its devastating and deliberate impact as a public relations weapon.

Chapter 1

"TO ROB CONSUMPTION OF ITS TERRORS"

Germ Theory, Hermann Biggs, and the "New" Tuberculosis

Of all the neighborhoods in early twentieth-century New York City, how did a four-acre parcel bounded by Cherry, Catherine, Hamilton, and Market Streets become recognized as a locus of tuberculosis infection? The answer, in part, rests upon two major scientific and medical developments that unfolded through the late nineteenth century: the advent of germ theory, which redefined tuberculosis as a bacterial, and potentially preventable, threat to public safety; and the corresponding rise of public health agencies, with their increasingly sophisticated and aggressive methods of intervention. In New York City—as in other large and well-established American cities during this period—these developments took shape against an inhospitable backdrop of municipal instability and corruption, as well as fierce resistance from within the medical community.[1]

A key figure standing at the nexus of these developments was Hermann Biggs, an ambitious New York City bacteriologist and public health administrator whose generation represented a dramatic break with nineteenth-century sanitarians and clinical observers. Having quickly grasped the significance of European microbiological breakthroughs and their implications for infectious disease prevention in America, Biggs spent much of his early career promoting the utility of the bacteriological laboratory through well-organized campaigns against cholera, diphtheria, and tuberculosis. Over the course of these campaigns, New York City's public health services expanded to include educating the community, analyzing culture specimens, manufacturing and distributing vaccines and antitoxins, examining schoolchildren, and closely monitoring the spread of infectious diseases. In later decades, Biggs's colleagues would praise these efforts to apply scientific advances to practical ends, bringing "bacteriology to the people."[2]

Biggs's success in converting bacteriological discoveries into public policy rested upon not just his professional expertise but also his talent for cultivating goodwill among municipal leaders, medical professionals, and the public.[3] For much of the twentieth century, historians attributed Biggs's tireless promotion of public health objectives to selfless, visionary civic ideals; recent scholars have approached his work more skeptically, emphasizing both his political shrewdness and the fact that his public health campaigns also advanced his own professional ambitions.[4] In this chapter, which places Biggs's antituberculosis efforts within the broader context of his medical training and early career, I argue that his efforts reflected the evangelical zeal of up-and-coming public health workers who now viewed infectious diseases as preventable—and subsequent deaths from these diseases to be morally inexcusable. In striving to alert political leaders, medical colleagues, and the public to the newfound dangers of tuberculosis, Biggs relied on biased surveillance and data-gathering methods that invariably aligned contagion with working-class populations and neighborhoods. When these methods revealed an alarming cluster of tuberculosis cases on Cherry, Catherine, Hamilton, and Market Streets, Biggs began including the block in his lectures and publications as a powerful argument for expanding the powers of public health in American cities: a promotional strategy that redefined the neighborhood as a "plague spot" requiring expert intervention.

FROM CONSUMPTION TO TUBERCULOSIS

Tuberculosis, as we know it today, is an airborne bacterial infection primarily targeting the lungs. Among healthy people, the immune system acts to "wall off" the bacteria by encasing them in lung tissue (tubercles). The bacteria can remain dormant indefinitely inside these tubercles, permitting their human hosts to lead active and productive lives. Among immunologically compromised people, the bacteria can breach these tubercles and begin spreading throughout the rest of the lungs and body. The course of active tuberculosis includes fever, night sweats, fatigue, diminished appetite, and internal hemorrhaging as the patient starts coughing up blood. In the days before the bacterial cause was known, people defined the disease in terms of its most common and visible effects. These effects, chiefly —paleness and emaciation, formed the basis of the disease's earlier names: phthisis, a Greek term meaning "to waste away"; consumption, which captured impressions of the illness consuming the victim from within; and the Great White Plague.[5]

Tuberculosis constituted the biggest killer in industrialized countries during the nineteenth century, most notably among people in their working and reproductive years.[6] It was believed to have infected between 70 and 90 percent of urban Europe and North America by the late nineteenth century, and accounted for one-seventh to one-quarter of all deaths: more than ninety-one thousand in 1880.[7] Yet until Robert Koch discovered the bacteria that caused tuberculosis in 1882, Europeans and Americans alike regarded the disease with little trepidation. The endemic nature of the disease across all classes of society, and its slow, gradual course in most active cases, conferred a dignified respectability upon consumption that contrasted favorably with fast-moving, "dirty" killers such as cholera or dysentery. "We have become so accustomed to [consumption]," lamented T. Mitchell Prudden, a bacteriologist and future associate of Biggs at the New York City Department of Health (NYCDOH), "that it is taken as a matter of course—one of the inevitable ills of life."[8]

In art, fashion, opera, and literature, the pale skin, flushed cheeks, and wasted physique of the consumptive embodied the gothic romanticism of the period, which assigned a redemptive, even transcendent quality to suffering and early death. As the material body wasted away, people believed that spiritual purification was taking place, liberating the individual's genius and creativity. Even the clinical descriptions in nineteenth-century medical textbooks conflated consumption with a fragile, translucent beauty and uncommon intelligence. One example from 1884 described the consumptive look as "tall, slim, erect, delicate looking," with "a pretty oval face, a clear complexion, bright eyes and large pupils"; the patient's skin was "very thin, soft and delicate," revealing the bluish veins underneath; the hair was "fine and silky, often light, the eyelashes being long." Consumptive types "cut their teeth early, and are generally precocious and clever, walking and talking soon. They are excitable and active in body and mind."[9]

Germ theory, a result of the efforts of Koch, Louis Pasteur, and other European scientists to forge direct connections between specific diseases and microorganisms, introduced a gradual shift in how people viewed the disease.[10] *Phthisis* and *consumption* were gradually replaced by *tuberculosis*, a term that conveyed microbial menace rather than romantic effect. The cultural allure of consumption began declining among middle-class Americans, in favor of a hearty athleticism promoted through cycling, tennis, the scout movement, and other forms of active, outdoor recreation.[11] For medical professionals, successfully diagnosing tuberculosis no longer required a thorough, intimate knowledge of the patient and his or her family and lifestyle; now it required only the presence of the bacillus, for which doctors needed access to cultures, microscopes, and other tools found only in laboratories.[12] These developments strengthened the authority of bacteriology and the public health establishment while at the same time accentuating generational and class divisions within the late nineteenth-century American medical community. At this critical juncture when medicine was completing the transition from trade to profession, younger, university-trained professionals shared the field with older, provincial healers who had acquired their education and credentials through on-the-job experience. This distinction mattered little throughout much of the nineteenth century, given the substandard quality of medical education as a rule.[13] One of Biggs's contemporaries in New England, William T. Sedgwick, recalled his medical training with a mixture of disdain and bemusement. "Even our best medical schools welcomed without any educational requirements whatsoever all students who could pay," he stated, adding that a standard degree reflected a year's worth of lectures, "the only laboratory . . . being the dissecting room."[14]

For Sedgwick and other young medical professionals, germ theory marked the true beginning of their professional training. "Before 1880 we knew nothing," Sedgwick declared. "After 1890, we knew it all; it was a glorious ten years."[15] During this brief span, dozens of feared and familiar maladies became detectable not just through their effects on human beings but by the microbial agents causing them: *Mycobacterium tuberculosis* (tuberculosis), *Vibrio cholerae* (cholera), *Corynebacterium diphtheriae* (diphtheria), *Salmonella Typhi* (typhoid fever), and *Streptococcus pyogenes* (scarlet fever).[16] With each new bacteriological discovery, the field of medicine transformed further from complex and uncertain clinical terrain into a hunting ground with clearly defined targets: a development that germ theory enthusiasts hailed as nothing short of miraculous. "The mysterious veil which has for so long hung over some of the most widespread and terrible of human diseases is gradually being drawn aside," Prudden rejoiced, revealing "particulate beings . . . things which we can see and handle and kill."[17]" Renowned pathologist Woods Hutchinson recalled decades later, "Our foe had come down out of the clouds and was spread out in battle array before us."[18]

HERMANN BIGGS, BACTERIOLOGY, AND THE PROFESSIONALIZATION OF MEDICINE

This dynamic decade of scientific advances and medical professionalization had profound influences on Hermann Biggs's professional training and career. Born in the industrial village of Trumansburg, New York, in 1859, Biggs hailed from a line of prosperous, old-stock merchants and manufacturers.[19] His active mind, coupled with a delicate physical constitution, helped mold the personality traits that later served him well as a public health administrator: patience, persistence, pragmatism with compromising and delegating tasks, and an understated charm that nevertheless exerted a powerful influence on people around him. Biggs "was never the least pushing nor self-assertive," recalled an old college friend; "nevertheless, he had the peculiar quality of making his presence felt . . . one always knew when he entered a room or any small assembly. And when any subject was under discussion, one instinctively turned to him for his opinion, which nine times out of ten was taken as final."[20]

Biggs followed Koch's research closely during his undergraduate years at

Cornell in the early 1880s, hailing the tuberculosis bacillus as "the grandest discovery of the age."[21] Later, at Bellevue Medical College in New York City, he witnessed firsthand the generational rift that germ theory wrought among faculty members. Biggs gravitated toward William T. Welch, a young professor recently returned from Europe who, along with Prudden, offered some of the first bacteriology classes in the United States.[22] Many of Welch's senior colleagues still viewed germ theory with skepticism, some dismissing it outright as an unsubstantiated hoax. "People say there are bacteria in the air, but I cannot see them," Bellevue professor Alfred L. Loomis once quipped to a tittering lecture hall of medical students—several of Welch's protégés among them.[23]

While most late nineteenth-century critics of germ theory no longer disputed the existence of bacteria, or the correlation of specific bacteria with specific diseases, accepting a direct causal link between microorganisms and disease was neither smooth nor automatic.[24] Their wariness toward "bacteriomania" stemmed from an impulse to defend not only their authority and expertise but also the validity of their own experiences with sickness and healing.[25] For clinicians who were accustomed to considering a host of variables before arriving at a diagnosis, focusing exclusively on microbes must have appeared appallingly reductionist—a shortsighted and reckless disregard for observation skills honed over centuries of practice.[26] By the same token, germ theory proponents dismissed clinicians' abilities as dangerously limited without a working knowledge of bacteriology. "The doctor who is ignorant on the subject is greatly handicapped from a practical standpoint," noted one editorial in a pioneering bacteriological journal; "a physician without a microscope," declared another commentator, "is like a man without eyes."[27] Within the next few years, Loomis and likeminded skeptics would move toward a cautious, measured acceptance of germ theory in their public statements; during Biggs's brief training at Bellevue, however, Welch and Loomis represented the medical profession's past and future competing side by side.[28]

BIGGS AND PUBLIC HEALTH IN NEW YORK CITY

Biggs cast his lot firmly with the bacterial revolution. After completing his undergraduate degree and medical training in only three and a half years, he joined a growing pilgrimage of American medical professionals to Germany for a firsthand look at the bacteriological research occurring there.[29] Many of these sojourners returned to help lead the bacteriology laboratories emerging among medical schools, universities, hospitals, and health departments. Biggs was among the first of these, taking control of Bellevue Hospital's bacteriology laboratory by 1886, at which point, by his own admission, "there was practically no bacteriological work being done in this country."[30]

By the early 1890s Biggs was working at the NYCDOH, one of the first municipal public health agencies to employ the "new science" against a wide array of contaminants lurking in food, water, and populations.[31] Its brand-new bacteriology laboratory had grown out of the cholera pandemic that threatened New Yorkers in 1892. By culturing bacteria from sick passengers aboard detained immigrant vessels, Biggs and his fellow bacteriologists confirmed that the passengers suffered from the same cholera strain ravaging Europe. Armed with this information, city officials moved quickly to disinfect and quarantine most of the passengers on a nearby island until the danger of contagion had passed. Of the 141 deaths resulting from the cholera outbreak, only nine took place within the city itself—an outcome that Biggs credited to the superior speed and accuracy of laboratory science over clinical observation methods.[32]

While Biggs and his laboratory received credit for helping New Yorkers avert a major public health crisis, the relative infrequency of cholera outbreaks meant that he would have to broaden the laboratory's objectives to ensure its long-term survival. New York's health department, like those of many other late nineteenth-century American cities, was overseen by a municipally appointed board of laypeople—often prominent businessmen whose priorities reflected those of the political party in power. In the early 1890s this power emanated from Tammany Hall, the city's largest democratic party. Controlled by boss Richard Croker, the party drew the bulk of its strength from the ever-growing immigrant population. In exchange for votes, an elaborate, far-reaching chain of command provided working-class newcomers with staples like food and coal, financial assistance in times of trouble, and access to steady jobs. In an era before these vital services became embedded formally within government agencies, funding usually came from graft: bribes that saloons, brothels, and other businesses paid to city inspectors and law enforcement in order to continue operating illegally. When mayoral administrations changed, so did the makeup of the city's workforce, as victorious candidates sought to reward their supporters with a place on the public payroll. This system of patronage, applied to the health department, sometimes resulted in skilled and seasoned professionals being pressured to move aside for less qualified people whose political connections outweighed theirs.[33]

To shield his laboratory from changing political fortunes, Biggs employed a combination of effective results, shrewd networking, and successful publicity campaigns.[34] After the cholera scare subsided, Biggs turned his attention to diphtheria, a common bacterial infection that killed more than a thousand New Yorkers each year in the 1890s. Biggs's campaign was threefold: offering free diphtheria screenings to physicians; tracking the spread of cases through disease maps and placards displayed in patients' homes; and adminis-

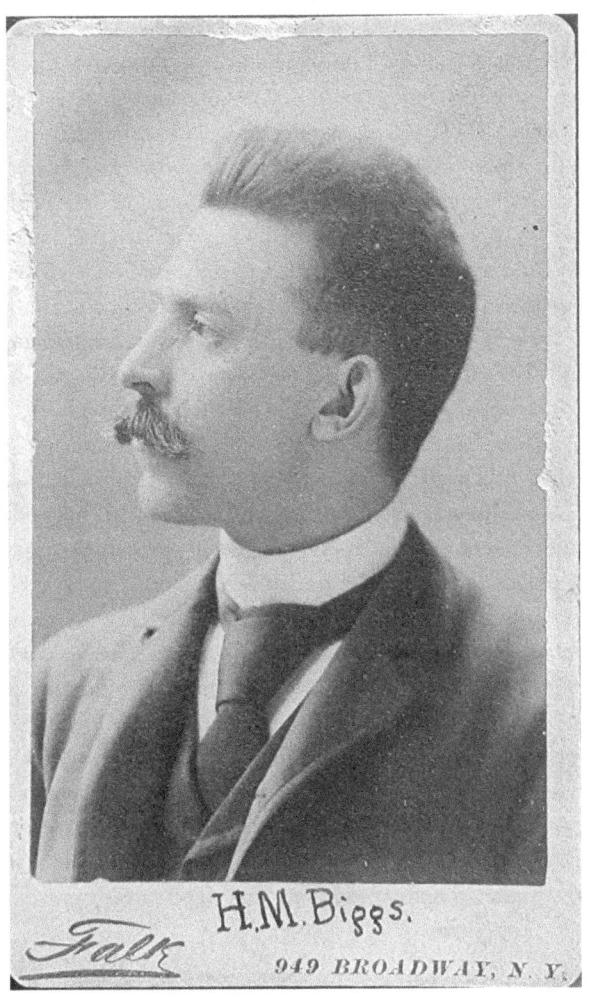

1.1. Hermann Biggs. Portrait taken by New York photographer Benjamin Falk, ca. 1880s. Photograph held in the collection of the author.

tering antitoxin, a recent European breakthrough that increased a diphtheria patient's chances of recovery if given in the early stages.[35] If cholera broke the ground for New York's municipal bacteriological laboratory, Biggs credited diphtheria with laying the foundations.[36] In 1896 his laboratory examined twenty-five thousand cultures for diphtheria, manufactured and distributed seventeen thousand vials of antitoxin, and performed countless house inspections and disinfections. These staggering numbers required larger facilities and a larger staff, which now included "25 physicians, 1 chemist, and 2 veterinarians, in addition to clerical and laboratory assistants and attendants."[37]

The fact that Biggs's diphtheria program experienced this rapid growth through a rapid succession of Tammany and anti-Tammany administrations reflects his aptitude for gaining the confidence of people in power, regardless of political affiliation.[38] "He was an excellent judge of human nature," remarked one of his associates, "and frequently seemed to know men better than they knew themselves."[39] Much of the program's success also stemmed from Biggs's initiative and willingness to take risks. Unwilling to wait until the city apportioned its next budget, Biggs secured much of the initial funding for producing diphtheria antitoxin through private donors. He then solicited public support through the New York *Herald*, which responded with a fundraising campaign that convinced city officials of the political expediency of supporting the program.[40] Within four years, Biggs publicly credited his laboratory's diagnostic procedures and antitoxin supply with lowering the city's diphtheria death rate by 40 percent. By then, the laboratory generated enough surplus antitoxin to sell to medical facilities across the country; this provided Biggs with a steady stream of independent funding, further insulating him from the political corruption that plagued his and other health departments during this period.[41]

Biggs's early years in the city health department demonstrated his enthusiasm for bacteriology and laboratory methods, his flair for cultivating the support he needed for his programs, and his belief in the ultimate authority of the public health establishment in preventing disease among New Yorkers.[42] As Biggs's prestige increased, so did the territorial hackles he raised among individual practitioners regarding "whose diagnosis of a private case of sickness is to stand—that of the physician . . . or that of the board whose examiners have made a bacteriological examination in connection with it."[43] Each of these patterns would figure prominently in Biggs's next campaign against a common killer: tuberculosis.

GERM THEORY ON TRIAL

Even though tuberculosis killed more Americans than any other disease during the late nineteenth century, Koch's discovery of the tubercle bacillus made little impact on the American medical community initially. Unlike fast-moving epidemics like cholera, influenza, or smallpox, the selectivity and gradual progression of active tuberculosis discouraged any direct associations with contagion: "In acute diseases," observed Philadelphia physician and antituberculosis pioneer Lawrence Flick, "it is comparatively easy to note the length of time which elapses between exposure and determining symptoms of the disease . . . but in chronic diseases [such as] phthisis, this is no easy matter."[44] Reluctant medical professionals demanded more compelling evidence before breaking with their traditional views of consumption as a product of internal imbalance and disharmony.[45] In the years immediately following Koch's discovery, critics continued to define the tuberculosis bacillus conservatively as a mere accompaniment to "certain deteriorative changes in organic matter . . . possessing no causative relations whatever." Cautioning their colleagues against a "too ready acceptance of the bacillus doctrine," they charged early germ theory proponents with being hasty, overzealous, and naïve, singling out younger pathologists for their "regular fanaticism" in sacrificing scientific method for "imagination and speculation."[46]

Meanwhile, these younger pathologists grew impatient with the reluctance of physicians and politicians to apply recent scientific breakthroughs to saving lives. "The germ theory—now no longer a theory in the case of tubercular consumption—tells us that we have to do with a contagious disease," argued Charles V. Chapin, superintendent of health for Providence, Rhode Island, in 1888. For Chapin and many other early public health crusaders, this now incontrovertible fact placed the power of prevention in human hands. "Now there is no theoretical reason why a purely contagious disease like tuberculosis cannot be exterminated," Chapin declared. "If we can prevent the spread of contagion at all, we can prevent it entirely."[47] Biggs, also convinced that "the most common and fatal disease which prevails in New York is both communicable and preventable," expressed similar frustrations six years later in the popular journal *Forum*. "There can be and is no difference of opinion among those who are conversant with the scientific facts," Biggs argued in his article, titled "To Rob Consumption of Its Terrors." He found particularly irksome the presumption circulating among germ theory detractors that "germs, as active agents in the production and dissemination of disease, really exist only as phantoms in the minds of over-imaginative and impractical bacteriologists."[48]

Biggs launched his campaign against tuberculosis in 1893 using the same multipronged strategy that he had employed successfully against diphtheria: surveillance, education, disinfection, and isolation.[49] To find the number and distribution of tuberculosis cases in the city, he proposed new measures requiring all public institutions to report the names and addresses of consumptive clients to the health department, and requested that private physicians do the same with their own patients. To encourage widespread cooperation, Biggs circulated informational pamphlets, wrote articles for popular publications, and offered physicians free screenings of sputum samples for arriving at a decisive diagnosis.[50]

Physicians responded less enthusiastically to these measures than they had during Biggs's diphtheria campaign, largely because they perceived little to gain from reporting a disease that not only lacked consensus on communicability but also an effective treatment in any case.[51] On the contrary, they perceived much to lose, both for themselves and for their patients. Early antituberculosis campaigns, in their efforts to purge the disease of all prior romantic associations, conveyed a degree of alarmism that effectively stigmatized "consumptives"as menaces to society.[52] This "phthisiophobia," as renowned specialist Sigard Adolphus Knopf once described it, discouraged such people from seeking help for fear of losing their jobs, homes, and relationships.[53] The prolonged and often terminal course of tuberculosis meant that patients endured this stigma indefinitely, making the implications of reporting different from "scarlet fever, diphtheria, and other infectious or contagious diseases which ran a short course," one doctor explained. "When we reported a case of tuberculosis, it was practically for life."[54] Moreover, the fact that many life insurance policies excluded tuberculosis from policyholders' coverage rendered an accurate diagnosis not only scandalous but also financially devastating for their families—and, by extension, their physicians.[55] Anxious to preserve the hopes, confidentiality, and steady business of their consumptive patients, many physicians avoided reaching a firm diagnosis for as long as possible; consequently, they complied with reporting their cases slowly and reluctantly.[56]

PLOTTING PATHOLOGY: BIGGS'S TUBERCULOSIS MAPS

Fully cognizant of his colleagues' skepticism and their reasons for it, Biggs employed a diplomatic blend of education, persuasion, and empirical evidence to gain their support in his speeches and writings on tuberculosis throughout the 1890s. Phrases he used often—"it has been proven without a doubt," "it has been abundantly established," "it has been shown experimentally," "it is a well-known fact," "it has become evident," "there is every reason to believe"— projected scientific authority and confidence in both the communicability of tuberculosis and the rightful place of public health departments at the head of community prevention efforts.[57] Meanwhile, Biggs plotted reported cases on sectional maps that included the block and house where tuberculosis sufferers lived. Biggs took his inspiration from Flick, who had mapped a variety of diseases in an impoverished ward of Philadelphia over twenty-five years. Over time, Flick discovered that tuberculosis cases appeared in clusters "identically the same as that of typhoid fever, smallpox, scarlet fever, and diphtheria," reinforcing the idea that tuberculosis spread only "by contact, by association, or by living in close proximity."[58] Following Flick's example, Biggs intended to drive home in visual terms the extent of tuberculosis's grip on the city. With the support generated from those results, he hoped to extend the reach of his tuberculosis-control program with tougher case-reporting policies and a taxpayer-funded sanitarium for isolating the city's poorest consumptives.

Biggs focused his surveillance efforts on the tenement districts, where tens of thousands of working-class New Yorkers lived in overcrowded rooms

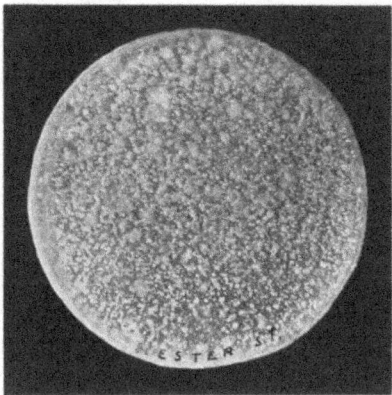 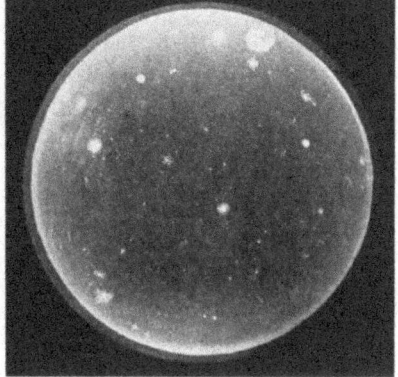

FIG. 18.—Hester Street, New York.   FIG. 19.—Madison Avenue and Sixty sixth Street, New York.

1.2. These photographs, published in a medical textbook from 1906, show the bacterial growth in Petri dishes containing samples from Hester Street on the Lower East Side (left) and a wealthier uptown neighborhood (right). "The former is a very unclean district," John Huber deduced from the comparison; "the latter, very salubrious." Reprinted from John B. Huber, *Consumption: Its Relation to Man and His Civilization* (Philadelphia: J. B. Lippincott, 1906), 83–84.

without sufficient air and sunlight.[59] This selective approach built upon recent experiments that found the tubercule bacillus could survive indefinitely in dark and ill-ventilated environments, which suggested that tenements provided ideal reservoirs for the disease.[60] Biggs's preoccupation with tenement districts also reflected the ongoing reluctance of private physicians to cooperate—a situation that resulted in most reported cases coming from public institutions frequented by the poor.[61] Aware of the skewed nature of his results, Biggs proceeded anyway, eager to make inroads in whatever direction offered the least resistance. "It was not deemed wise at first . . . to make it obligatory for physicians to report cases," he explained to colleagues the following year; by contrast, "it was comparatively easy to obtain reports from public institutions, which would give the most numerous class of patients and those whom it was most important to instruct."[62]

From a logistical perspective, restricting public health oversight to areas believed to contain the largest numbers of cases represented a pragmatic and efficient use of resources. Strategically, it allowed Biggs to pursue his ambitious agenda without arousing the ire of private practitioners and their wealthier patients. In practical terms, this meant that Biggs's early tuberculosis-control efforts depended upon the involuntary participation of consumptives who could not afford to hire their own physicians. While Biggs later admitted to colleagues that such unequal treatment would be "undemocratic,

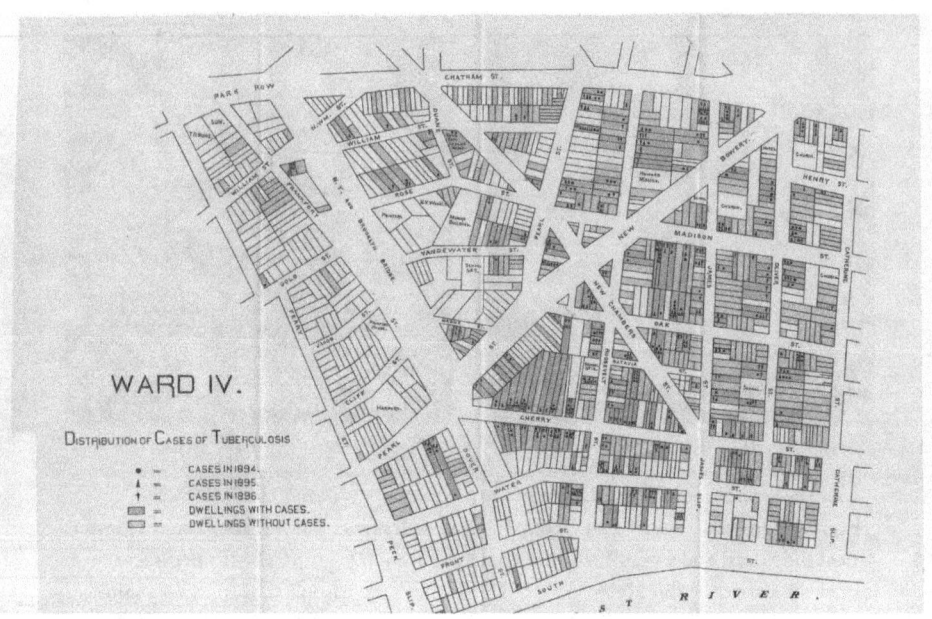

1.3. An early example of a tuberculosis map from New York's Lower East Side, compiled from case reports gathered under the direction of Hermann Biggs, New York City's chief bacteriologist. Each dot represents one tuberculosis death occurring between 1894 and 1899. Reprinted from NYCDOH, *Annual Report of the Board of Health of the Health Department of the City of New York for the Year Ending December 31, 1896* (New York: Martin B. Brown, 1897). Courtesy of the New York City Municipal Library.

and probably illegal" if coded into official policy, he nevertheless maintained that "sanitary authorities may use their discretion . . . depending upon the danger which they conceive exists as far as the public is concerned."[63] In his urgent quest to eliminate needless deaths, Biggs clearly viewed working-class consumptive people as more of a public menace than wealthy ones, and consequently less entitled to having their autonomy and privacy taken into account. Other compulsory notification advocates viewed this dual, class-oriented approach as sensible and fair. "The wealthy are abundantly able to take care of themselves," argued Flick. "The poor are not, and it will be no hardship to them or interference with their private rights to help them to protect those near and dear to them against so fatal a disease."[64]

Within several years, the case dots accumulating on Biggs's maps formed clusters bearing strong resemblances to Flick's in Philadelphia.[65] Skewed data gathering ensured that these clusters appeared only in tenement districts, where "the lowest class of Italians, Irish, Russian Jews, Greeks, [and] Chinese" lived in "overcrowded houses, rear tenements and dilapidated buildings." Biggs's maps, forged in the pre-germ-theory belief that "ignorance, poverty, and filth furnish[ed] a suitable soil for all infectious diseases, as well as tuberculosis," had succeeded in reinforcing that belief using scientific, post-germ-theory methods.[66]

By 1897, when Biggs estimated the number of active tuberculosis cases in New York to be twenty thousand, he felt the time had come for more aggressive tactics. Seizing upon the telltale clusters generated from the disease maps as irrefutable evidence that tuberculosis was contagious, he called for the NYCDOH to "assume a more complete and comprehensive control" over tuberculosis prevention, starting with making case reporting universal and compulsory for all physicians.[67] Representatives from New York's medical community responded swiftly, rejecting compulsory notification of tuberculosis as "mistaken, untimely, irrational, and unwise." Their subsequent complaint—that the health department "had only to declare a disease infectious in order to take charge of it"—reveals their uneasiness about germ theory's power to shape public policy in ways that undermined their own autonomy.[68] Mandatory tuberculosis case reporting introduced additional levels of government oversight into the traditional patient-healer relationship; it also placed public health officials "in the rather equivocal position of dictating to the profession . . . and of creating a suspicion of an extra bid for public applause by unduly magnifying the importance of its bacteriological department."[69] The city's medical societies called upon state legislators to formally restrict the powers of public health officials.[70]

Biggs, using his time-tested approach of education, persuasion, and empirical evidence, overcame this organized resistance to compulsory notification within a matter of months. In prominent medical talks featuring the most heavily case-spotted disease maps, which "argue[d] more forcibly for the infectious and communicable character of this disease than could any words," he defended the NYCDOH's imperative to act against tuberculosis.[71] Meanwhile, his steady assurances of gradual and selective enforcement enabled leaders of New York's leading medical organizations to reach a compromise that left the new compulsory notification policy unchallenged, provided that public health workers continued to apply it gently.[72]

TRANSITIONAL ETIOLOGIES IN TUBERCULOSIS

As Biggs harnessed his tuberculosis maps to promote more aggressive public health policies, the dot clusters forged powerful visual associations between tuberculosis and the structures housing the people infected with it. "Tuberculosis is not uniformly diffused through a community," observed Arthur Guerard, one of Biggs's subordinates who helped compile the maps, in 1896;

instead, it was "confined within . . . certain streets and within the walls of certain houses."[73] Like many tuberculosis experts, Knopf attributed these clusters to a vicious circle of transmission between "careless tuberculous patients [who] have lived for years in these houses," and "the soil on which these houses have been built, or the manner in which they have been constructed . . . [being] of a nature to retain the tuberculous infection indefinitely."[74] Flick, whose block-by-block disease maps of Philadelphia gave rise to the theory originally, also came to envision houses as passive receptacles and incubators of contamination. "Consumption may well be termed a house disease," he declared in 1904; "without the house, it would not exist."[75]

Two critical, related elements fueling the house infection concept were sputum and dust. Prudden explained in 1889, "Thousands of consumptives are walking about the streets . . . who discharge the infectious material coughed up from the lungs upon the pavements or floors. This dries . . . and takes its place among the rest of the floating dust of the air."[76] Many late nineteenth-century tuberculosis specialists believed this dust to be dangerous, citing recent laboratory findings and anecdotal examples in which tuberculosis bacilli remained active in dried sputum for weeks and even months.[77] Some, like Boston physician Edward O. Otis, became preoccupied with people spitting in public places. In 1898, he recalled counting "193 expectorations in less than an eighth of a mile; in another locality where fewer people pass I counted 211 in rather more than that distance."[78] Other experts focused on the dangers that tuberculosis bacilli presented inside the home. In *Dust and Its Dangers*, Prudden speculated on the "living and virulent germs . . . clinging to the walls and furniture and bedding and handkerchiefs of consumptive persons, and in the dust of the rooms in which they dwell."[79]

The perceived pathological dangers of dust and spit began receding in significance by the 1900s, as researchers refined their understanding of how tuberculosis transmission worked.[80] During the 1880s and 1890s, however, sputum and dust provided common ground for sanitarians and germ theory proponents alike. Both groups regarded human bodies as sites of contamination; the germ theory model merely superimposed living bacteria upon the same filth that sanitarians had long associated with disease, ignorance, and weakness of character.[81] Likewise, both groups advocated higher standards of cleanliness and hygiene, which imposed harsh new layers of scientific authority over individual behavior in ways that disproportionately targeted the poor. Convinced that "the sputum alone . . . is the source of danger," Biggs urged New York to outlaw public spitting—the first of many American cities to do so.[82] Although violators of antispitting ordinances hailed from all classes, the poor were least likely to be able to afford a typical fine of two dollars, and thus most likely to go to jail.[83] These new and exacting standards of cleanliness also increased the physical and emotional strain on housekeepers; for tenement dwellers struggling to keep deadly germs at bay in dark, close quarters without running water, the task was difficult if not impossible.[84]

The NYCDOH had multiple opportunities to observe the role of structural deficiencies in "infected houses." Its own Sanitary Bureau, created in 1866 to detect and eliminate public health hazards anywhere in the city, conducted thousands of tenement inspections and disinfections every year.[85] In 1896, Guerard suggested that current public health tactics did not go far enough in tenement houses with multiple cases of tuberculosis. "Such houses would seem to be permanently infected," he observed, citing multiple anecdotal examples of healthy people contracting tuberculosis after moving to a dwelling where multiple cases had already occurred. He advocated their full-scale renovation, "or, better[, that they be] condemned and torn down. They are old houses, in bad sanitary condition, some of them rear tenements, and densely packed with the poorest and filthiest class of people."[86]

This progression from "house infection" to "permanent infection" reflected public health workers' growing awareness of the true scope of the tuberculosis problem. Disinfection measures could wipe out the tubercle bacillus, but not the crowded, substandard living conditions favoring its transmission from person to person. Informational pamphlets and lectures, however expertly presented, still foundered on barriers of language, culture, and education. Isolation proved elusive in a city with few hospital beds set aside for impoverished tuberculosis patients, and an unstable municipal leadership more concerned with dispensing patronage than with building sanitariums.[87] Faced with these limitations, public health leaders began expanding their tuberculosis-prevention campaigns to include broader social and environmental concerns. This shift would bring them into an alliance with the housing reform movement, the growth of which paralleled the rise of public health throughout the 1890s. In the absence of an immediate cure for tuberculosis, both groups agreed that the bacillus needed to be targeted at its source; authoritative, objective-looking statistics and maps, all compiled from tenement districts, ensured that this source would be pictured as squalid, overcrowded slum dwellings.[88]

When viewed within a broader context of late nineteenth-century developments, the concept of lung blocks first emerged from the etiological confusion, political instability, and medical professionalization occurring in large American cities. All three of these trends manifested most visibly in New York. As newly minted bacteriologists pursued the tubercle bacillus in the air, on the street, and inside buildings, they projected new and invisible dangers onto common and familiar patterns of daily life. When communicating these newfound threats to their colleagues and the public, germ theory proponents often fell back upon sanitarian models that linked disease with miasmas, filth, poverty, and moral failings. This engrafting of new knowledge on to older mindsets created favorable conditions for the theories of tuberculous dust and house infection to take shape. By the 1900s several influential public health leaders had begun calling the dangers of dust into question. "We know that the germs themselves are much more rarely air borne than had been thought [previously]," Chapin observed in 1902; he discredited the idea altogether several years later, citing insufficient evidence.[89] The decades immediately preceding this shift constitute a brief window in which the filth and germ theories of disease competed for legitimacy and dominance. During this fluid period of transition, public health agencies began expanding their powers on the belief that tuberculosis could be prevented and even eradicated through education, isolation, and disinfection campaigns of unprecedented scale and scope. These efforts required generous resources, which in turn depended upon the shifting allegiances and priorities of municipal leaders. They also depended upon the cooperation of private physicians, many of whom resisted state-sponsored intervention as a threat to their autonomy and livelihoods. In this unstable and politically charged environment, forging a successful public health career with the city required proficiency in adapting to changing power structures as well as changing technologies.

Hermann Biggs navigated this complicated terrain successfully through a combination of savvy public relations, astute behind-the-scenes diplomacy, and pragmatic willingness to make the most of every opportunity for advancing his agenda. A close examination of Biggs's early career, and his tuberculosis campaign in particular, suggests that his actions stemmed not from personal ambitions but rather from the deep-seated conviction that germ theory constituted a mandate for taking immediate action to save lives. Biggs saw it as only reasonable that the individual autonomy of physicians and patients should begin yielding to the superior knowledge, resources, and coordination of state-funded institutions: a powerful idea grasping hold in all aspects of European as well as American society.[90] "The Government of the United States is democratic, but the sanitary measures adopted are sometimes autocratic," Biggs remarked to members of the British Medical Association in 1897. "We are prepared, when necessary, to introduce and enforce . . . measures which might seem radical and arbitrary, if they were not plainly designed for the public good, and evidently beneficent in their effects."[91]

This notion of the "public good" provided the strong moral imperative behind Biggs's bold and innovative measures against infectious diseases. By the turn of the twentieth century, his efforts had transformed the New York City Department of Health into a model of national and international importance, providing inspiration to European cities and attracting the admiration of Robert Koch himself. "My dear Biggs," Koch told him in 1908, "[while] most bacteriological and serological discoveries have come from Germany . . . we in Germany are years and years behind you in their practical application.

You have done marvelous work!"[92] Throughout his steady rise in power and prestige, Biggs's fundamental personality remained unchanged. "We loved him for himself," recalled a Columbia medical professor who had known Biggs for thirty years, citing "his quiet, modest manner, his freedom from all pretense and self-seeking, and his genuine quality of heart."[93]

The darker, more problematic side of Biggs's legacy stemmed from his notion of "the public good" being universal and absolute. "Once [Biggs] made up his mind," observed his biographer and former colleague, Charles-Edward Winslow, "he moved straight forward and did not desist until he had attained what he had set out to attain, fully and completely . . . [H]e knew he was right and he used the resources of the law wisely but fearlessly."[94] In his quest to eliminate needless deaths, Biggs promoted increased public health oversight as the only reasonable solution; in this characterization, those who did not share his vision acted out of ignorance, error, or stubborn opposition to enlightenment and progress. His singlemindedness manifested repeatedly in his writings, speeches, policies, and fundamentally skewed research, all of which reinforced preconceived associations between pathology and place. By literally mapping disease onto buildings, Biggs reduced brick-and-mortar neighborhoods to two-dimensional symbols of dirt and disorder; by compressing the experiences of lower-class tuberculosis sufferers into uniform, impersonalized dots, he discouraged any further attempts to see and relate to them as individuals.[95] From the late 1890s onward, these dot clusters would assume their own forward momentum, providing housing reformers, settlement workers, and muckraking journalists with a powerfully effective focal point for their own determined crusades to improve society. In the process, they literally blotted out one working-class neighborhood's ability to forge its own collective identity forever. Years after Biggs had died, his legendary status assured, New Yorkers continued to regard the area bounded by Cherry, Catherine, Hamilton and Market Streets as "a black blotch on the tuberculosis map."[96]

Chapter 2

"CITY OF THE LIVING DEATH"

Tuberculosis, Lawrence Veiller, and the Tenement House Commission of 1900

If late nineteenth-century developments in disease etiology and public health forged the link between tuberculosis and crowded tenement neighborhoods, how did that link transform the block bounded by Cherry, Catherine, Hamilton, and Market Streets into a target for social reform campaigns by the early 1900s? The answer rests upon a series of large-scale economic shifts transforming American society and culture. Manufacturing and commerce, both of which expanded dramatically during the Civil War, drew millions away from their traditional agrarian lifestyles to work in urban factories. As industrialization generated enormous wealth for employers and investors, the intensified competition for jobs and housing generated lower wages, higher rents, and substandard living conditions for wage workers and their families. Nowhere were these patterns more prevalent than in 1890s New York, where the number of tenements in Manhattan nearly tripled, from fifteen thousand in the 1860s to forty thousand, and its tenement population from five hundred thousand to 1.8 million—most of them recent immigrants from southern and eastern Europe.[1]

As this skyrocketing growth tested the limits of municipal governments and infrastructures, the tenement became a potent symbol of the dangers that industrialization, immigration, and urbanization posed to traditional American democratic ideals. High rents and low wages, concerned citizens argued, created a permanent underclass who would look to political machines and radical causes for the advancement opportunities denied to them under a free landholding republic. As these voices grew in number and strength over the next decade, tenement spaces descended in public opinion from a substandard home to an anti-home: "a synonym for degradation and unwholesomeness," constituting "a menace to a republican form of government."[2]

Germ theory provided these social critics with a potent metaphor for the threat that tenements represented to their way of life. While varying in specifics, their imagery often suggested a condition that was progressive, debilitating, and fatal: "a social cancer," "blotches of disease upon the civic body," "an evil gnawing at the vitals of the country." Amid these rising concerns, the tuberculosis dots on Hermann Biggs's disease maps encouraged reform-minded activists to reconceptualize tuberculosis from a moral judgment on unworthy individuals to a symptom of larger social ills. Abandoning moral suasion for social-scientific methods, social workers from settlement houses and organized charities banded together to stamp out the "tenement-house evil" from a variety of angles: regulating new construction, improving existing buildings, and clearing the worst slums to create "breathing spaces" in the form of parks and playgrounds.[3]

The man tying these developments together was Lawrence Veiller, a young housing activist whose 1890s settlement work alerted him to the overcrowded, unhealthy conditions in New York tenement districts. His innovative Tenement House Exhibition of 1900 further amplified the associations between tenements and tuberculosis by placing Biggs's arguments and disease maps before a wider audience; the subsequent outcry led to a state commission that lobbied successfully for stricter building and maintenance regulations. In the process, Veiller united social and public health activists in a common cause of eliminating "diseased houses," flagging the block bordered by Cherry, Catherine, Hamilton, and Market Streets as one of several "city wildernesses" demanding immediate intervention.

FORMATIVE INFLUENCES IN VEILLER'S REFORM CAREER

Most accounts of Veiller's career begin with his sudden emergence in New York housing reform circles as a youthful and determined firebrand, armed with an unnerving mastery of municipal housing codes and an eagerness to battle shady builders and their political allies from City Hall to Albany.[4] Historians also tend to present Veiller as being cast from a different mold than other reformers of his generation; even as he pursued humanitarian objectives central to their overall agenda, he did so purportedly from the standpoint of a coolheaded technician, motivated more by a desire for social order and state-dispensed justice than personal stirrings of compassion or altruism.[5] A closer look at Veiller's early career suggests that these deviations from the prototypical reformer—cynicism, preoccupation with restrictive legislation, and pragmatic willingness to work within the corrupt Tammany system—did not constitute hardwired personality attributes but rather strategic responses to setbacks he had encountered while pursuing reform with the same idealism as his comrades. These deviations enabled Veiller to parry more successfully with political and entrepreneurial opponents of housing reform, and achieve concessions where previous generations of social activists had failed.

Born in 1872, Veiller grew up in New Jersey, Chicago, and New York, his childhood backdrop shaped by the boom and bust of his father's entrepreneurial ventures.[6] He was a precocious and highly motivated student, entering the City College of New York and earning multiple academic awards there before graduating at eighteen.[7] From there, he joined the settlement house movement to study and alleviate the effects of immigration and industrialization on working-class urban neighborhoods. Over the next decade, these settlements increased from a handful in Chicago, New York, Philadelphia, and Boston to more than one hundred across the United States.[8]

At the University Settlement on New York's Lower East Side, Veiller joined a community of concerned activists who closely resembled him in many respects: young, single, college educated, and descended from prosperous, US-born Protestant families.[9] Disillusioned by the materialism and social unrest that accompanied the industrialism of the Gilded Age, these activists sought to transcend their insulated upbringings in settings "where all classes of society meet on a common ground."[10] Settlements nevertheless signified upper-class privilege in that workers often relied upon their families for financial support. "The fact that [residents] were able to enter settlement work at all," noted one historian, "especially during the early years, was often an indication that they did not have to earn a living."[11]

Veiller worked at the University Settlement during the Panic of 1893, a severe economic depression in which approximately three million, or one-fifth of the American workforce, lost their jobs due to a combination of overproduction, low crop prices, and several major railroad failures. The downturn hit New York manufacturers especially hard, resulting in tens of thousands of Lower East Side factory laborers put out of work.[12] In his own account of the crisis, published in a popular national magazine the following summer, Veiller shared powerful impressions of his impoverished neighbors "crying out from want and hunger, and some going insane, inflamed to acts of violence by the speeches of anarchistic demagogues."[13] The immediate effects of the economic downturn clarified to Veiller the role of wealth in dividing those who lived "in the midst of broad streets with pure air and sunlight . . . their children shielded from every sorrow," from "thousands of struggling people, fighting for a mere chance to keep alive . . . grinding themselves out in the treadmill of ceaseless toil; without rest, without joy, without hope—only a dull, smoldering existence."[14]

Notably, Veiller's grim depictions of working-class life overlook the value of his subjects' homegrown support networks and recreational outlets. "For music, many have only the occasional hand-organ, with its groups of dancing children," Veiller observed. "For art they have the chromos of the corner grocery-store . . . for literature, the sensational newspaper and the cheap 'novel.'"[15] Fellow settlement workers echoed Veiller's descriptions of the Lower East Side as a cultural wasteland with "no museums and art galleries, no libraries . . . no fine stores encouraging discriminating tastes, scarcely one in fact of all those elements which encourage a wholesome and intelligent living."[16] Such remarks underscore the class tensions delineating two competing visions of settlement work: one that pursued democratic inclusiveness through reaching out to working-class neighbors as equals, and another, more paternalistic vision that sought to "improve" their neighbors through an agenda of intellectual, cultural, and moral uplift.[17]

Veiller responded to the crisis by joining the East Side Relief Work Committee (ESRWC), a joint project administered through the Charity Organization Society of the City of New York (COSCNY). The ESRWC reflected COSCNY founder Julia Shaw Lowell's mission to avoid the pauperizing effects of direct relief by linking it with moral uplift and social control. "No greater injury can be done to a human being," remarked Lowell in 1890, than to "induce him to give up the use of his self-supporting faculties."[18] Funded through private donations, the project provided paying work to keep families together "in self-respecting independence."[19] The project eventually employed nearly five thousand people for several-week stints as tailors, street cleaners, and tenement whitewashers.[20] In order to restrict these jobs to "deserving" applicants, organizers worked with selected churches, unions, settlement houses, and charities to assess job seekers' character and level of financial need. These methods reflected the influence of "scientific charity," an emerging brand of social welfare that emulated the emerging corporate model by stressing efficiency and a businesslike detachment toward helping others.[21]

Settlement workers, as a rule, rejected the deliberating, arm's-length approach of organized charities as counterproductive to building interclass harmony. Robert Hunter, a settlement worker from Chicago who took charge of the University Settlement in 1902, classified organized charity workers as "Hamlet" types whose moral anxiety over whether "to do or not to do" constantly impeded their efforts. By contrast, he saw settlement workers as "Don Quixote" types who were "constantly pressing forward, sometimes tilting at wind-mills, often making mistakes, at times, doubtless, doing injury, but filled with earnestness and warmth of purpose, and with not too much of question."[22] By the same token, organized charities dismissed the fraternizing methods of settlements as aimless, impractical, and unproductive. "You settlement folks remind me," began one such critique, attributed to a prominent charity worker, "of a man who found a drunkard lying in the gutter . . . [and] said to the wayward one, 'I can't help you up my friend, but I will sit down in the gutter beside you.'"[23]

As a settlement house resident who worked closely with COSCNY during the Panic of 1893, Veiller absorbed these clashing perspectives, bringing his sympathy toward the poor into direct conflict with the business principles driving scientific charity. "It is often so very hard to act contrary to one's feelings and emotions," he remarked, "when men kiss your garments, begging not to be discharged, and with tears in their eyes tell heart-rending tales of the sufferings of their families." However, he concluded that yielding in such cases endangered "the self-respect of the workingman" and represented "the first step toward the demoralization of the community."[24] Nevertheless, Veiller's public approval of scientific charity did not prevent him from issuing harsh critiques of its practices in private. In an eleven-page handwritten document, composed during the same period and presumably intended for COSCNY leaders, Veiller cited multiple patterns of "discrimination between the rich and the poor" that he had observed during his brief involvement with the organization. Singling out its interrogations of charity applicants as "unjust, unnecessary, and cruel," he suggested bluntly that the COSCNY rename itself "Society for the Detection and Suppression of Frauds."[25]

Veiller's brash, outspoken style quickly earned him a reputation among prominent New York reformers for being an "idealist and a great worker" who required delicate handling and close supervision to be fully effective.[26] Much of this idealism stemmed from his belief in the potential of social work projects to expand the "common ground" between classes. "When the poor see thousands of dollars spent for their relief," Veiller observed in his account from the Panic of 1893, "and see men and women working far into the night, giving everything they have for them, they begin to have a better opinion of the rich." Veiller's statement—notably lacking in supporting evidence—illustrates the naiveté and noblesse oblige that fueled settlement workers' efforts and the passive roles they envisioned for their charges. Still, the Panic of 1893 had awakened Veiller and his settlement cohorts to the larger social and economic patterns shaping the lives of New York City's poor. "We have at last awakened to a sense of our responsibilities, and are beginning to realize that this life of ours is full of very real and vital problems," Veiller wrote. "'Hard times' and financial panic will pass away, but the problems of the city will remain . . . shall it be so always?"[27]

The Panic of 1893 also marked a key turning point for organized charities, the leaders of which had begun to question the culpability of individual moral failings in Gilded Age poverty patterns. "The present acute distress may be said, broadly speaking, to be among men and women who have always supported themselves . . . and their families," Lowell observed. Rather than attributing their hardships to "moral or intellectual defects on their own part," Lowell now considered the role of "economic causes . . . which were as much beyond their power to avert as if they had been natural calamities of fire, flood, or storm."[28] Lowell's shifting views on poverty changed the course of the COSCNY and influenced other chapters in major cities, inspiring subsequent historians to refer to the ESRWC as "a bridge linking the past and the future of social welfare."[29]

Throughout the remainder of the 1890s, the COSCNY—and organized charities in general—transitioned from a calling of Christian-inspired volunteers to a profession staffed by social workers.[30] Employing an increasingly sophisticated arsenal of statistics and survey methods, its in-house committees sought to uncover and investigate the deeper socioeconomic roots of urban "evils" like intemperance, disease, and crime.[31] This shift in approach brought organized charities and settlements closer together, prompting a University Settlement head worker in the early twentieth century to observe that "each has come to value the work of the other in a way that would not have seemed probable a decade ago."[32] This fluid, transitional environment provided opportunities for Veiller, who emerged from the Panic of 1893 with the personal conviction that "the improvement of the homes of the people was the starting point of everything."[33]

HOUSING REFORM IN NINETEENTH-CENTURY NEW YORK CITY

New York's housing situation had reached a crisis point by the 1840s, when thousands of Irish and German immigrants poured into the Lower East Side in search of low-wage jobs in the shipbuilding and mercantile industries.[34] As prosperous merchant families left to seek more fashionable addresses uptown, speculative builders carved up the vacated houses into apartments; adjoining yards and gardens gave way to hastily assembled multifamily dwellings of three to four stories, unhampered by legal restrictions.[35] As they waited for the value of their holdings to rise and attract more lucrative commercial development, landlords charged exorbitant rents while maintaining the dwellings as cheaply as possible. Slums and enormous profits were the result.[36]

The earliest cries for housing reform issued from New Yorkers working among the poor: physicians, missionaries, and social reformers who perceived a physical and moral connection between derelict houses and their inhabitants. John H. Griscom, the city's health inspector in 1842, became its first housing crusader when he published a report highlighting the escalating disease mortality in tenement districts. Through physicians' testimonies, mortality statistics, and his own searing commentary, Griscom challenged mainstream attitudes toward impoverished tenement dwellers by attributing their illnesses to environmental hazards beyond their control, rather than moral shortcomings.[37] He argued that restricting tenants' access to fresh air, clean water, and adequate living space brought about their moral and physical degradation by encouraging an "indifference to the common decencies of life," which exerted "a depressing effect upon the physiological energies" governing their susceptibility to disease.[38]

Griscom continued his crusade through the New York Association for Improving the Condition of the Poor (NYAICP), a private charitable organization that he cofounded in 1843 with temperance activist Robert Hartley. While the organization sought to eradicate poverty through individual moral uplift, its annual reports revealed a growing recognition of environmental contributors to the "destitution and misery" its volunteers witnessed.[39] By the 1850s the NYAICP reached the same conclusion as other social outreach groups that had tried, unsuccessfully, to prioritize their charges' moral redemption: "Vain will be the effort to elevate their character, without first improving their physical condition."[40] Early housing reformers sought solutions within the laissez-faire economy by urging landlords to strike a better balance between their profit-seeking imperatives and their humanitarian obligations. Conceding that cleaner, safer accommodations generated smaller profits, Griscom exhorted "the benevolent capitalist" to consider "the increased happiness, health, morals and comfort of the inmates, and good order of society, which cannot be estimated in money."[41] The NYAICP also created "model tenements" like the Working Men's Home, which offered modern amenities such as lighted hallways and indoor plumbing in exchange for adherence to a strict code of behavior.[42]

Although reluctant to challenge property rights directly, Griscom perceived increased government regulation as critical to safeguarding the health and welfare of all New Yorkers. Inspired by the work of English sanitarian Edwin Chadwick, Griscom called upon city leaders to provide clean water, construct sewers, and remove public "nuisances" such as slaughterhouses from crowded residential areas. Accomplishing such sweeping changes, in his view, required replacing politically appointed officials with "a well-regulated and efficient Health Police" to inspect and, if necessary, condemn dwellings as unfit for habitation.[43] When Griscom's suggestions resulted in his removal from public office, he continued appealing to well-heeled New Yorkers' sense of self-preservation through the NYAICP.[44] In the days before germ theory, the group warned of "poisonous miasmas" capable of spreading from tenement districts to the "splendid squares and spacious streets of this metropolis."[45] Maintaining that "physical evils produce moral evils," it also promoted housing reform as a way to prevent "a vast amount of pauperism, crime, and wretchedness" that increased New Yorkers' tax burden for public support services and jails.[46]

Despite the city's escalating population growth through the 1850s, tenement house conditions remained essentially unchanged until the 1863 draft riots highlighted the role of substandard housing in fueling working-class discontent. "As long as New York disregards the home life of this class of the poor," warned city physician Stephen Smith, "she nourishes in her bosom a viper which any day may inflict a fatal wound." With the same environmental determinism and civic self-preservation that Griscom and the NYAICP had promoted for decades, Smith recommended "radical reform of the homes of the poor," replacing "the old rookeries in crowded and filthy districts" with "new and convenient houses." He also echoed Griscom's call for "a clean Board of Health" to implement these measures, convinced that conditions would not change "until compelled to do so by the rigid enforcement of law."[47]

The following year, Smith led the privately formed Citizens Association in investigating sanitary conditions in the city's tenement districts. The final report, which included detailed inspections of every street, alley, court, and building of the city, confirmed a close link between filthy, overcrowded buildings and deadly contagious illnesses. Citing statistics that showed New York's death rate to be well above other major cities, the report reiterated the preventive suggestions that had been offered since the 1840s: clean streets, improved drainage and ventilation, elimination of "public nuisances" like slaughterhouses and fat-boiling establishments, and a sanitary police force to monitor and respond to disease outbreaks.[48] Broad popular acceptance of sanitarian principles by the 1860s ensured that these suggestions were no longer limited to professional circles but circulated and reinforced by prominent citizens.[49]

This postriot wave of reform agitation, bolstered through fears of an imminent cholera epidemic, convinced state legislators to establish a permanent municipal board of health with broad powers of sanitary regulations and enforcement.[50] The city also enacted its first comprehensive housing law in 1867, a measure more valuable for the precedent it set than for its ability to effect meaningful change. First, its minimum standards were quite modest. For example, it required that one water closet serve no more than twenty tenants.[51] Second, its flexible language regarding room dimensions, ventilation, and fire prevention created ample opportunities for evading these requirements.[52] Third, it failed to restrict lot coverage, enabling builders to continue blocking air and sunlight in order to accommodate as many renters as possible.[53] Ultimately, then, the chief significance of the Citizens Association's report lay in the blueprint it established for future housing reform campaigns: thorough, systematic investigations employing empirical methods, accompanied by proposed mechanisms for implementing and enforcing the new regulations.[54]

Throughout the late nineteenth century, New York City housing reform efforts remained remarkably static in their easy conflation of environmental, physical, and moral contamination, their heartfelt entreaties to those who profited from tenements, and their repeated calls for increased government oversight. These efforts assumed a heightened urgency as Gilded Age industrialization transformed urban populations, vastly expanding the proportion of wage earners and increasing the "foreign element" among them. New Yorkers' fears of class warfare, ignited during the draft riots, continued to flare as working-class discontentment percolated upward through union organization, violent railroad and factory strikes, and radical political movements.[55]

While Gilded Age philanthropists, evangelical ministers, and sanitary reformers approached the "tenement-house evil" from different perspectives, all of them agreed that the detached, one-family, middle-class Protestant home formed the standard unit of American civilization. Held to this exacting standard, tenements often suffered unflattering comparisons to "dens," "rookeries," and "hives"—subhuman shelters fostering subhuman values.[56] "These black holes in the wall are not the homes you and I know and love," *New York Evening Post* editor Parke Godwin declared at a public meeting in 1879. "They are the homes where intemperance is nursed, crimes are nourished, the modesty of girlhood is crushed, and the innocent instincts of childhood are stifled in their birth."[57] Clergyman S. Parkes Cadman maintained that tenements "could not be dignified by the sacred name of home, for not one of the virtues that go to make that name are inculcated, practiced, or even understood."[58]

Housing reformers' preoccupation with working-class filth and immorality only intensified as their advocacy intersected with the lurid sensationalism gaining popularity in mainstream publications and urban guidebooks.[59] "You crawl like a spider up a black, narrow, slimy stairway," began a typical you-are-there example, "squeezing past ill-smelling persons [who] live in filth . . . breathe it, are saturated with it." This filth, accumulated through overcrowding and constant turnover of tenants, "is never fully removed; the walls and floors become saturated with it; the vaults are clogged, and reeking with foul odors; the light is shut out and the air is shut in."[60] Descriptions often included references to a distinctive smell: a "familiar stench . . . almost as sharp to the nostrils as a whiff of pure ammonia."[61] Physicians, reformers, and journalists used the term *tenement-house rot* to describe the pale, wizened appearances they associated with prolonged exposure to these dark, damp, and foul conditions. This state of premature decay left "infantile life . . . nipped in the bud," remarked journalist and sanitary engineer Charles F. Wingate; "youth is deformed and loathsome; decrepitude comes at thirty."[62]

As housing reformers gravitated slowly toward the empirical methods employed by Smith and the Citizens Association, their early attempts often revealed a cavalier, even haphazard approach toward statistics and source attribution. Citing anonymous "experts," Wingate alleged that "probably seventy-five percent of the maladies of the cities . . . arise from the tenement-houses [and] ninety percent of the children born in these dens die before reaching youth."[63] Meanwhile, their continued reluctance to challenge tenement owners' property rights left housing reformers vacillating between private philanthropy and government for solutions. "If our capitalists were content with five per cent interest on their money," argued an 1888 editorial, they could provide "homes for men and women who are now housed with less regard to comfort or even decency than many a well-stabled horse."[64] Felix Adler, of the Society of Ethical Culture, who would chair the state Tenement House Commission

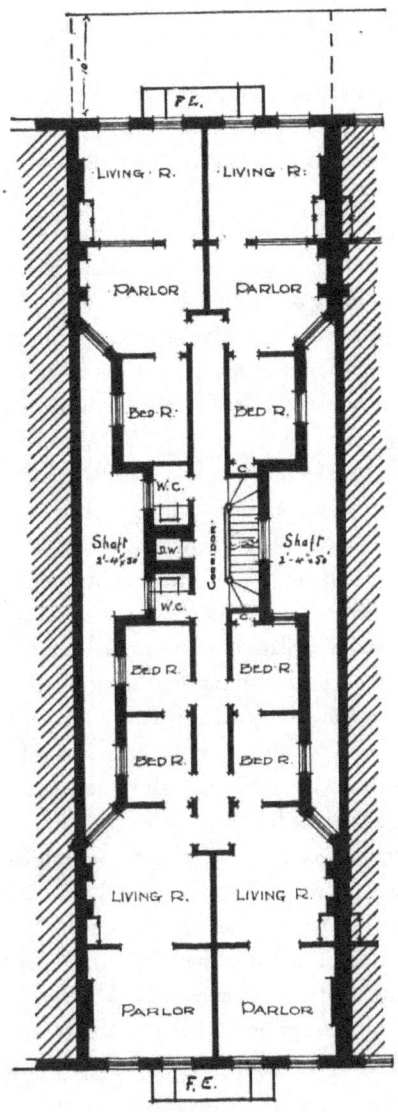

Typical Dumb-bell Tenement, built under the present law.

2.1. A floor plan sketch of a typical "dumbbell" tenement building, which appeared in the New York State Tenement Commission report of 1900. Reprinted from Robert Weeks de Forest and Lawrence Veiller, eds., *The Tenement House Problem: Including the Report of the New York State Tenement House Commission of 1900* (New York: Macmillan, 1903), advance sheets.

of 1884, echoed previous reformers' calls for government to step in. "Common decency," he remarked, "binds the government to see to it that these houses shall not prove fatal to the lives and morality of the inmates. . . . [I]t must compel a reduction of the number of inmates, enforce renovation at the expense of the landlord . . . [or else] dismantle the houses and remove them from existence."[65] Mounting public pressure, channeled through the efforts of Smith, Wingate, Godwin, Adler, and others, resulted in amendments to the 1867 tenement house law regarding lot coverage and access to light, ventilation, and plumbing facilities. However, builders and landlords still found ample opportunities to circumvent these requirements.[66]

By the 1890s housing reformers in New York City faced a daunting scenario: tens of thousands of unsanitary and unsafe tenement buildings housing 1.7 million people, or more than half of the city's population.[67] Most recent construction reflected the late-1870s "dumbbell" model, which featured five to seven stories and four apartments per floor. While dumbbells provided air and direct sunlight through windows facing the street or back yards, interior bedrooms opened on to narrow shafts running along the sides of the building. Incapable of providing sufficient light and air, these shafts sealed the dumbbell's fate among reformers as "the one hopeless form of tenement construction . . . it cannot be well ventilated, it cannot be well lighted; it is not safe in case of fire."[68] While some tenement families shared hallway toilets, many still relied upon outdoor privies that had evaded municipal scrutiny for years.[69] Four different municipal departments shared responsibility for monitoring these conditions, all but guaranteeing that construction and maintenance issues would remain unresolved.[70]

While late nineteenth-century reformers credited "strong-willed intelligent people" with the ability to transcend squalid and demoralizing tenement house environments, they feared that "the weak-willed, the careless, and the unreflecting" would only perpetuate them.[71] Left unmanaged, the tenement would continue producing future generations of "dependents, defectives, and delinquents" to undermine traditional American values and institutions.[72] Reformers' concerns centered especially on recent immigrants from southern and eastern Europe, most of whom resided in tenement neighborhoods near their jobs on the docks and in nearby factories.[73] Reflecting the rampant nativism of the period, reformers often interpreted poor housing conditions as reflections of the intelligence, lifestyles, and cultural practices of these immigrant groups. For example, Wingate singled out "Italian, Poles, Russians and Bohemians" as "ignorant, filthy and debased" for their apparent willingness to crowd "six and seven persons of all ages and of both sexes . . . in one or two rooms."[74]

Convinced that proper homes were essential to transforming immigrants into Americans, reformers viewed tenements as retarding and even derailing that process. This rising tide of public anxiety proved critical in propelling the housing reform movement forward. No one communicated the danger that tenement-dwelling foreigners posed to traditional American values more effectively than Jacob Riis, a Danish immigrant and journalist who had acquired an intimate knowledge of urban housing conditions through his police-beat reporting for major New York newspapers. He galvanized public opinion in 1890 with *How the Other Half Lives*, a grim and arresting portrait of working-class city life that blended the moral suasion, sensationalism, and empirical methods that had defined housing reform up to that point. In a series of vivid literary sketches, Riis captured the teeming squalor in which tenement dwellers lived, the grueling sweatshop labor they endured, the temptations they encountered in saloons and on the street, and the downward spiral that many of them traveled toward almshouses, public hospitals, prisons, and unmarked paupers' graves. Riis attempted to jolt readers out of their complacency by interspersing sentimental anecdotes with the hard-boiled police and public health statistics he had grown comfortable with in his reporting work. He also used innovations in flash-lighting technology to gather indisputable photographic evidence of the dark and dirty environments in which thousands of New Yorkers lived.[75] Like many reform-minded contemporaries, Riis feared the potential implications of continuing to neglect these problems. "The sea of a mighty population," he warned, "held in galling fetters, heaves uneasily in the tenements."[76] By merging older arguments with newer evidence-gathering methods, Riis's *How the Other Half Lives* represented a significant bridge between nineteenth- and twentieth-century housing reform models.

The resulting groundswell of popular interest from Riis's work triggered a series of newspaper investigations, which in turn convinced state legislators to appoint another Tenement House Commission in 1894. Led by Richard Watson Gilder, editor of *Century* magazine, and advised extensively by Riis, the commission produced an exhaustive survey of 8,500 tenements, packed with statistical data on immigration, population density, overcrowding, fire safety, sanitary and plumbing arrangements, disease mortality, and the need for parks and playgrounds in Lower East Side neighborhoods.[77] Using photographs and maps that revealed population density and nationalities, the report confirmed New Yorkers' fears of their tenement districts being "the most crowded on the face of the earth," with some blocks approaching the unparalleled density of Bombay, India.[78] The report also confirmed that previous restrictive legislation had had little effect: of the tenements included in the report, only a fraction provided tenants with bathtubs and toilet facilities in their apartments, and many still had windowless bedrooms.[79]

Despite the dizzying amount of new evidence that the commission compiled in favor of effective housing reform, it remained consistent with its predecessors in failing to hold builders and landlords accountable for providing the basic necessities of air, water, and sanitation. Instead, it called for the city to provide more public bathhouses, drinking fountains, toilets, and parks in the tenement districts. Likewise, it addressed overcrowding by reinforcing statutes that set minimum space requirements per person, rather than examine the larger socioeconomic forces fueling the problem.[80] However, the Tenement House Commission of 1894 managed to make progress in one key area: demanding revisions to existing housing laws that would give the Board of Health "unquestioned power" to condemn and destroy private property, when it was deemed hazardous to people's health.[81] Commission members presented this measure as necessary for avoiding a civic catastrophe. "New York is breeding a mob in her tenements," warned *New York Press* publisher Edward Marshall, consisting of "the offscourings of every nation under the sun."[82] Architect Ernest Flagg concurred: "The tenement-house evil is staring us in the face . . . a desperate disease needs a desperate remedy."[83] He supported educating landlords while subjecting them to government oversight. "Show them how they can build good houses for less than it now costs to build bad ones," he declared. "Then let the Board of Health do its part to bring about the change . . . [making] use of the powers which years ago were vested in it for this very purpose."[84]

Less than a year after state legislators passed the slum-clearance measure in 1895, the Board of Health condemned eighty-seven buildings.[85] While most of these remained vacant, several dozen—including the "rookeries" of Mulberry Bend, which Riis had denigrated in *How the Other Half Lives*—vanished to make way for improved housing and parks.[86] Despite the modest scale of these changes, the 1894 state commission had compelled politicians to consider limiting property rights in order to protect the public: a crucial precedent for Veiller to build upon.

VEILLER, THE CHARITY ORGANIZATION SOCIETY, AND THE TENEMENT HOUSE EXHIBITION

When Veiller began taking his first professional steps beyond the University Settlement, his associates knew him as a short, stocky, and bearded "storm trooper of reform." Supremely confident in his own knowledge and abilities, the young man often found it difficult—if not impossible—to defer graciously to older and more influential reform figures. Veiller's absence from the 1894 state Tenement House Commission, for example, stemmed from his unwillingness to work with Marshall, whom he later accused of exploiting reform causes to sell newspapers.[87] Finding Marshall's manner "ungentlemanly and dictatorial" and his objectives "unnecessary and foolish," the twenty-two-year-old activist agreed to join the commission only if Gilder, the chairman, allowed him "a free hand" in planning and executing the investigation. Veiller promoted his daring idea, which evidently did not find acceptance, as a superior alternative to undertaking the work "in a slip-shod, careless, sensational way."[88]

Shortly afterward, Veiller underwent civil examinations to become a clerk at the city's Department of Buildings—an opportunity that exemplified the nonpartisan professionalism that the incoming reform mayor, William L. Strong, intended to bring to city government.[89] Over the next two years, superiors rewarded Veiller's "executive ability and accuracy" with more and more administrative responsibility behind the scenes.[90] As he examined builders' plans for compliance with existing codes, Veiller developed a keener appreciation for how structural design affected the lives of the working-class people he had encountered through the University Settlement. In the meantime, he also grew adept at detecting the shoddy techniques, secondhand materials, and shady subcontracting arrangements that speculative builders often used to maximize their profits.[91] Veiller's first immersion in municipal affairs, though brief, arguably left him with a deep skepticism of human nature that would continue to set him apart from other reformers.[92] Rejecting moral suasion as useless with unscrupulous profiteers "who build only what they are forced to build by law, and seek upon all occasions to evade even these requirements," Veiller came to regard power—more than love, faith, or a sense of common brotherhood—to be the key to regulating human affairs.[93] From this point on, Veiller focused on curbing the power of tenement builders and owners through stricter housing codes and enforcement—both outgrowths of increased government oversight, which housing reformers had been championing for decades.[94]

Using the COSCNY as a base of operations, Veiller began assembling a pressure group of philanthropists, lawyers, architects, and social workers to lobby for improved housing conditions.[95] This Tenement House Committee (THC) reflected an early manifestation of the larger shifts within the COSCNY toward addressing the root causes of poverty, already under way since the Panic of 1893.[96] It attracted the support of contemporary housing reform advocates, including Adler, Gilder, Flagg, Riis, and Elgin R. L. Gould of the US Bureau of Labor Statistics.[97] The THC began by offering suggestions to a municipal commission that was revising the building code in anticipation of the city incorporating Brooklyn and Staten Island. These measures limited the maximum height of new buildings and set standards for lighting, ventilation, and fire safety.[98] The municipal commission adopted none of these suggestions—an outcome that Veiller attributed to the disproportionate influence of builders on the revision process.[99] The municipal commission members "were, I think, on the whole amused at the thought that this bunch of 'reformers' could seriously present these proposals to them," Veiller recalled later, "knowing as they did how firmly entrenched the Building 'ring' was politically in the government at that time."[100] The final code revisions not only weakened existing housing regulations even further but also placed corrupt building officials in charge of interpreting and following them: the precise opposite of what Veiller and the THC had envisioned.[101]

Now firmly convinced that effective housing reform required bypassing the corrupt business-political arrangements he had witnessed at the Department of Buildings, Veiller sought to convince the public that "in New York City the workingman is housed worse than in any other city in the civilized world . . . [and] pays more for such accommodations than is paid anywhere else."[102] Doing that required new ways of stimulating awareness among prosperous and influential New Yorkers who were unlikely to visit the slums themselves, and who had grown complacent with the literary sensationalizing of Riis and other reformer-authors. With the Columbian Exposition and other large-scale commercial ventures drawing great crowds in other cities, Veiller conceived of hosting a similar event that would bring "the so-called slums to the people uptown, instead of trying to take the uptown people down to the slums."[103]

The Tenement House Exhibition opened in February of 1900 in an elegant Fifth Avenue banquet hall that immersed its visitors in the tenement experience with papier-mâché models, more than a hundred maps, a thousand photographs, and "many charts, diagrams and tables of statistics" filling two entire floors.[104] The event broke new ground not just for the sheer amount of information compiled but also for Veiller's innovative methods of integrating the information into an effective argument for housing reform. Riis's heart-rending photographs of tenement life, stripped of his literary flourishes, now appeared alongside investigative data that settlement workers had collected regarding population densities, death rates, nationalities, occupations, income and expenditures, overcrowding, fire hazards, and health conditions. From the walls, two sets of multicolored street maps displayed each New York tenement building's height, shape, number of stories, and small amount of land left vacant for light and air.[105] Through rows of uniform, color-coded dots, the first set of maps related the number of contagious illnesses reported from each building to the Department of Health; the second, directly below the first, indicated the number of families who had applied for charity within the past five years.[106] Using these new modes of visual presentation, Veiller built upon the work of previous reformers who had asserted, but not proved direct associations, among environment, poverty, and disease. In the process, Veiller remained remarkably true to their traditional themes of environmental determinism and middle-class morality. Declaring that "the tenement-house problem is at the root of most of our social evils" when promoting the exhibition, Veiller charged "the inconvenience and unattractiveness of the homes" with

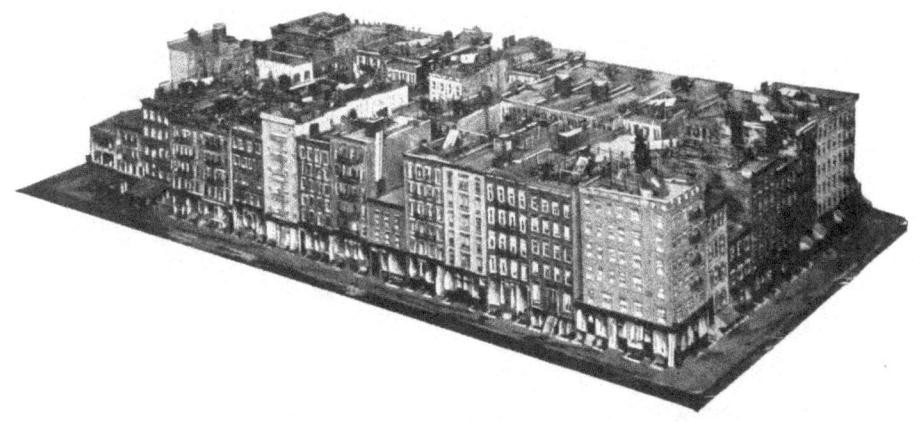

An existing Block of Tenements, Chrystie, Bayard, Forsythe and Canal Streets.

2.2. A three-dimensional papier-mâché model of an overbuilt tenement Lower East Side block, manufactured for the Tenement House Exhibition of 1900. Reprinted from de Forest and Veiller, *Tenement House Problem*, advance sheets.

encouraging the immorality, disease, and drunkenness that made its tenants a financial burden and source of danger to the city at large.[107]

The two-week event, covered in mainstream publications, reportedly drew ten thousand visitors "from the millionaire to the poorest, unskilled laborer."[108] Not unpredictably, the most vocal and effusive praises emanated from reformers. Settlement worker Lilian Betts hailed it as "one of the greatest contributions, if not the greatest . . . [toward] a proper understanding of the subject of the housing of the poor." A central point of attraction was the map displays, where experts found abundant empirical evidence to confirm tenements as the source of a host of social dangers. The maps convinced Gould that poverty was "a contagious disease . . . spread[ing] through a house just as tuberculosis might."[109] Physician Sigard Adolphus Knopf pointed to the maps for scientific proof that dark and dirty surroundings, poor and ignorant consumptive tenants, and tuberculosis-laden dust transformed tenement buildings into "infected houses."[110] Then governor Theodore Roosevelt detected in these maps the roots of political corruption. Instructing exhibitgoers to align the thickest concentrations of disease and poverty dots with the thickest concentrations of voters, he then posed to them that they "ask how you can expect the political stream to rise . . . when its very sources are polluted."[111]

The exhibition's impact on rank-and-file New Yorkers remained more elusive. One week before the event closed, a reporter from the *Commercial*

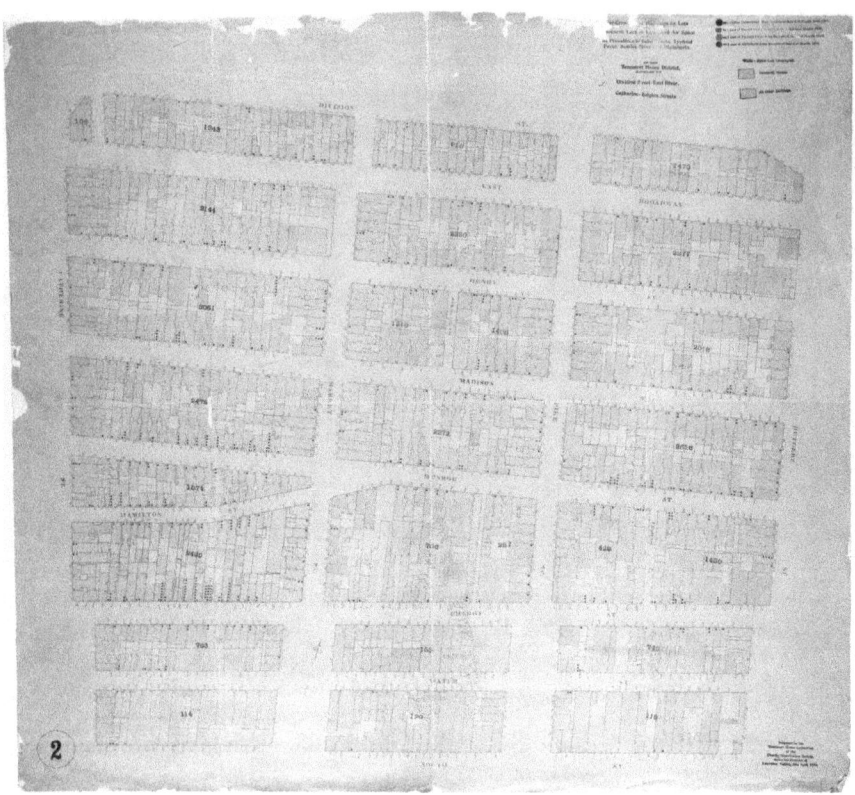

2.3. This disease map, one of at least forty created by Lawrence Veiller for the Tenement House Exhibition, shows the distribution of tuberculosis, scarlet fever, typhoid fever, and diphtheria cases reported to the NYCDOH across a portion of the Lower East Side between 1895 and 1899. It includes the block bounded by Cherry, Catherine, Hamilton, and Market Streets (third up from bottom on the left, block no. 2429). Original held in the collection of the New-York Historical Society.

Advertiser remarked that "the maps, charts, models, [and] photographs, do not always speak plainly to the layman." Without experts on hand to personally guide them, the "constant though rather meagre stream of visitors" resorted to "prowling about the exhibits, first with a puzzled and then with a bored air," eventually leaving "without apparently understanding or caring to understand the meaning of the entire undertaking."[112] Even among the uninitiated, however, the maps made the connection between tenement neighborhoods and contagious diseases glaringly apparent: "The red-colored squares representing the tenement houses are all but covered with dots," the reporter observed from the maps, while the green spaces representing private houses "were almost free from them."[113]

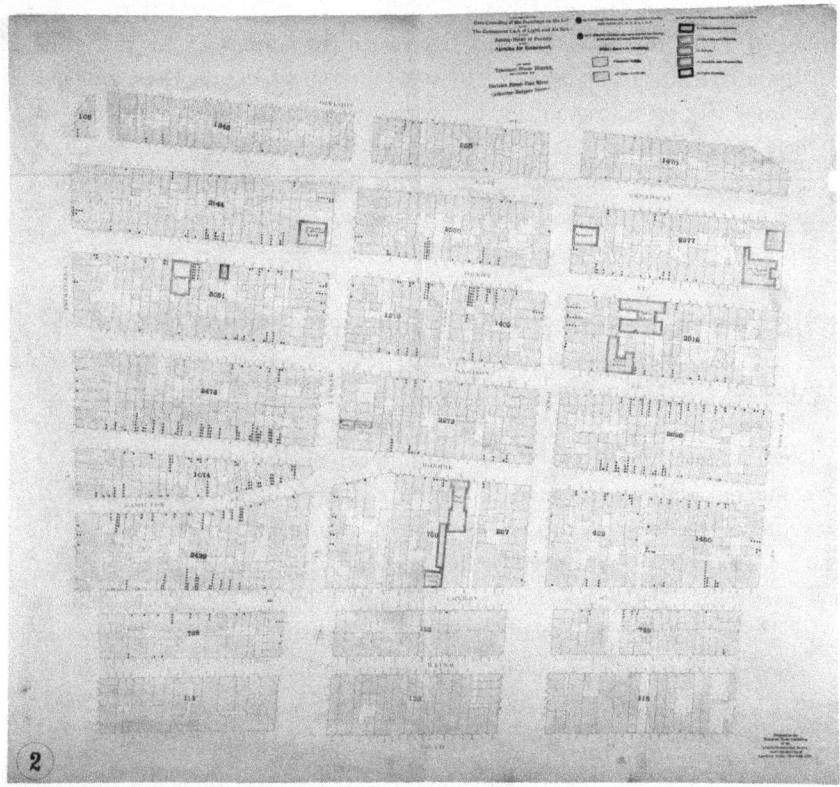

2.4. This poverty map, one of at least forty created by Lawrence Veiller for the Tenement House Exhibition, shows the distribution of families who applied for assistance from COSCNY, NYAICP, and United Hebrew Charities within a five-year period (presumably ending in 1896). "It seems beyond belief," Veiller recalled later in his Reminiscences, "that there was hardly one tenement house in the entire city that did not contain a number of these dots, and many contained as many as 15 of them, indicating that 75 different families had applied for charity from that house in 5 years (15). The map includes the block bounded by Cherry, Catherine, Hamilton, and Market Streets (third up from bottom on the left, block no. 2429). Original held in the collection of the New-York Historical Society.

Veiller, who had invested "about 16 hours a day for months, and almost killed myself" during the preparation stages, asserted the exhibit's originality and significance. He predicted that the maps alone, by linking tenements with disease "in accurate, scientific form" that few could fail to understand or acknowledge, "might well earn for New York . . . the title of 'city of the living death.'"[114] He later claimed, with some justification, to have "invented the Social Exhibition as a mechanism in civic and social work."[115] After traveling to Boston, Chicago, and Hartford, Connecticut, portions of the exhibit earned a gold medal at the Paris Exposition that summer.[116] In the immediate aftermath, the exhibition's most significant achievement was its galvanizing effect on Roosevelt. Publicly lauding Veiller and the COSCNY for their "effort to cut at the root of the diseases which eat at the body social and the body politic," the governor threw his support behind tenement-house reform. "Tell me what you want from Albany," he told them, "and I will do everything I can to help you get it."[117]

THE NEW YORK STATE TENEMENT HOUSE COMMISSION OF 1900

After his exhibition closed, Veiller introduced a bill establishing a state commission to "study the whole subject from A to Z" and propose solutions. Despite Governor Roosevelt's strong support, the bill faced a "gauntlet of Tammany opposition" emanating from the city's building interests.[118] As Veiller outmaneuvered these interests to ensure the bill's passage through the state assembly, he continued honing the shrewd pragmatism and technical prowess that distinguished him from his moralizing reform contemporaries.[119] Successfully manipulating politicians, he realized, did not involve tugging at heartstrings but applying "the right pressure, in the right place, at the right time, in the right way, by the right person."[120]

The resulting New York State Tenement House Commission of 1900 (NYSTHC) included lawyers, physicians, architects, fire prevention experts, builders, and housing activists from the city's settlements and organized charities.[121] These diverse professional perspectives were intended to act as checks upon one another in order to generate the most practical and effective reforms possible.[122] Leading the effort was COSCNY president Robert Weeks de Forest, an attorney and career philanthropist whose brand of patrician diplomacy inspired confidence and loyalty among his associates.[123] Arguably, de Forest's appointment said less about his housing reform expertise than it did about Veiller's reputation for abrasiveness and confrontation—the same traits that curtailed the settlement worker's participation in the 1894 commission.[124] As de Forest's executive officer, Veiller nevertheless supplied the driving force behind the investigation, organizing and carrying out most of the work.[125]

For the better part of a year, NYSTHC members reviewed previous housing reform efforts, compared New York's housing situation and building laws with those of other American and European cities, and probed the extent of dangers associated with tenement neighborhoods: overcrowding, sanitation, disease, fires, and prostitution. Previous reform campaigns, the commission surmised, had done little to prevent working-class housing conditions from deteriorating. The dumbbell tenement, which lax code enforcement rendered capable of occupying up to 75 percent of a standard 25-by-100-foot lot, provided "less light and less ventilation, less fire protection and less comfortable surroundings, than the average tenement of fifty years ago," their final report observed.[126] With the work of inspecting the city's 82,652 tenements—which together housed 2.4 million people—falling to only sixty-one public health workers, NYSTHC members concluded, "It is not to be wondered at that grave evils exist . . . it is obviously a physical impossibility for so small a corps of men to make the slightest pretence of adequately inspecting such buildings."[127]

In order for NYSTHC members and the media to "see and smell at first hand the conditions that existed," Veiller led several well-publicized walking tours into Lower East Side neighborhoods.[128] Dressed in elegant suits, ties, and bowlers, the commissioners squinted into dark rooms, descended into putrid cellars, inched up staircases so narrow and winding that "each man had to keep in touch with the one in front," and trod gingerly across rooftops to peer into narrow air-shafts.[129] "The eyes of the commissioners seemed always to be for light," observed one reporter.[130] Everywhere they went, the party noted flagrant health and building violations: overbuilt lots, horse stables kept in narrow alleys, condemned buildings still crammed with tenants, and cluttered, poorly constructed fire escapes.[131] "The laws are as little respected . . . by builders and owners," concluded the *New York Journal*, "as if they had never been placed upon the statute-book."[132] Veiller later credited these tours with generating the public indignation he wanted, recalling one newspaper editor who told him ten years afterward that he "hadn't gotten the stink of those privy vaults out of [his] nostrils yet."[133]

More difficult to recapture is how tenement residents themselves regarded the commissioners' "slumming tours." Based on reporters' observations, locals' initial reactions were of curiosity, tinged with apprehension. "Windows blossomed with faces" as the men made their way down the narrow, crowded streets filled "with yelling vendors and gaping slum folk."[134] As they filed into the houses, residents flooded the hallways to gaze upon them "in open mouthed astonishment, wondering what it all meant." Many associated the gentlemen's sudden appearance with trouble: a fire, sanitary inspection, or condemnation proceedings.[135] Once assured that nobody faced the threat of injury or eviction, residents received the newcomers in different ways. Some women invited them in with smiles, eager to put their homes and children on display; others appeared "half-frightened," or "in a bad temper," slammed their doors.[136] Still others hailed the visitors contemptuously as "dudes."[137] Gaudily dressed prostitutes amused themselves by taunting the commissioners from their windowsills as "hosts of hooting children" trailed them below.[138]

These varied reactions—politeness, hostility, fear—confirmed locals' perception of Veiller, his bowler-wearing band of commissioners, and accompanying flock of reporters as outsiders. In several instances the party's attempts to engage residents in conversation only accentuated this perceived gap. When de Forest advised the janitor of a derelict rear tenement that "it would pay you to improve," the janitor replied that "it would, if we had the money to make improvements."[139] Another janitor, after listening to the visitors criticize the darkness of his rooms, responded to their questions about his health with, "I never felt better in my life." The journalist recording this exchange did not attempt to discern whether the man, who had a "pallor like that of an inmate of a prison," actually felt well, or simply refused to discuss personal matters with strangers who clearly disapproved of his home.[140]

After the slum tours came public hearings in which commissioners grilled experts and government officials on the relationship between tenements and physical, moral, and civic decline.[141] With cholera outbreaks now under control through improved sanitation and public health surveillance, NYSTHC members devoted the first hearing to tuberculosis, a disease fast gaining in notoriety through germ theory, Biggs's recent public health campaigns, and the recent Tenement House Exhibition maps. Physicians and public health officials provided testimony that reframed in microbial terms the vague claims of "tenement-house rot" that reformers had made for years. Biggs supplied commissioners with statistical evidence suggesting that tuberculosis had infected as many as twenty thousand New Yorkers, striking down up to one-third of them between the ages of fifteen and sixty-five. Bolstering Knopf's house-infection argument, he cited experiments showing tuberculosis bacilli to remain viable for years in houses deprived of fresh air and sunlight.[142] Biggs's assistant, Arthur Guerard, then stressed the daunting prospect of ridding these buildings of bacilli-laden dust that settled into carpets, the woodwork, and even the wallpaper. "It may be impossible to disinfect and renovate the premises without practically rebuilding them," he warned.[143]

Drawing heavily on these experts' arguments, the NYSTHC's final report placed tuberculosis at the heart of its case for the urgency of tenement house reform. Declaring that the disease had become "practically epidemic in this city," with an unknown number of houses "permanently infected with tuberculosis," the commission declared that "the connection between this disease and the character of the tenement houses in which the poor people live is of the very closest."[144] As it had during the exhibition, up-to-the-minute scientific and statistical evidence ushered the moral indignation of past generations into a new century: "The tenement districts of New York," the report concluded, "are centres of disease, poverty, vice, and crime, where it is a marvel, not that some children grow up to be thieves, drunkards, and prostitutes, but that so many should ever grow up to be decent and self-respecting."[145] Newspapers provided steady coverage of the commission hearings and reports, some of them with rising alarm and indignation at the dangers that lax code enforcement had unleashed on New York.[146] "We take the greatest precautions against smallpox, yellow fever and cholera," the *New-York Tribune* argued, "yet we permit to exist in the heart of this city a standing source of infection . . . which causes greater misery and money loss in a year than would one of the epidemics the mere rumor of which drives people into a panic."[147] The *Evening Post* traced the "veritable plague in our midst" to greed and corruption: "Wherever a landlord has a pull," it declared, "he is given a free hand to violate health ordinances and overcrowd infected tenements." Fixing the situation would require "wholesale condemnation of tenements and impartial enforcement of the law."[148]

Rather than challenge the market forces underlying tenement conditions, the NYSTHC concluded that "the chief evil to be remedied is the tenement house itself"—an environmentally deterministic notion amply reinforced through street maps depicting poverty and disease as stationary and rooted in structures, rather than people.[149] Commissioners proposed new restrictive legislation that outlawed the dumbbell model; mandated renovations to older tenements providing more light and air, more sanitary toilet facilities, and improved fire safety; and new levels of government supervision to ensure compliance.[150] Veiller drafted the legislation himself, citing his "encyclopedic knowledge of all such legislation . . . enacted in New York State from 1647 to 1900," as well as his "complete familiarity with the technical aspects of the subject."[151]

Applying the lessons he had learned about navigating bills through a boss-controlled state legislature, Veiller did not begin at the committee level. Instead, he approached Roosevelt's successor, Governor Benjamin Odell, a Republican "boss" whom Veiller admired for his "clear, cold mind" and "[lack of] hesitation in making decisions and seeing that they were carried out."[152] Although NYSTHC members had anticipated Odell's opposition, "imagine our astonishment and delight," Veiller remarked, "when [Odell] said that he was very familiar with our work; that he had kept in touch with it as it had been reported in the press . . . that he was heartily for our recommendations and would see that they were enacted into law." Veiller's skillful use of publicity, and his willingness to work within the prevailing power structure, enabled him to harness the Tammany machine in favor of his reform agenda. "The mistake . . . too often made," Veiller learned from the experience, "is in assuming that the boss, because he has an unsavory reputation politically, has ceased to be a human being . . . that he is the enemy of all good things." A boss eventually could be groomed into an ally of reform: "especially," Veiller added dryly, reforms that "will be a source of political capital and incidentally secure for him the commendation of public-spirited citizens."[153]

The resulting New York Tenement House Law of 1901, passed by both houses of the state legislature, imposed stricter lighting, sanitation, and fire and safety standards on tenement house builders. From that point on, new tenements would be limited to six stories, taking up no more than 70 percent of the lot; shafts and stairwells would be fireproofed, and water closets provided in each apartment. For older tenements, the law mandated renovations that increased tenants' access to light and air, improved bathroom facilities, provided fire escapes and lighting for dark hallways, and waterproofed cellar floors.[154] To ensure that builders and property owners followed these requirements, the law consolidated code-enforcement responsibilities into a separate municipal agency: the Tenement House Department.

As the driving force behind the COSCNY Tenement House Committee, the Tenement House Exhibition, and the 1900 Tenement House Commission, Veiller possessed excellent qualifications for leading this new municipal enterprise. Moreover, a series of Tammany-related scandals had encouraged voters from both major parties to unite behind a new reform mayor, Seth Low, who pledged to value expertise over political connections when filling important positions. However, Veiller's zeal and unflinching honesty throughout the publicity, investigation, and reporting phases of his tenement house reform campaign had alienated enough people on both sides of the issue to render him a potential liability as an administrator.[155] He had disappointed settlement workers—many of whom had assisted in all aspects of the project—by backing out of an agreement to bring the exhibit to the Lower East Side working classes, citing a lack of time to prepare for higher-profile events in Chicago, Boston, and Paris.[156] Meanwhile, supporters who had assumed active roles in the 1880s and 1890s housing reform campaigns bristled at Veiller's reluctance to credit their past efforts.[157]

Anticipating harsh resistance from builders and landlords over the new regulations, Veiller's allies perceived the importance of choosing the fledgling Tenement House Department's battles carefully.[158] Based on Low's concerns that Veiller was—in Veiller's own words—"too radical . . . and might get his administration into trouble," de Forest once again stepped in to take official leadership of what would be in reality Veiller's organization.[159] This arrangement, replicated from the Tenement House Commission a year earlier, continued to provide Veiller with the public "face" he needed for organizing and running the department as de Forest's assistant. Moreover, through collaborating on the tenement house reform campaign, the unlikely pair had become friends. "I felt toward [de Forest] very much as if he was a fond and much loved elder brother," Veiller recalled, "though he was of an age when he could have been my father."[160] He also noted with wry amusement that reformers who shied away from his youthful, "radical" persona eventually came to regard him as "a conservative and reactionary," concluding, "Such is life."[161]

While late nineteenth-century medical and scientific developments laid the groundwork for slum-demolition campaigns by redefining tenements as permanently diseased, late nineteenth-century social developments supplied the necessary traction for moving the campaigns forward. As New York swelled with unskilled immigrants to meet the escalating demand for cheap factory labor, social activists squared off against the environmental, physical, and moral dangers that industrialization had unleashed on their city—dangers that converged most visibly and alarmingly in the tenement house. As their methods shifted from moral suasion to empirical investigation, from intermittent activity to sustained pressure applied through permanent organizations, and from moral appeals to calls for government intervention, these activists continued believing in the power of the environment to shape human beings' destinies. Germ theory, disease maps, and "house infection" superimposed a new urgency and authority on this longstanding environmental determinism by the 1890s, inspiring reformers to assert new levels of surveillance and control over tenement spaces.

Lawrence Veiller and his housing-reform campaign stood at the center of these developments. His early activities with settlement houses and organized charities instilled in him a keen awareness of how class divisions shaped the circumstances in which people lived and died in New York City. Later, working in the Department of Buildings brought him face to face with the profiteering, corruption, and weak legislation that had sustained the "tenement-house evil" through five decades of failed reform attempts. Throughout the course of his campaign, Veiller's settlement house ideals receded in favor of the cynicism and technical prowess that enabled him to pursue decisive change within a corruption-riddled system. These attributes solidified Veiller's image among fellow reformers as "a man of indomitable energy, keen intelligence and level-headed judgment"; among building and real estate interests, they made him a formidable adversary whose "mere presence at a hearing was wont to cause panic" because he "knew too damned much."[162]

By the late 1890s Veiller's chief housing reform objectives—adequate restrictive legislation and state-sponsored enforcement mechanisms—were not new. Neither was his belief that environment held the key to maintaining social and moral order. What enabled Veiller to succeed where decades of predecessors had failed were his hard-boiled realism, his innovative methods, and the groundswell of public interest in housing conditions that provided favorable conditions for his work and propelled it forward. As industrialization, immigration, and urbanization placed people and their dwellings in ever-closer proximity, housing reformers became more vocal in acknowledging the necessity of curtailing personal liberties as natural, even inevitable. "We are merely readjusting to changing conditions," de Forest explained, "as our ancestors have done."[163] Veiller's pathbreaking Tenement House Exhibition showcased and channeled these sentiments, cultivating the public and political support he needed for creating new restrictive legislation—and a new municipal agency to enforce it—in just three years.

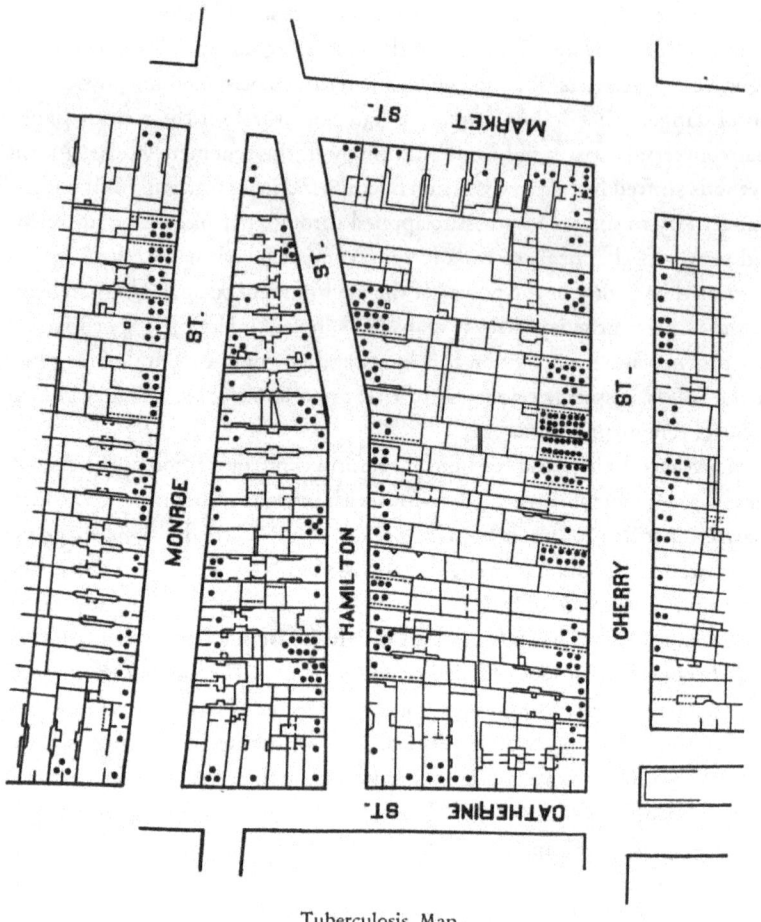

Tuberculosis Map.

Each dot represents one case of Tuberculosis reported to Health Department in 5 years.

2.5. This disease map, which covers a small portion of a larger map that Lawrence Veiller created for the Charity Organization Society Tenement House Committee's Tenement Exhibition of 1900 (Fig. 2.3), was eventually published in 1901 as part of the New York State Tenement House Commission's report titled *The Tenement House Problem.* The greater number of dots in this map suggests that Veiller had been working from an older data set for the exhibition; while his maps were completed in 1899, the total tuberculosis cases for 1895–1899 may not have been available for some time after that. Likewise, given that this map represents tuberculosis cases reported over five years without identifying a specific span, it's possible that these maps do not line up chronologically. Courtesy of the New-York Historical Society.

Arguably, one of the most significant achievements from Veiller's tenement house reform campaign was the opportunity it created for social activists and public health advocates to engage each other on common ground. This fateful development reflected the newfound power of tuberculosis to illustrate the dangers of poor housing conditions, and the cross-disciplinary association of the tenement with physical and moral degradation. Likewise, it reflected notable parallels between the campaigns' respective visionaries. Veiller and Hermann Biggs shared prosperous, old-stock, educated, Protestant backgrounds; they monitored tenement populations with similar combinations of pity, disgust, and fear. Each worked relentlessly, driven by the unshakable conviction that tenements nurtured the seeds of New York's most pressing problems; each sought a solution in increased government oversight that valued expertise above party loyalties, disarming or circumventing opposition through a deft combination of politicking and publicity.[164] Ultimately, each of their campaigns created blueprints for other cities, inspiring national movements in housing and public health.[165] The chief difference between them lay in their unequal legacies, a product of fundamental differences in their personalities. Where Biggs's ways were smooth, amiable, and winning, Veiller's were abrasive, supercilious, and blunt, impairing the latter's professional advancement and obscuring the true impact of his contributions.[166] Yet Veiller's tenacity, buttressed with support from key power figures at key moments, enabled him to press forward despite these handicaps. "If it had not been for my unwillingness to accept defeat," Veiller related with characteristic self-importance, "there would have been no Tenement House Reform for countless years, and New York and other cities would have gone on with their dark rooms and all the other evils. . . . I have always had great satisfaction in 'doing the impossible.'"[167]

Throughout this eventful first decade of Veiller's career, the block bordered by Cherry, Catherine, Hamilton, and Market Streets inched closer to notoriety. At the Tenement House Exhibition, its tuberculosis- and poverty-riddled street maps hung passively alongside those of other blocks; however, its heavy dot concentrations signaled to visitors that it ranked easily among the worst trouble spots in the city. Veiller described it to exhibitgoers as "a sort of pest block" containing nearly 2,500 people, "many of whom are prostitutes."[168] Biggs later singled out the block along with two others in his NYSTHC testimony, noting that it had accumulated a tuberculosis death rate of 144 out of 1,000 in the past four years; on Cherry Street alone, sixty-six people had died in three houses within 150 feet of one another. As the city's daily newspapers placed these details prominently in their stories, the men, women, and children living on this "pest block" continued with their daily lives, their well-dressed visitors having receded—for the moment.[169]

Acknowledging public health experts' observations that many similar problem spots existed, Veiller nevertheless returned to the question, "What shall we do with the Cherry street block?"[170] By way of an answer, he included it among more than a dozen overcrowded "city wildernesses" that he judged to be in desperate need of outdoor recreational space. Transforming these "waste spaces," as Veiller expressed it, into additional "lungs" for the city was "absolutely indispensable, not what is desirable or ideal . . . if it expects to have decent citizens."[171] The block's disease map and "city wilderness" status then appeared in the final commission report, a two-volume set titled *The Tenement House Problem*. Now a matter of public record, it framed all aspects of the problem and outlined solutions for future reform campaigns.[172]

By 1901, then, all the major elements had shifted into place for the neighborhood bordered by Cherry, Catherine, Hamilton, and Market Streets to be transformed into a target for reform. New and more powerful building restrictions, enforced by new and more powerful municipal agencies, aimed at numbering the days for the block's "permanently infected" old law tenements. Organized charities and settlement houses supported the work of these agencies through public education, surveillance, and continued political pressure, all of which promoted a scientifically validated link between slums and tuberculosis. Over the next several years, these efforts would fuse into a joint crusade against "the white plague in its stronghold."

Chapter 3

"THE PLAGUE IN ITS STRONGHOLD"

Lilian Brandt, Ernest Poole, and the Committee on the Prevention of Tuberculosis

"There are but few masters in the lessons of tuberculosis; one well versed in the medical aspects of the disease has much to learn from one acquainted with social problems and *vice versa*."[1] This observation, offered by leading specialist Arnold Klebs in 1904, marked a critical turning point for early antituberculosis activism in the United States. Over the previous twenty years, tuberculosis had become recognized as the terrain of medical and public health professionals—a shift paralleling the disease's gradual reconceptualization from innate hereditary phenomenon to preventable bacteriological scourge.[2] Although bacteriologists had created an effective antitoxin for diphtheria by the 1890s, their attempts to develop a similar remedy for tuberculosis met with repeated failures, leading another specialist, Edward O. Otis, to conclude in 1898 that "exterminating the elusive and ubiquitous bacillus appears now to be a chimerical fancy."[3] Instead, he promoted its containment through aggressive public health policies that included mandatory case reporting, disinfection, crackdowns on public spitting, and hospitalization.[4] Additionally, in light of new diagnostic methods suggesting that most Americans already had been exposed to the bacillus, Otis urged the public to maintain its natural defenses through nutritious diet, exercise, fresh air, and rest.[5] Not surprisingly, these generalized strategies failed to stir ordinary Americans into taking preventive action against the "yearly holocaust" of tuberculosis deaths, with Otis lamenting several years later that "we have become so inured to it that it no longer startles us, like some sudden catastrophe which destroys a few hundred lives."[6]

Tuberculosis evoked similar discouragement among social reform organizations, which had broadened their focus over the late nineteenth century from material aid and moral redemption to larger-scale social and economic developments. Throughout the 1890s and 1900s, the Charity Organization Society of the City of New York (COSCNY) called public attention to the devastation that tuberculosis wreaked upon hundreds of struggling families.

"It was the same story in each case," COSCNY officials reported: "the chief bread-winner . . . at last giving way to the consumption which had been making work for him more and more difficult, even while it made wages which might buy necessary food and decent lodgings more than ever essential."[7] At the district level, caseworkers substantiated these patterns with vivid descriptions of working-class Lower East Side neighborhoods where "the very air seem[ed] to be infected with the plague."[8]

While public health crusaders focused on containing and destroying the bacillus, social workers took aim at the crowded tenements where tuberculosis case dots accumulated on Hermann Biggs's disease maps. Guided by Lawrence Veiller, the New York State Tenement House Commission (NYSTHC) eventually secured legislation in 1901 that mandated more light and air in tenement buildings. Now in command of the city's brand-new Tenement House Department (THD), Veiller and Robert de Forest faced the Herculean task of applying these new standards to more than eighty thousand preexisting "old law" buildings—housing more than three million New Yorkers—on a skeletal budget. They also faced bitter opposition from builders, suppliers, lending institutions, architects, and tenement owners regarding the expenses of bringing the houses in compliance with the new code.[9] "Even with a materially increased force," Veiller and de Forest forecast gloomily, "it will necessarily be several years before all of the changes . . . can be accomplished."[10]

As New York social activists incorporated antituberculosis talking points into their agitations for housing reform and poor relief, they came to share their public health counterparts' sense of futility regarding the magnitude of the tuberculosis problem and their limited powers for addressing it. For both sets of activists, reform candidate Seth Low's mayoral victory in 1901 provided a valuable window of opportunity for expanding municipal efforts in tuberculosis prevention and control. Collaborating on Veiller's recent housing reform campaign had familiarized these groups with each other's stake in the fight, as well as the advantages of pooling their efforts. Through the COSCNY's new Committee on the Prevention of Tuberculosis (CPT), these professionals worked together to convince New Yorkers that tuberculosis was "communicable, preventable, and curable" through increased public investment in education, sanitariums, and other large-scale social improvements.

With their resources limited and the territory vast, the CPT sought to identify areas and populations where intervention would yield the swiftest results. Lilian Brandt, the statistician they recruited in 1902 to determine "the size of the enemy" and "strategic points for attack," occupied the edge of several important social trends.[11] One of the first American women to earn a graduate degree in economics, and among the first to complete the courses offered at the COSCNY's New York School for Philanthropy, the thirty-year-old Brandt stood poised to make her mark in one of the newest professions open to women: social work. While her statistical analysis for the CPT amply demonstrated the value of women's intellectual powers applied outside the home, it also highlighted the social biases that continued to influence early twentieth-century approaches to tuberculosis, even as germ theory found wider acceptance.

When CPT leaders looked for a writer in 1903 to provide "human-interest material" to make their antituberculosis message more broadly appealing, they found what they were seeking in Ernest Poole: a young, well-to-do University Settlement worker who had come of age with germ theory and the urban-industrial development driving reform movements.[12] Hard-working, personable, and eager to make his name in literary circles, Poole viewed the Lower East Side as a training ground for honing the evocative storytelling techniques of Jacob Riis and other "muckraking" journalists. For his CPT assignment, Poole would not have to look far for material; rows of uniform case dots, accumulated during recent public health and tenement house reform campaigns, led straight to the block bounded by Cherry, Catherine, Hamilton, and Market Streets. His emotionally gripping account breathed life into the committee's medical facts and statistical analysis, completing the transformation of the neighborhood's public image into a "stronghold" of deadly contagion.

COMMITTEE ON THE PREVENTION OF TUBERCULOSIS

As the first wave of tuberculosis fighters took stock of their accomplishments at the turn of the twentieth century, many of them did so with a degree of satisfaction. Tuberculosis in 1900 still ranked among the three leading killers in the United States, claiming 10 percent of all deaths; however, mortality had remained on a downward trend for decades. It was declining most sharply in cities, and in New York most of all, plummeting to 256 per 100,000 from 428 per 100,000 in 1870. This downward trend persisted despite exponential increases in population and case reporting during this time span.[13] Public health experts embraced these figures as confirmation that tuberculosis was not only preventable but eradicable given enough manpower, resources, and time.[14] However, these elements remained in critically short supply.

Biggs estimated that ten thousand New Yorkers still perished from tuberculosis annually in the early 1900s, with an additional thirty thousand sick.[15] With only eight health inspectors to handle these cases and fewer public medical facilities to isolate and treat them, New York City public health officials considered themselves "far behind other [European] cities, both great and small" in their ability to cope with the problem. They despaired of making further progress "until the City provides a place where its consumptives . . . may cease to be a menace to the health of their associates."[16] Despite their impassioned pleas, the wheels of government—and public opinion—remained largely intractable on the subject. "Statistics . . . have been quoted so frequently as to have almost lost their force," Biggs fumed in 1902, "and still the people, the legislators, the sanitary authorities, and even the medical profession, have remained indifferent to the vast expenditure unnecessarily made by the human race to this evil."[17]

Organized antituberculosis agitation, already under way in Philadelphia since the early 1890s, gained a foothold in New York when physician Sigard Adolphus Knopf assembled a coalition of medical professionals from private practices, hospitals, sanitariums, and public health departments who were ready to take decisive action against "the white plague."[18] Hampered by internal disagreements over leadership, Knopf asked COSCNY official Edward T. Devine to recommend a layperson "of influence, prestige, and public spirit" to fill the role.[19] Devine, his own organization's recent tenement house reform victories still fresh in his mind, invited Knopf to pursue the group's objectives within the COSCNY. Both sets of professionals recognized the advantages of such an alliance: the COSCNY offered public health activists a structural network for expanding their support base into the community, and its own social workers gained access to the scientific knowledge and authority they needed for making their public appeals more persuasive.[20] Likewise, both parties perceived the interdependence of their causes: as long as improved tenement housing occurred independently of additional sanitariums for containing the sick, controlling tuberculosis would remain impossible.[21] Lastly, both causes required significantly more resources and public backing to succeed. "The sanitary authorities," Biggs argued, "however enthusiastic and efficient, and the medical profession, however influential and numerous, cannot grapple with this problem [without] the hearty support of the people and the administration of the city."[22]

Using the representative character of COSCNY's Tenement House Committee as a template, the CPT included a variety of professionals familiar with different aspects of the tuberculosis problem. It included sixteen medical and public health experts, most notably Knopf; Biggs and Commissioner Ernst J. Lederle of the NYCDOH; tuberculosis specialists E. G. Janeway, T. Mitchell Prudden, and Abraham Jacobi; and Edward Trudeau, founder of Adirondack Cottage Sanitarium at Saranac Lake. Joining them were sixteen laypeople active in organized charities, settlement work, and municipal government, among them Devine; COSCNY president and THD commissioner de Forest; University Settlement head worker Robert Hunter; and Lillian Wald, public health nurse and director of the Henry Street Settlement.[23] Formed in June of 1902, the committee aimed to provide authoritative guidance for professionals, practical information for the public, and political pressure for securing legislation and resources that furthered its goals. In the process, it sought to define the most pressing aspects of the tuberculosis problem and arrive at a clearer understanding of how social, economic, and environmental factors interacted to promote the spread of disease.[24]

CPT MEDICAL PROFESSIONALS AND THE FACTS ABOUT TUBERCULOSIS

During its first year, the CPT sponsored more than eighty public lectures in churches, settlement houses, and schools, where thousands of New Yorkers learned about tuberculosis in English, Italian, Yiddish, German, and French. The CPT also printed and distributed tens of thousands of informational pamphlets based on these lectures.[25] Participating tuberculosis experts agreed on several main points: the disease was caused by living germs; these germs multiplied outside the laboratory only under certain conditions; and human beings provided these favorable conditions only under certain circumstances. Nevertheless, considerable differences emerged among these experts as they related the facts of tuberculosis to CPT audiences. One such difference concerned the favored mode of transmission. While Prudden continued ruminating on the perils of tuberculous dust, Knopf promoted new research favoring direct droplet infection from close-proximity coughing; Jacobi cautioned mothers to avoid meat and milk from tubercular cows, even as Biggs cited recent studies calling these sources of danger into question.[26] In a similar vein, CPT physicians agreed with Prudden that the bacillus "[did] not flourish equally well in the bodies of all human beings"; while most declined to speculate further on the nature of this susceptibility, Knopf classified "predisposed individuals" into several categories, reserving one of them for issuing harsh invectives against the degrading effects of alcoholism.[27]

These differences among medical experts regarding causative factors for tuberculosis also extended to the solutions they proposed. While each stressed the importance of containing and destroying the bacillus, Prudden advocated proper household dusting methods; Knopf devoted nine full pages to cuspidors and spittoons; Jacobi discussed the finer points of boiling milk; and Biggs promoted his longtime objectives of surveillance, education, disinfection, and isolation.[28] Confusing matters further, each CPT physician declared that interacting with consumptives was perfectly safe, provided that his own exacting precautions were followed. At times, the precautions themselves contained fundamentally conflicting messages. After Knopf cautioned people with tuberculosis to "never kiss, no matter whom, on the mouth," to sterilize their eating utensils in boiling water, and to "associate as little as possible with young children," he hastened to reassure his audience that "a clean, conscientious consumptive is as safe a person to associate with as anybody."[29] Likewise, Biggs stressed that "the most intimate contact with a tuberculous

patient may, under proper conditions, be quite free of danger"; when eluci-
dating upon those "proper conditions," he relied upon lengthy excerpts from
Knopf's instructions to consumptives.[30]

CPT medical experts' attempts to provide clear and concise information
revealed not only their conflicting ideas about tuberculosis but also their limited awareness of the hardships governing working-class New Yorkers' lives.
For example, one CPT tuberculosis prevention pamphlet advised readers to
get adequate nourishing food and rest, maintain clean homes and bodies,
seek fresh air at every opportunity, and consult physicians promptly with any
troubling symptoms.[31] Such instructions implied that most New Yorkers possessed sufficient control over their time, budgets, and environments to assume
full responsibility for their health, which CPT physicians knew from their
own experiences to be false. Prudden, for example, interspersed his dusting
tips with frustration at the "choking dust clouds" that resulted from careless
street cleaners, as well as the overcrowded conditions that compromised air
quality in tenements.[32] His colleagues voiced similar frustrations: "We are
hardly entitled to call ourselves a civilized community," Jacobi declared, "when
fifty thousand families at least, with three or six children each, live each in one
light room and one or two small dark holes . . . [that] breed tuberculosis."[33]
"Would that I could take some of our philanthropic friends to our densely
crowded tenement districts," Knopf lamented, "and show them . . . the poor
consumptive, who must die, not because his disease was incurable, but because
there was no place to cure it."[34]

Knopf and his colleagues called for municipally funded hospitals and
sanitariums, along with large-scale prevention and treatment programs that
built upon the work of Biggs and other public health crusaders. They justified
these costly ventures chiefly by appealing to the public's self-interest. People
with consumption posed a significant drain on the economy, they argued,
both through lost wages and growing dependence on social services; thus,
investing more public funds in tuberculosis prevention and treatment would
actually save taxpayers money over the long run.[35] The CPT also drew upon
imperialist rivalries by presenting sanitariums as one more way in which the
United States lagged behind England, France, and Germany, whose governments provided tubercular citizens with free treatment as a matter of course.[36]
Matters of self-interest aside, CPT members agreed with Prudden that states
and municipalities "owe [consumptives] at least a shelter and a place to die."[37]

CPT SOCIAL PROFESSIONALS AND THE RISK FACTORS FOR TUBERCULOSIS

To arrive at a clearer understanding of who was at most risk for contracting
tuberculosis and why, the CPT recruited Lilian Brandt to analyze New York

City Department of Health (NYCDOH) statistics for illuminative patterns. Despite a growing awareness of Brandt's importance as an early American female social statistician—with one recent historian claiming that "no one wrote about poverty with more authority and insight"—a dearth of primary-source material limits researchers to vital records, college rosters, faded newspaper clippings, and occasional flashes of wry commentary in her publications.[38] While these fragments contain only fleeting glimpses of Brandt's personality and perspectives, examining them against a broader contextual backdrop reveals a path to the Lung Block park campaign that was significantly more competitive and uphill than those of her male colleagues. Taken together, these fragments evoke the narrow window of opportunity that social work professions provided college-educated women for brokering a socially acceptable compromise between traditionally feminine domesticity and traditionally masculine ambition and self-reliance. As Brandt committed her social-scientific expertise to the CPT's battle against tuberculosis, she was engaged in her own battle for credibility in what was still very much a man's world—an important consideration when assessing her statistical research and its impact on her working-class subjects.

Born in 1873 in Indianapolis, Lilian Brandt was the eldest surviving child of John Baughman Brandt, a Presbyterian minister from Ohio, and Emily Greene, a former teacher from Illinois.[39] Such parents were likely to instill a deep respect for education, charity, and public service—the same values driving many of Brandt's reform contemporaries.[40] Unlike previous generations of ministers' daughters, Brandt headed east to attend Wellesley College; this placed her among a growing number of middle- and upper-class women seeking more rigorous academic training amid the modernizing forces transforming America after the Civil War.[41] Early proponents argued that higher education would equip women to be more effective domestic helpmeets and nurturers, as well as "municipal housekeepers" for the growing health, educational, and philanthropic needs in their communities.[42] By 1890, this private-to-public shift in women's involvement prompted one contemporary female scholar to observe that "in the schools . . . churches . . . charity organizations, [and] even in the state charitable institutions, women serve on boards of management and fill positions of executive responsibility to a degree that would have astonished our grandmothers."[43] As the spectrum of possibilities for college-educated women widened, so did the range of missions and curricula among the colleges admitting them. Where early nineteenth-century institutions like Mount Holyoke began as seminaries that emphasized religion and restraint in preparing women to become teachers, missionaries, and wives, late nineteenth-century institutions like Bryn Mawr emphasized self-reliance in preparing women to compete directly with men in the professions. Founded as a women's seminary in 1870, Wellesley fell somewhere in between these two templates, molding its students into cultural hybrids who were "intelligent and capable of direct action yet never mannish."[44]

By the time Brandt arrived at Wellesley in 1890, American college-bound women were seeking greater autonomy as well as personal self-improvement. "Nine-tenths of the girls at college are there for the purpose of fitting themselves to earn a livelihood," an early twentieth-century article noted.[45] Brandt's undergraduate career at Wellesley paralleled this larger shift in college women's objectives. After following a traditional nineteenth-century curriculum of music, religion, and the classics, she set a course for the social sciences with economist Katharine Coman, the first female college professor of statistics in America; and historian Elizabeth Kendall, whose forward-thinking, global approach reflected her upbringing as an American diplomat's daughter.[46] These recent faculty arrivals showcased how Wellesley itself was changing to embrace new models of womanhood based on hard work, expertise, and steady persistence against widespread discrimination.[47] While women's suffrage remained an open question, Coman and Kendall prepared their students for responsible citizenship by encouraging independent research and critical thinking. Many of Coman's course topics—"the nature of competition and its power for good and evil, the causes of pauperism and methods of relief, the uses and abuses of public and private charity"—would frame Brandt's research efforts for decades to come.[48]

After graduating from Wellesley in 1895, Brandt navigated the bleak landscape of occupations open to college-educated single women. Competition among the growing ranks of her fellow graduates rendered teaching, the most traditional option, low-paying and unstable; nevertheless, Brandt secured a position at the all-female Lindenwood College in Missouri, where she was promoted to principal within three years.[49] She then joined the faculty of an elite women's boarding school in Massachusetts, a decision likely driven by her desire to pursue graduate research at her nearby alma mater.[50] Brandt's return to Wellesley placed her in the orbit of Emily Greene Balch, an economist of "intense, driving energy coupled with a devastating intellectual curiosity" whose research agenda had taken her from Bryn Mawr to Harvard, the University of Chicago, the Sorbonne, and the University of Berlin by the age of thirty.[51] Having lived at Hull House and cofounded Denison House in Boston, Balch also frequently included fieldwork at nearby settlements in her courses.[52] Under Balch's tutelage, Brandt acquired a thoroughly integrated understanding of statistics, economic theory, and industrialization's impact on society, along with grounding in practical applications through firsthand encounters with urban poverty.[53] She then followed her coursework with ten months' travel through Great Britain, France, Belgium, the Netherlands, Germany, Switzerland, and Italy. This transatlantic exposure offered bountiful opportunities for investigating a wide range of state-sponsored approaches to social problems that were reaching crisis levels in the United States.[54]

While Brandt appeared to be following in the footsteps of her academic mentors, her research—coinciding with the growing professionalization of social work—would take her in a different direction. Her master's thesis, completed in 1901, employed statistics to examine the "negro problem" in her hometown of Saint Louis, a city ranking second only to Baltimore in its relative number of African American inhabitants.[55] Deeply influenced by W. E. B. Du Bois's sociological research on African Americans in Philadelphia, Brandt's study measured African Americans' upward mobility across a broad range of health, social, and economic categories. With the eagle-eye of the statistician, Brandt identified inconsistencies and inaccuracies in municipal data gathering that rendered decade-by-decade comparisons problematic. Through the long gaze of the historian, she set her analysis within a broader framework of national developments affecting race relations before and after the Civil War. With the earnestness of a budding social reformer, she weighed the roles of biology and environment in shaping African Americans' access to health, resources, and justice. While Brandt's thesis traced the poverty, disease, and crime associated with Saint Louis's "Negro Problem" to her subjects' ignorance and moral failings, it also cited the virulent white racism that excluded African Americans from industrial opportunities and restricted them to squalid, overcrowded housing in segregated neighborhoods. Despairing of any change in white attitudes, Brandt promoted the social and economic self-help efforts already under way in African American communities. "It is what [the Negro] does for himself and by his own efforts," Brandt concluded, "in the face of opposition, that will win for him salvation."[56]

While "The Negroes of St. Louis" established Brandt's place in the social-scientific community, embedded within it were several notable weaknesses that would later influence her analysis of tuberculosis in New York.[57] First among these was her use of sweeping generalizations that anticipated a likeminded, sympathetic audience. For instance, Brandt first defined the "Negro Problem" as "the degree of difference between it and the prevailing national type," modified by "the strength of the forces at work within and without . . . to bring [African Americans] in touch with what is best in American civilization." Using German immigrants as a counterexample, she noted, "There is no German problem . . . because they are already in line with American ideals before they come over, and quickly become assimilated." Brandt's direct juxtaposition of American and Germanic cultures confirmed her image of "the prevailing national type" to be white, Anglo-Saxon, and Protestant: groups with which she and her presumed readership self-identified, and from which African Americans had been systematically excluded.[58] By framing the "Negro Problem" in terms of one group's compliance with an external set of cultural standards, Brandt established parameters that not only placed responsibility for Saint Louis's "Negro Problem" squarely upon her study's subjects but also failed to recognize the cultural standards operating internally within this group.

A second weakness in Brandt's analysis was a tendency to base the validity of her findings on how closely they mirrored her preexisting assumptions. In part, this pattern reflected social scientists' frustration with turn-of-the-century recordkeeping: "The interest and importance of vital statistics," Brandt observed dryly, "are equaled only by the difficulty of getting any that are reliable."[59] This skepticism often led researchers to rely upon their personal experiences and observations when determining which statistical findings carried more weight. For example, Brandt rejected Saint Louis figures that placed the late nineteenth-century African American death rate below that of white Americans, on the rationale that "there is always an abnormally high death rate among Negroes in cities." She then charged faulty recordkeeping with underreporting African American deaths over the previous decade and overreporting their population size, even while conceding that the city's African American population did in fact increase dramatically during that period.[60] While faulty recordkeeping could and did pose significant obstacles for early statisticians, Brandt's easy dismissal of data that did not support her preconceptions risked undermining the integrity of the larger project.

Similarly, Brandt bridged informational gaps with anecdotal evidence filtered through a combination of unidentified "expert" testimony and her own perceptions. Sometimes this practice put her personal biases in direct competition with her observations of the disproportionate hardships and discrimination that African Americans experienced. When discussing the health effects of overcrowding, for instance, Brandt assigned equal weight to tenants' "faults and incompetence" and the impact of significantly higher rents in African American sections of the city.[61] While maintaining that African Americans were not biologically more vulnerable to diseases than other racial groups, Brandt attributed their higher prevalence to collective risky behaviors. "Negroes," she stated, "go insufficiently clothed in cold weather, are careless about wet clothing, are unwilling to call for medical attendance until the last moment, are ignorant of the laws of hygiene and sanitation, and live in surroundings that favor the spread of bacteriological diseases." Brandt would have considered such judgments within professional bounds, given that they reflected standard practice in prominent medical journals from the period.[62] These judgments also may have reflected the cultural biases of her local informants, whom she described as "teachers, clergymen, doctors, lawyers, and political leaders . . . [who were] interested in the progress of the Negroes as a race and to have well defined theories of the reasons for their present conditions and the ways in which they should be helped."[63] This description suggests a lack of direct communication with the working-class African Americans who made up the bulk of Brandt's investigation. Whether this decision reflected concerns about logistical constraints, protecting subjects' privacy, maintaining protocol in a fiercely segregated city, or something else entirely, it influenced Brandt's work by removing additional opportunities to test her interpretations.

Ultimately, Brandt's "Negro Problem" assumed the form of a vicious circle that traced the problem's chief symptoms—"enormous waste of life and vitality . . . imperfectly developed moral sense and . . . lack of control that bear fruit in alarming amount of crime"—back to perceived African American failings, "their ignorance and inefficiency that go hand in hand with poverty, at once reasons for it and results of it."[64] Despite having cited white discrimination at various points throughout her study, Brandt did not assign it a clearly defined role in this circle. Having grown up in white Saint Louis, she accepted its racism as an unfortunate and unalterable reality—the uniform background upon which the circle existed.

BRANDT AND "THE SOCIAL ASPECTS OF TUBERCULOSIS"

When Brandt arrived in New York in the summer of 1902, social work was fast acquiring the rough contours of a profession. In keeping with its ongoing mission to legitimize charity through scientific and business approaches, COSCNY now offered formal training through its Summer School in Philanthropy, which preceded the Chicago School of Civics and Philanthropy by several years.[65] Scholar and social activist Kate Holladay Claghorn described early cohorts as a "heterogenous" assortment of college graduates lacking on-the-job experience and veteran caseworkers lacking systematic methods. "Our chief qualification," Claghorn remarked, "was our interest in the subject."[66] Within six years of the school's opening in 1898, more than two hundred students were reported to have earned certificates.[67] As Brandt attended classes with future reform colleagues like Frances Kellor and Paul Kellogg, she appreciated the groundbreaking significance of their activities. "The idea that any training was desirable to prepare men and women—chiefly women—to minister to the poor, was [still] a novel idea," Brandt later recalled, "and to many a preposterous and distasteful idea."[68]

While scientific charity represented a conscious departure from older conceptualizations of philanthropy as emotionally charged "women's work," traditional gender patterns persisted within social work's power structures. Women's involvement at COSCNY, while welcomed, was relegated to casework and clerical roles while men assumed the administrative responsibilities. Nevertheless, women were working from within those power structures to assert their own authority and independence.[69] When Devine recruited

Brandt in 1902 to compile and analyze statistics for the CPT, he thus offered her one of the earliest and most visible opportunities to date for applying a woman's expertise to an organization and field still decisively dominated by men. As Brandt prepared to take on this new project, much lay at stake beyond her future prospects: her teachers' reputations, her family's investments in her education, and the largely untested professional capabilities of women at large.

Reminiscent of her master's thesis, Brandt's tuberculosis study established credibility by appealing to the presupposed Western biases of her readers. She opened with a popular anecdote in which a Turkish ruler dismissed his European friend's request for statistical information as not only "difficult and useless" but also dangerous, citing Islamic teachings equating such curiosity with the desire to transcend God's wisdom and ultimate authority. Using the ruler's objection as an analogy for contemporary critics of statistics and germ theory, she attributed their passivity and skepticism to an "Oriental habit of mind"—the tacit implication being that readers who upheld the legitimacy of her project without hesitation were more worldly, progressive, and civilized by comparison.[70]

Drawing on national census and NYCDOH records, Brandt weighed the significance of social factors such as age, sex, occupation, race, nationality, and population density in determining tuberculosis mortality. The preliminary results of her analysis revealed that tuberculosis killed more men than women; that it affected both sexes most between the ages of fifteen and forty-four; and that it exacted proportionately heavier death tolls in cities.[71] Domestic servants, as well as those who worked in dusty and confined spaces, stood a higher chance of getting sick. African Americans, Native Americans, and Chinese immigrants were nearly three times more likely to die of it than white Americans; among European immigrants, the Irish fared worst, with Italians and eastern European Jews faring better.[72]

Having established that "there is no feature in the composition of a population which does not affect the prevalence of consumption," Brandt then attempted to determine more precisely how each feature contributed to the complex web of variables she had uncovered.[73] As with the Saint Louis study, complicating her efforts were questions that her original sources could not answer. With most cities and towns trailing behind New York in public health infrastructure and medical training, to what extent could their death records be relied upon when comparing tuberculosis mortality from different areas?[74] Other questions involved correlation versus causation: Did occupational mortality figures reflect the risks of contracting tuberculosis in each line of work, or merely the concentration of people with consumption in each field?[75] Moreover, if tuberculosis flourished in densely populated areas, as medical and housing reform experts had maintained for years, why were some of the

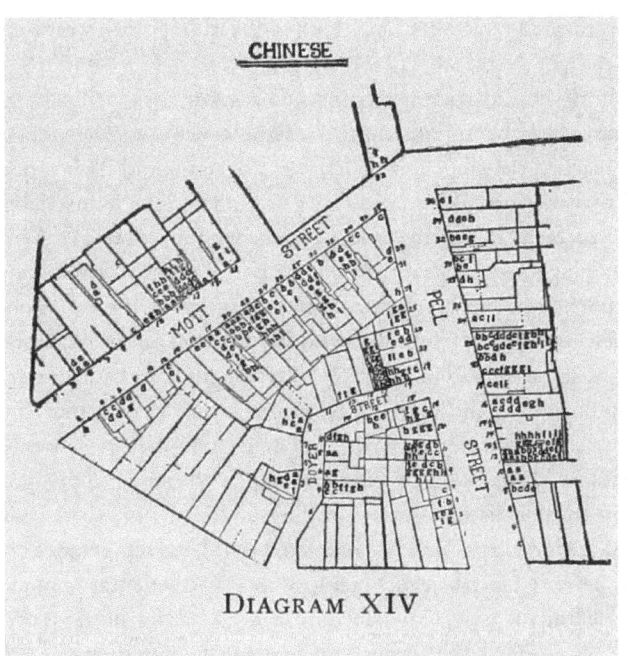

CHINESE

DIAGRAM XIV

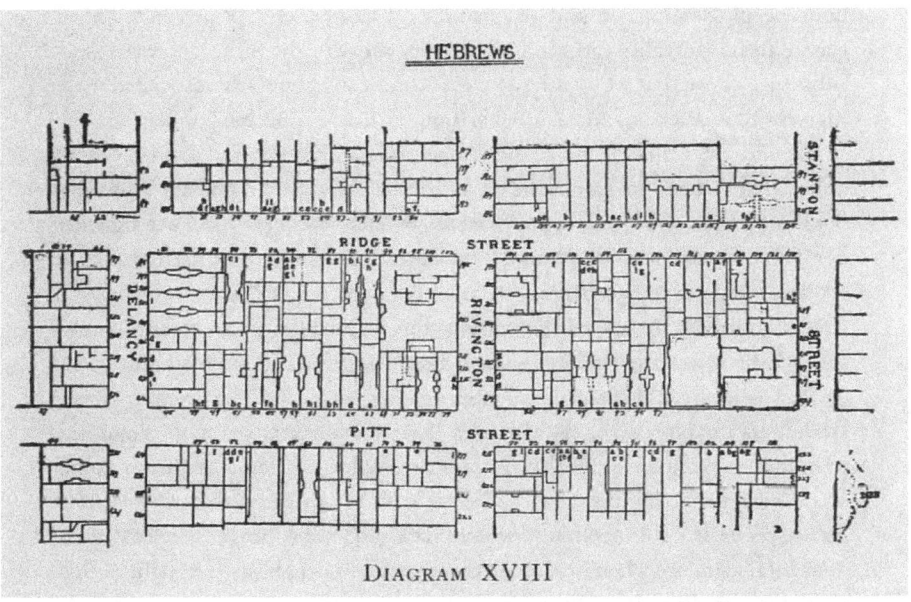

HEBREWS

DIAGRAM XVIII

3.1A AND 3.1B. Disease maps showing the distribution of tuberculosis cases reported to the NYCDOH from predominantly Chinese and Jewish immigrant neighborhoods from 1899 to 1902. Reprinted from Lilian Brandt, "The Social Aspects of Tuberculosis Based on a Study of Statistics," in COSCNY, *A Handbook for the Prevention of Tuberculosis* (New York: Charity Organization Society, 1903), 89, 91.

most overcrowded New York neighborhoods yielding the lowest tuberculosis death rates?[76]

Much as she did with her Saint Louis study, Brandt dealt with these uncertainties by either minimizing their significance or resolving them in ways that overreached the empirical evidence at her command. When her analysis revealed higher tuberculosis mortality rates outside the industrial northeast region—a pattern challenging post-germ-theory definitions of tuberculosis as an "urban" plague—Brandt dismissed this pattern as a probable combination of overreporting in rural regions and underreporting in registration-area cities.[77] Likewise, when attempting to explain the uneven prevalence of tuberculosis that she observed in New York's tenement districts, Brandt fell back upon popular racial and ethnic stereotypes rather than comparing income levels or housing conditions. Noting that many high-density, low-tuberculosis areas contained large numbers of Italian or Jewish immigrants—groups that public health officials and several leading physicians associated with lower tuberculosis mortality—Brandt postulated that Jews' temperance and kosher diets compensated for their physical weakness and sedentary indoor occupations, while Italians' easygoing temperaments and active, outdoor occupations evidently outweighed the hazards of inadequate nutrition, "less hygienic" housekeeping standards, and overcrowding.[78] Conversely, she attributed high tuberculosis mortality rates in high-density areas to the filth, ignorance, and substance abuse that white middle-class Americans popularly associated with high concentrations of African American, Irish, and Chinese populations.[79]

Brandt then illustrated these associations with several of Biggs's tuberculosis-riddled block maps, labeled by ethnic group to emphasize what she held to be the crucial determining factor in each instance.[80] In keeping with her Saint Louis research, many of her bases for comparing different ethnic groups—degrees of cleanliness, "occupation, housing, and temperament, and habits governing forms of dissipation, food, clothing, and exercise"—correlated directly with their projected assimilability into white mainstream society, what Brandt termed "our high-grade civilization."[81] However, where Brandt had explored the connections between poverty, poor housing, and prejudice in Saint Louis health disparities, she largely demurred from doing so in New York, claiming that "sufficient data for authoritative explanations do not yet exist." This newfound reluctance belied her willingness to rely upon anecdotal evidence when broaching these topics in her thesis.[82] In light of this inconsistency, Brandt's decision to forgo deeper, more critical socioeconomic analyses may have reflected tight deadline restrictions; CPT members' priorities; or her sources, limited to rows of numbers and the overlapping perspectives of medical and social professionals.

Based upon a combination of crude death rates and speculation, Brandt's study concluded that the demographic profile most vulnerable to dying from tuberculosis was male, of prime working and reproductive age, urban, working-class, and foreign-born or African American. Given the inconsistencies among Brandt's original sources, these conclusions reveal more about the power of confirmation bias than about the social aspects of tuberculosis. She accepted without criticism the statistical patterns supporting middle-class preconceptions of tuberculosis as "a disease of the tenements," even though uneven reporting methods in New York City ensured that tenement districts yielded the highest tuberculosis death rates; likewise, she did not hesitate to discredit patterns challenging these preconceptions. Having arrived at the most promising targets for intervention using these methods, Brandt declared that "the campaign can be conducted economically—attacks can be made where the minimum of effort will result in the maximum of success."[83] As with the subjects of her thesis, the subjects of her tuberculosis study—people whose lives Brandt judged to be most at risk—remained confined to the aggregate in charts, tables, and maps, their individual perspectives uncharted.

Given Brandt's precarious status as an early-career female statistician, to what extent did her tuberculosis analysis reflect her own views, and to what extent did they reflect the objectives of the CPT, which had recognized her potential and offered her a valuable opportunity to enter a male-dominated field?[84] Likewise, to what degree did Brandt's detachment from working-class subjects represent a personal bid for legitimacy in a profession striving to divorce itself from older models rooted in feminine moral authority and compassion? Whatever the precise mix of factors shaping her interpretative approaches, what remains certain is her successful reception. Brandt's work on "the Tuberculosis Problem" appeared in newspapers, lecture halls, professional journals, and public expositions, eventually earning her a gold medal for her contribution to the COSCNY exhibit at the Saint Louis World's Fair in 1904.[85] As the CPT study opened professional doors for Brandt, it continued reproducing and reinforcing popular assumptions about tuberculosis before wider circles of professionals and the public—many of whom had already subscribed to them in the first place.[86]

ERNEST POOLE, A MUCKRAKER IN THE MAKING

Having compiled information on tuberculosis prevention, identified cross-sections of society in need of intervention, and outlined potential solutions, CPT members now looked outside their circle for a gifted writer to generate powerful popular appeals from their arsenal of facts and statistics. Where Lilian Brandt supplied the rationales for their publicity campaign, the young and aspiring journalist Ernest Poole would deliver the emotional pull. As Poole would soon discover, converting abstract clusters of case dots back into human beings demanded skills that extended far beyond writing.

While his path to antituberculosis activism contrasted with Brandt's in many respects, Poole was also a staunchly private individual whose inner life and personality eluded decades of frustrated biographers.[87] Born in Chicago in 1880, Poole hailed from the same urban, well-to-do backdrop as many of his future reform contemporaries. His father, a stockbroker like Lawrence Veiller's, lived by the fluctuations of "the wheat pit" at the Chicago Board of Trade. After accumulating and losing three fortunes in ten years, he secured a fourth that enabled him to raise seven children amid abundant opportunity and material comforts.[88] Largely insulated from the city's rising class warfare, Poole's childhood featured private schools, music and dancing lessons, summers in the country, and steady circulation among Chicago's wealthy and prominent families.[89] Despite their prosperity, Poole's parents instilled a blend of tolerance and humility that discouraged him from identifying fully with upper-class aristocracy. His father, descended from small-time Dutch farmers and merchants in New York, still espoused the solid bourgeois values of hard work, thrift, and practicality.[90] Likewise, his devout Presbyterian mother often took him along when visiting local families living in humbler circumstances.[91] Both sets of parental influences encouraged Poole to remain receptive to different lifestyles and viewpoints—traits that later became indispensable to him as a writer.[92]

Poole's instinctive gravitation toward common ground sometimes blinded him to the wealth and privilege distinguishing him from most Americans. When his family hosted a group of disadvantaged children at their summer home while he was growing up, he never forgot one plucky boy who suddenly grew somber and blurted out, "Jesus Christ, but it's hell to be poor!"[93] When Poole later joined a gang of working-class youths who played in the dumps and lumberyards around Chicago's waterfront, some of the rough characters he encountered left him feeling frightened and even disgusted.[94] Others sparked his imagination, such as the "junkman," with "his harsh guttural croaking voice, his dirty face with ragged beard and his strange deep tragic eyes," who "came from a world I knew nothing about . . . even then, I loved to explore into all that was strange in this queer big human adventure of ours."[95] Later on, Poole's vivid portrayals of the poor would continue bridging the warm sympathy of the insider with the voyeuristic curiosity of the outsider.

Poole's early worldly exposures, facilitated through his status as a boy of wealth, prepared him for dealing directly with people of different classes and cultures in ways that Brandt, the minister's daughter from Saint Louis, would have found much less accessible. These stark differences in their backgrounds then carried over into their college experiences. Where Brandt used her time at Wellesley to hone her intellectual abilities with socially conscious mentors, Poole—dubbed the "most useless man" in his class at Princeton—struggled to remain motivated through the "genial ease or utter boredom" of lectures that failed to address the modernizing forces transforming the world around him.[96] The Columbian Exposition, which had transformed Poole's hometown into a gleaming electric wonderland several years earlier, inspired him to envision a new world that supplanted the "grime, disorder and haste" of Gilded Age industrialism with clean and orderly scientific design.[97] Poole was hardly alone in his restless anticipation: "That the world was preparing to take a new step in social advance," recalled one of his literary contemporaries, "most men I knew agreed in feeling."[98] Assuming command of his own education, Poole immersed himself in late nineteenth-century Russian realism, in hopes that the insights of Leo Tolstoy and Ivan Turgenev would give him a clearer perspective on the social developments unfolding around him in his own time. "What were the forces here and now," he kept asking himself; "could I get close to them and see them in terms of human life?"[99]

At this critical juncture, one of Princeton's newest faculty additions, Woodrow Wilson, emerged as a role model for Poole. Lecturing on history and politics to packed halls of four hundred, Wilson urged his students to take an active part in reforming American society and institutions; outside class, his informal chats about current events gave Poole "an exciting sense of new life stirring in our land."[100] When Wilson instructed him to read Riis's *How the Other Half Lives*, its vivid descriptions of tenement life restimulated Poole's memories of the working-class people he had encountered in Chicago. "Tenement life appealed to me as a tremendous new field," Poole remarked later, "scarcely touched by American writers yet."[101] By the early 1900s this "new field" had already provided ample material for Riis, William Dean Howells, Abraham Cahan, Lincoln Steffens, and a host of other authors, making Poole's statement more remarkable for its naïveté than for its accuracy.[102]

When Poole arrived at New York's University Settlement in 1902—having, like Brandt, just spent months studying social reform methods in London, Paris, and Berlin—his fellow residents hailed from elite backgrounds, as when Veiller lived there ten years earlier.[103] Likewise, they still aimed to tackle urban problems by engaging their working-class neighbors on equal terms, "not [as] uplifters but mixers and explorers."[104] However, the settlement had begun a more radical shift under its new head worker, Robert Hunter, a recent transplant from Chicago's Hull House who shared Veiller's interest in housing reform as well as his forceful and abrasive personality.[105] Many of Poole's fellow residents went on to become outspoken agitators in socialist and labor circles, most notably philanthropist James Graham Phelps Stokes and journalist William English Walling.[106]

For Poole and other aspiring writers, settlements provided not only the opportunity to take action on pressing social issues but also a "human gold mine" for digging stories "hot out of life."[107] At first, however, Poole's attempts only highlighted the class and cultural chasms that separated him from his subjects. "Their shrill harsh voices spoke in tongues that were completely strange to me, and strange their faces, strange their eyes!" he lamented. "How ever get close to such people as these, to write about them?"[108] Settlement life put Poole in circulation with muckraking journalists like Ray Stannard Baker and Steffens, who offered him valuable advice for conveying his subject matter to a wider audience. Baker urged Poole to keep his focus trained outside himself: "When I'm at work," Baker told him, "I keep in mind a dozen Americans I've known . . . who seem to me to represent my million readers everywhere, and never for a minute do I forget 'em while I write." Steffens, by contrast, advised Poole to rely upon his own judgment. "Dig hard for hunks of life just as it is," Steffens told him, "and write 'em down just as they come . . . choose your side, your personal angle, and then warm up to it! Don't just see it—feel it, feel it hot and strong!"[109]

Poole threw himself into writing about the Lower East Side, where "the great pot seethed and boiled and new Americans were made."[110] Hunter, observing Poole's popularity with the local boys, recruited him for a child labor investigation taking shape across the city's settlements and social work organizations.[111] Drawing on his early experiences playing with street children, Poole spent the next months working among the "wise tough little guys" who formed the ranks of the city's newsboys, messengers, and bootblacks. Just like the "street Arabs" whom Riis had profiled more than a decade earlier, many of these boys still slept in doorways and under bridges, sustaining themselves through "hastily bolted meals, with often double a man's portion of coffee, cigars, and cigarettes."[112] Where Riis delighted in portraying these boys as shrewd and enterprising little scamps, Poole revealed a darker picture by disclosing their off-hours activities, where they squandered their scant earnings—often supplemented through petty theft—on gambling, opium, and prostitutes.[113] Citing common dysfunctional patterns among the hundreds who passed through the city's wayward-boy institutions, Poole argued that the "irregular life" of street trades sowed future generations of tramps and criminals. "The street is making a man of him—swiftly," Poole offered as a counterpoint to Riis's plucky "street Arab"; "but when the man is finally made he has long since passed from our attention. And if a failure, we lose all connection between him and the bright, attractive little newsboy who has taken his place."[114]

Poole's lurid depictions of working boys' lives appeared in a variety of popular magazines throughout the spring of 1903, helping Hunter and his allies secure state legislation regulating the hours and conditions of "street trades" for children.[115] They also cemented Poole's reputation as an up-and-coming muckraker, eliciting flattering comparisons with the author who inspired his interest in tenement writing. "[Poole] writes extremely well," Hunter wrote to COSCNY president de Forest when recommending Poole to write for the

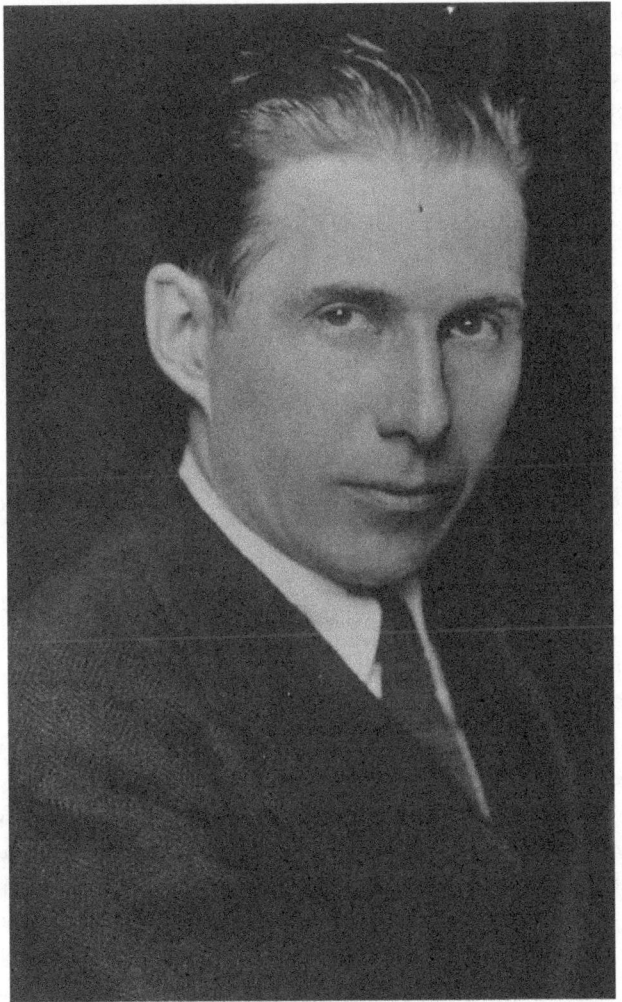

3.2. This undated portrait of Ernest Poole, taken by Harris & Ewing, is held in the Library of Congress Prints and Photographs Division, Washington, DC.

CPT, adding that "[he] has done for the child labor agitation what Jacob A. Riis has done for the tenement house agitation."[116]

"THE PLAGUE IN ITS STRONGHOLD"

In theory, Poole's next assignment appeared simple enough: go to the block bordered by Cherry, Catherine, Hamilton, and Market Streets, "where the Plague had left deadlier records than in any other block in town . . . trace down the stories behind them and so give a picture in human terms that could be featured in the press."[117] In practice, achieving these objectives required him to push beyond the exotic colors and cacophony that engulfed him on Lower East Side streets, rising and receding daily from the "common ground" of the University Settlement. Accompanied by public health and tenement inspectors, Poole spent a month of long days and nights ascending rickety staircases, fumbling down dark hallways, and venturing across thresholds that assailed him with "the heavy, foul odor from poverty, ignorance, filth, disease."[118] Streamed through Poole's privileged aesthetic filters, the rows of dotted rectangles on tuberculosis maps resumed the three-dimensional contours of "a block packed close with huge grimy tenements . . . honeycombed with rooms." "These rooms," Poole added incredulously, "are homes for people."[119]

Through detailed, heartrending vignettes—set inside buildings sporting local nicknames like "the Bucket," "the Morgue" and "the Ink-Pot,"—Poole made the block his focal point for conveying CPT talking points about New York's tuberculosis problem, and the need for organized, collective action. His opening scene captured the last moments of a dying Jewish tailor "in a room only ten feet square, where six people lay on the floor packed close," with four children sleeping in a nearby closet. Poole highlighted the environmental hazards of this cramped, overcrowded space. "From his soiled bed he could touch and infect the table where the two families ate," Poole noted; "the cooking stove was but six feet from his; the cupboard, just above his pillow; he could even reach one of the cradles, where his baby girl lay staring."[120] Like generations of reformers before him, Poole maintained that these environmental hazards paved the way for moral failings, weakening people's resistance to infection even further. "Foul air, darkness, wretched surroundings—these work on the home by day and by night," Poole declared. "So come squalid homes and wretched meals. So comes the humorous, shattered old chap who told me, 'I ain't never sober but when I gits out of bed.' So come hundreds of others, men and women, young and old; drunk, bestial, vile, forever steadily sinking."[121]

Despite such dismal character appraisals, Poole reassured his readers that "the good outnumber[ed] the bad eight to one" in this block, and included "some of the kindliest good people that ever lived."[122] For Poole, the source of the block's deadly contagion lay not in the residents themselves but in the inanimate structures housing them. Citing material from recent public health and housing reform campaigns, he pointed out how air shafts, ill-ventilated bedrooms, and dark hallways provided efficient pathways for germs to circulate. In houses where "things and people—good and bad—have only partitions between them," he warned that even the most virtuous people risked exposure to contamination. To illustrate this point, Poole rattled off a list of the block's "innocent" tuberculosis victims: an Irish woman who "drank not a drop" and kept her home "as neat as wax," but nevertheless shared hallways with a saloon; a teenage girl who supported her family for months "on bread and tea alone" after her alcoholic father died; a "gentle little girl of seven" who cared for her younger siblings and dying father in rooms where "foul air arose from the cellar, the [court], the halls, the closet."[123]

Citing the "house-infection" arguments of Knopf, Biggs, and other public health professionals, Poole explained that the coughed-up germs from successive waves of tenants compounded inside tenements over time, transforming rooms into permanent repositories of tuberculosis with that "held death ready and waiting for years." Tracing more than one hundred reported cases of tuberculosis to six buildings, Poole described the succession of tenants who sickened and died in one apartment over a seven-year span: "a blind Scotchman . . . [and] his little daughter"; a Jew who died the following summer; a German woman who died in the autumn; an Irish father "[who] was a hard, steady worker, and loved his children."[124]

In demonstrating that tuberculosis did not restrict itself to derelicts and sinners, Poole reaffirmed the CPT's core message that "hundreds of thousands from every class in the city are in constant danger." From this block, he warned, "the Plague is constantly spreading out all over the city—to rich and poor alike."[125] He jolted his readers' complacency with descriptions of consumptives laboring over clothing to be sold in uptown department stores, or handling and dispensing food from the nearby markets, fruit carts, and bakeries. After recounting a prostitute's slow demise, Poole added provocatively, "Thousands like her have been sick of this Plague in New York. How many have infected their patrons?" After appealing to his readers' fears with stories of contagion, and then to their purses with Biggs's estimates of how much tuberculosis was costing the city, Poole then called for New Yorkers to attack "the plague in its stronghold" by supporting expanded public health services, parks and playgrounds, public baths, and sanitariums. Such large-scale improvements would put New York on the same footing as other European cities, where "thousands of lives have been saved." Poole concluded by appealing to his readers' hearts: "Millions must be spent—because we are human," he pleaded.[126]

In many respects, *A Plague in Its Stronghold* exhibited the strong guiding influence of Riis's *How the Other Half Lives*, the book that first alerted Poole to the "tremendous new field" of tenement writing. Both authors delivered their message through colorful impressions of rough but decent people making the best out of bad situations. Likewise, both grounded their arguments with statistics and expert opinions, embellishing them with samples of "street" dialect, humorous asides, and biblical references to brotherhood. Poole's photographs of the block also revealed a remarkable similarity to Riis's style in terms of staging and subject matter. Squalid tenement interiors, a "little mother" hold-

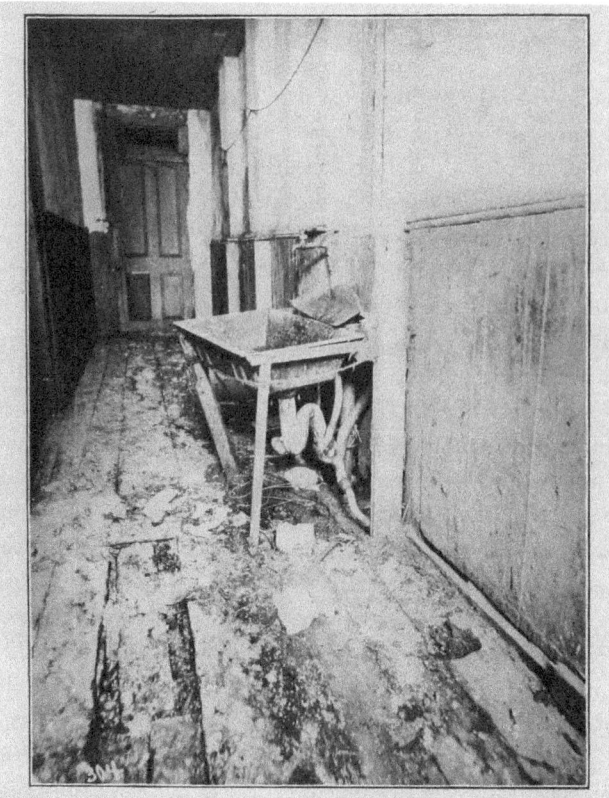

" It is in Halls Like These that the Germs Can Live Two Years or Longer."

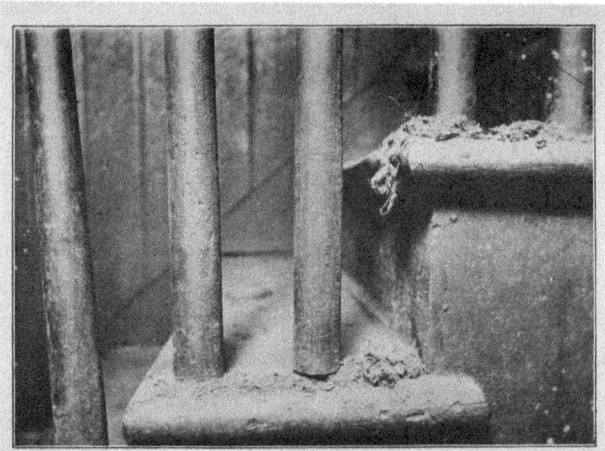

"The Stairways in the Rear House are Low and Narrow, Uneven, and Thick with Dust Piled in Every Nook and Corner."

3.3A AND B. The photographs accompanying Ernest Poole's first-person observations in *A Plague in Its Stronghold* reflected early twentieth-century conceptualizations of tuberculosis as a "house disease" that flourished in darkness, dust, and disorder. Reprinted from COSCNY, *Handbook for the Prevention of Tuberculosis*.

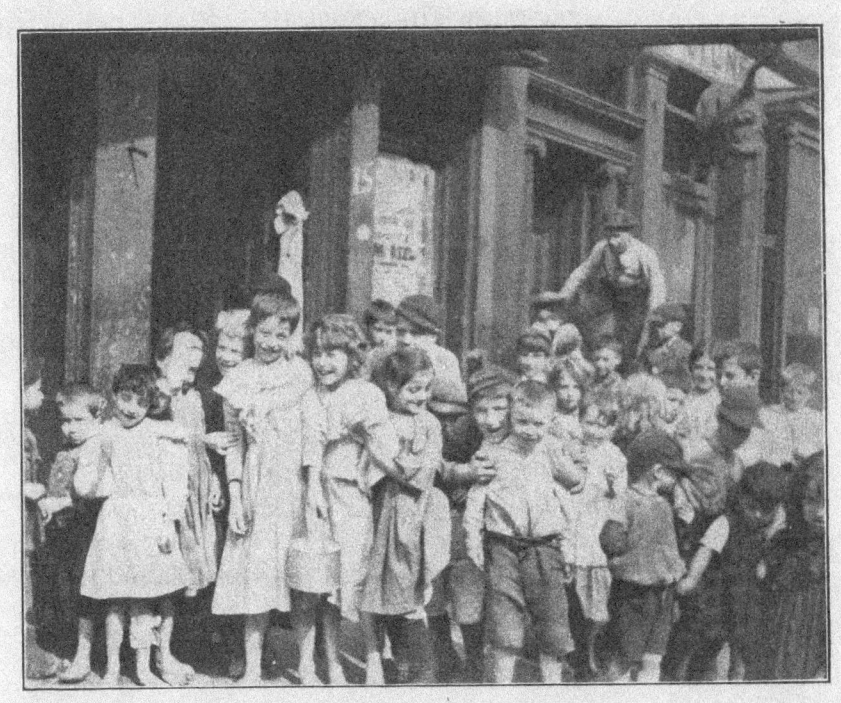

A GROUP OF "LUNG BLOCK" CHILDREN

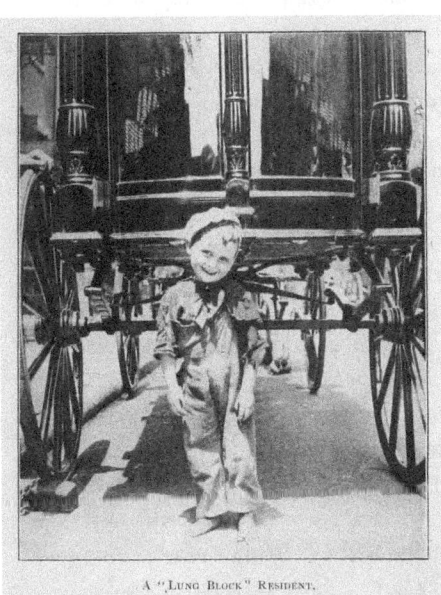

A "LUNG BLOCK" RESIDENT.

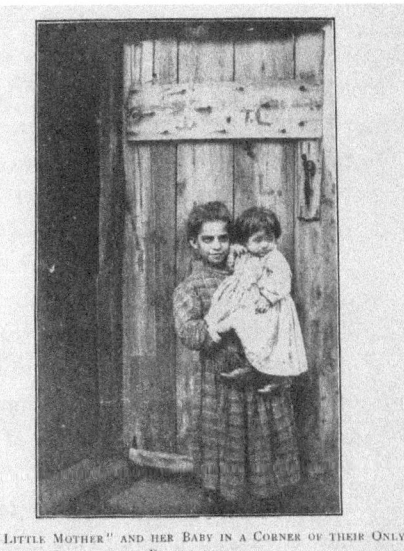

A "LITTLE MOTHER" AND HER BABY IN A CORNER OF THEIR ONLY PLAYGROUND.

3.4A–C. In ways strikingly reminiscent of Jacob Riis's reform writings, Poole's *A Plague in Its Stronghold* included photographs intended to convey the innocence and vulnerability of children growing up in contaminated, unwholesome environments. Reprinted from COSCNY, *Handbook for the Prevention of Tuberculosis*.

ing her baby sibling protectively, dozens of school-aged children gathered near a day nursery on the street, a lone, barefooted toddler grinning impishly in front of a hearse—all appeared carefully calculated to elicit disgust as well as sympathy. When explaining the uneven distribution of tuberculosis cases throughout the block, Poole cited Irish alcoholism, Italian superstition, and Jewish adherence to ancient custom—the same ethnic stereotypes so prevalent in Riis's work.[127] Lastly, Poole followed Riis's example in portraying the block as a strategic battlefront in an ongoing war for the nation's physical, moral, and civic wellbeing.[128]

Poole's most notable departure from *How the Other Half Lives* involves his attitude toward his working-class subjects, who appeared not as amusing, vicious, or pathetic caricatures but autonomous human beings with their own legitimate perspectives on the issues at hand. "Go tonight through this same block," Poole instructed his readers; "you will find no one sick. They must know you first. What is your business there, how can you help?"[129] These descriptions reflect Poole's efforts to relate to his subjects directly; by gradually earning the locals' trust, he acquired the ability to observe them from a closer vantage point. As was the case during his Chicago childhood, being male made connecting with strangers in rough neighborhoods an option more accessible and less fraught with danger than for Brandt. Notably, what he learned through these encounters challenged the prevention and treatment strategies that his CPT colleagues promoted with such aggressive urgency. Most families on this block could not afford to hire a private physician, Poole reported; public health services, while free, resulted in automatic registration, loss of privacy, and possible coercion into accepting treatment elsewhere. Many of the tuberculosis sufferers Poole interviewed shouldered responsibilities that could not accommodate even a temporary leave from work or caretaking at home. Likewise, they feared hospitals, notorious for their lack of space, as simply places to die. Even death offered little relief from their cares; because most life insurance companies refused to cover tuberculosis, an accurate diagnosis could devastate their survivors financially as well as emotionally.[130]

Taking these grim realities into account, *A Plague in Its Stronghold* yielded a dramatically different profile of working-class tuberculosis from Brandt's. Poole's subjects resisted CPT intervention measures not out of ignorance but from a combination of tenacity, self-reliance, and shrewd assessments of the meager treatment options available. When offered a short stay in the country, one mildly consumptive woman said, "'It's got to come anyway, an' we'd get homesick for the block, so I guess we'll stay.'" Another told Poole that "work was too rare to be given up; what if she could find no other work in the fall and so go on charity? Anyway, she wasn't yet sick. . . . No arguments from visitor, doctor or friends could change this decision." Despite his frustration with his subjects' refusals to seek treatment, Poole had come to understand that in a

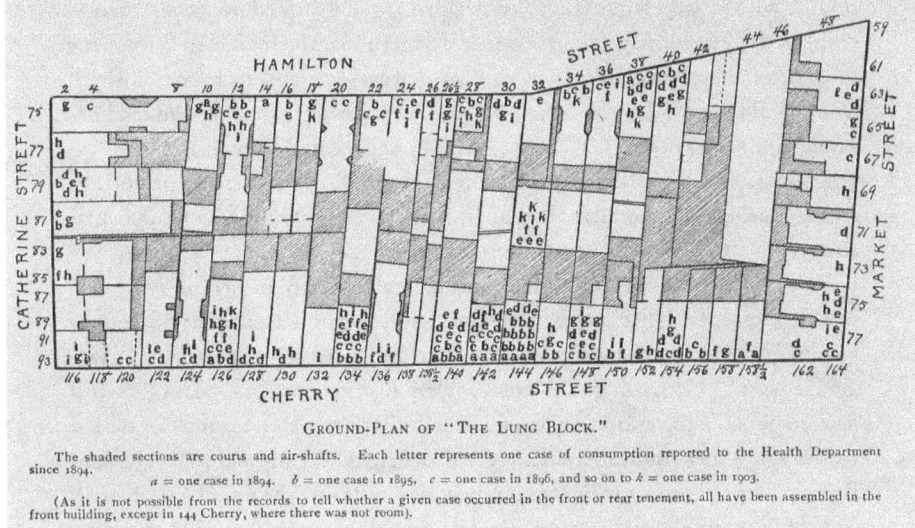

GROUND-PLAN OF "THE LUNG BLOCK."

The shaded sections are courts and air-shafts. Each letter represents one case of consumption reported to the Health Department since 1894. a = one case in 1894. b = one case in 1895. c = one case in 1896, and so on to k = one case in 1903.

(As it is not possible from the records to tell whether a given case occurred in the front or rear tenement, all have been assembled in the front building, except in 144 Cherry, where there was not room).

3.5. A tuberculosis map of the block bordered by Cherry, Catherine, Hamilton and Market Streets, compiled from New York City Health Department reports from 1894 to 1903. Reprinted from COSCNY, *Handbook for the Prevention of Tuberculosis.*

hand-to-mouth existence where nothing was guaranteed, "they want[ed] to live today, not after six months of tedious, doubtful recovery."[131] Poole's quest to trace the stories behind the dots had yielded truths about tuberculosis that had long eluded public health and social work professionals, suggesting that any serious campaign to eradicate the disease required listening more closely to those living in its "stronghold."

Shortly after discovering the tubercle bacillus in 1882, Robert Koch predicted that when enough physicians came to accept consumption's status as an infectious disease, "the question of an adequate campaign . . . will develop by itself."[132] Twenty years later, these campaigns had taken root in American cities, the most active among them being COSCNY's Committee on the Prevention of Tuberculosis. During its ambitious first year alone, the CPT distributed thousands of educational pamphlets, sponsored hundreds of public lectures, and commissioned a far-ranging statistical study, all with the goal of increasing support for sanitariums and broader social improvements. By late summer of 1903 its furious agitations had set New York's state and municipal machinery in motion to provide additional medical facilities and contributed directly to the growth of a national antituberculosis movement.[133]

The CPT's early years constituted a significant moment when early twentieth-century American public health and social activists overlapped briefly within the same frame. Both groups subscribed to germ theory, employed the same mapping and statistical methods, and looked to Europe for inspiration when promoting government-driven solutions for tuberculosis.[134] While CPT medical professionals emphasized the need for state-funded hospitals and sanitariums, CPT social workers advocated providing consumptive people and their families with financial assistance and fresh-air outings to the seashore and country.[135] Remaining true to COSCNY's broader mission, they also promoted the importance of large-scale social improvements in reducing tuberculosis morbidity and mortality: more healthful living and working spaces, higher wages, and outdoor recreation areas that offered an alternative to saloons, dance halls, theaters, and other forms of working-class amusement.[136] Conceding that "the problem would soon disappear of itself if it were possible for everybody to breathe fairly pure air, to keep clean with a reasonable effort, and to have enough of the right sort of food to eat," Lilian Brandt echoed her European contemporaries' calls for "the mobilization of all social forces, public and private, official and voluntary" to fight tuberculosis, adding that "complete eradication is only a matter of time if the public can be roused to a sense of its responsibility."[137]

As CPT physicians attempted to provide clear and concise information about tuberculosis, the considerable inconsistencies and contradictions among them undermined their effectiveness. Meanwhile, CPT researchers like Lilian Brandt struggled to define relationships between social factors and tuberculosis mortality amid uncertain data gathering. Both sets of trained experts navigated uncertain terrain by relying on abstract methods and their personal perceptions, which linked tuberculosis with impoverished tenement populations. These perceptions, when sprinkled among precise-looking maps, charts, and tabulations of numbers, took on a scientific legitimacy that rendered them self-fulfilling. Assumptions shaped evidence and evidence reinforced assumptions, creating closed circuits of investigative inquiry that etched the certainty of fixed and permanent "strongholds" of tuberculosis ever more firmly into the public consciousness.[138]

As Brandt's work became more widely known, it fulfilled Katharine Coman's and Emily Greene Balch's aims to challenge popular assumptions about women's intellectual capabilities. While statistics were "commonly supposed to bristle with terrors for the feminine mind," a New-York Daily Tribune interview with Brandt opened, "once in a while a woman arises who gives the lie to this absurd theory by taking statistics as her life work, for better or worse, for richer or poorer." These jocular remarks touched upon another popular assumption: that women could excel at marriage or a career, but not both. This assumption applied even more starkly to women working in the social sciences, whose commitment to dispassionate objectivity signaled a rejection of the "feminine" values traditionally ascribed to them. Brandt, like her Wellesley mentors, never married.[139] As the newly elected head of COSCNY's Committee of Social Research in 1904, Brandt issued calls for more rigorous and systematic reporting to improve the quality of statistics compilation. With more—and more reliable—quantitative data, she anticipated a time when it would "be possible to arrive . . . at a knowledge of causes which shall be based on facts and not on impressions."[140] In advancing the CPT's antituberculosis agenda using the data and methods available to her in 1902, Brandt nevertheless took decisive steps toward advancing her career at a transitional moment when women's professional advancement, while possible, was neither guaranteed nor smooth.

Ernest Poole emerged on the New York muckraking scene at precisely the moment that CPT professionals required a colorful writer to synthesize their evidence and objectives for a popular audience. Educated, well-to-do, and receptive to modern trends, he embodied a generational bridge between cutting-edge bacteriological concepts and age-old moral judgments regarding the sick poor. In highlighting the humanity behind the case dots of Biggs's and Veiller's disease maps, he fulfilled the CPT's mission of "[taking] the warfare against consumption away from the private domain of the medical profession and [making] it of vital concern to every member of society."[141] Poole's youth, lack of professional training, and loose class affiliation had left him with fewer preexisting assumptions than his CPT colleagues held about the poor; these attributes facilitated more direct connections with tenement dwellers, enabling him to challenge different angles of the antituberculosis campaign from their perspectives.

These attributes also left him more psychologically and emotionally vulnerable as he encountered "case after case of brave, unceasing effort, of kindness, devotion, and death."[142] Nearly forty years later, Poole still recalled the agony coursing through him as the dying Jewish tailor from his opening scene "begged us to kill him . . . begged until I thought I'd go mad!" Poole's sense of helplessness only increased as "records kept piling in on me from the living present as from the past, and I met so many men, women and kids who appealed to me, yet were doomed to die."[143] In desperation, Poole began accompanying sick residents to hospital clinics, or arranging for short stays in the country. "For a few, there was hope," he remembered; "for most there was none."[144] After completing the assignment, Poole sought escape at his family's country estate in Lake Forest; yet even this familiar retreat, "so clean and comfortable, pleasant and safe . . . seemed so different now, for I couldn't forget what I had seen."[145] On returning to New York, Poole's promotional work for the CPT revealed a growing sense of helplessness and rage at the larger social and economic forces that permitted such deadly conditions to exist. This discontentment colored Poole's future literary projects, steering him down the radical paths of Hunter, Stokes, Walling, and other University Settlement residents whose disgust with working-class conditions had turned them into avowed "class traitors."[146] "The Lung Block," Poole later reflected, "had made of me a rebel, too."[147]

In time, Poole's assignment would exact a far more devastating impact on the block and its inhabitants. Originally, he approached the neighborhood as a powerful example of a much larger problem; referring to it as "a single block [that] can be paralleled in every crowded quarter of the city," he included a substantial list of similarly disease-ridden neighborhoods.[148] Nevertheless, he succeeded in distinguishing this block from all others with a stigmatizing moniker that he later claimed to have invented himself. "'The Lung Block' has well earned its name," he remarked when introducing the neighborhood to his readers."[149] Having reduced New York's tuberculosis problem to a specific point in space, Poole then spelled out in uncompromising terms what Biggs's and Veiller's disease maps only suggested. "It is here among the crowded poor that the Plague feeds fat on ignorance and poverty, in dark halls, foul rooms, dark closets," Poole declared; "It is here that unceasing danger lies for the whole community."[150] In his zeal to drive home the dangers of tuberculosis to his readers, Poole fulfilled only too well the CPT's objective of highlighting specific areas and populations for immediate intervention. His anecdotes of "sick rooms" in which entire families perished lent damning weight to the "house infection" arguments circulating among public health and social work professionals; his lurid images of sin and squalor appeared to confirm what their maps and statistics stopped short of avowing openly. When the CPT published *The Plague in Its Stronghold* as a pamphlet in September of 1903, major city newspapers would seize upon these powerful notes of alarm and disgust, leaving Poole's compassionate glimpses of working-class consumptives further and further behind.

That same month, an abridged version of Poole's essay—retitled "The Lung Block"—appeared in the COSCNY journal *Charities*, just before Brandt's impassioned call for introducing more parks into the Lower East Side.[151] The back-to-back placement of these stories, far from coincidental, marked the precise point where New York antituberculosis activism intersected with its parks and playgrounds movement. Where one set of reformers framed tuberculosis as a problem of permanently infected houses, the other promoted a solution through the introduction of "breathing spaces." In crowded tenement districts, such projects could occur only through clearing the land of existing buildings: a step that both groups had come to embrace as both essential and desirable. Years earlier, Biggs had proposed that "permanently infected" houses should be completely renovated, "or, better, condemned and torn down"—an idea with which many colleagues agreed.[152] As housing reformers fought to regulate the environment inside tenements, small groups of settlement workers focused on improving the landscape outside tenements by replacing notoriously crime-ridden neighborhoods with parks.

By the early 1900s this idea had gained ground among a wider circle of reformers, with one COSCNY official remarking that "the razing of large areas in . . . plague centres, together with the establishment of new parks, is a policy which both justice and expediency demand."[153] Even before Poole finished his damning portrait of the neighborhood, he confided to a friend that "we mean to raise hell with the politicians till they get busy and tear the whole stinking damned block down!"[154] To Poole and his CPT colleagues, the neighborhood bounded by Cherry, Catherine, Hamilton, and Market had come to signify more than disturbing concentrations of tuberculosis in Biggs's and Veiller's maps. It now embodied tuberculosis itself, its black case dots and dark, diseased rooms projecting literal infection upon an otherwise healthy and vigorous city. With the "Lung Block," Poole ignited a long-awaited flashpoint for multiple branches of reformers anxious to reclaim their city from dirt, disease, mismanagement, and corruption, providing them with both a battleground and a rallying cry.

Chapter 4

"LUNG BLOCK OR PARK-PLAYGROUND—WHICH?"

Jacob Riis, "City Wildernesses," and the Crusade for "Breathing Spaces" on the Lower East Side

Once the Charity Organization Society's Committee on the Prevention of Tuberculosis identified the block bounded by Cherry, Catherine, Hamilton and Market Streets as the epicenter of New York's tuberculosis problem, why did they seize upon replacement with a park as the ideal solution? The answer lies in the overlap between two popular interrelated ideas driving urban reformers and sanitarians throughout most of the nineteenth century: their perception of environment as key to determining people's health, characters, and destinies, and their belief in the redemptive powers of nature. If darkness and "bad air" in tenement houses caused physical and moral degeneration, they reasoned, sunlight and fresh air would reverse these effects and prevent them from recurring.

How to introduce these natural elements into working-class New Yorkers' lives then became the question. With unimproved, unoccupied land fast disappearing in the industrial development following the Civil War, and weak housing laws that encouraged overbuilding as well as overcrowding, parks shifted in significance from private aesthetic retreats for the wealthy to functional "lungs" that powered and purified the whole city.[1] By the 1890s, as changing demographics and disease etiologies focused public anxiety on tenement neighborhoods, small parks and playgrounds had emerged as a solution that multiple branches of social activism could agree upon. Public health and housing reformers hailed them as safety valves that relieved high crime and death rates in surrounding areas; settlement workers welcomed them as extensions of their common-ground approach, where immigrant children could begin forging American identities and values through play. In a larger sense, small parks and playgrounds also came to represent strategic defenses against the political corruption, capitalist greed, and Old World ignorance that many civic-minded New Yorkers tied to the slum districts. During a period when the Western frontier was closing and new opportunities for expansion beckoned in the Caribbean and Far East, small-parks supporters' interest in appropriating and taming these "city wildernesses" paralleled a broader national agenda of empire building amid the world's "waste spaces"—as did their breezy paternalism toward those already inhabiting the places they wished to transform.[2]

As an immigrant, reporter, and reformer, Jacob Riis was uniquely positioned to embrace these events and to propel them forward. Growing up in rural Denmark imparted to him a deep reverence for nature and the power of environment to mold human beings, putting him on a common footing with Frederick Law Olmsted and the romanticism of previous urban reform movements. Later, he harnessed groundbreaking developments in public health, photography, and social science to communicate the dangers of tenement life to late nineteenth-century audiences. Thus, his reform writings, lectures, and community activism form a bridge between older and newer perspectives on urban parks advocacy, as well as a key intersection linking reform movements in his own time period.[3] While Riis viewed urban social problems in the same spatial terms as his contemporaries, he often infused them with romantic, even sensational elements that contrasted sharply with the more systematic and technical orientations of a rising generation of social work professionals.[4] Ramshackle tenements, dark alleys, and trash-strewn rear yards loomed before him as active agents of evil to be vanquished in a "battle with the slum."[5] While younger colleagues such as Lincoln Steffens and Lawrence Veiller sometimes scoffed at Riis's unapologetic idealism and subjectivity, they nevertheless incorporated many of his strategies into their own projects, sharing his conviction that professional experts were best qualified to reimagine working-class urban spaces.

Since his death in 1914, Riis's publicly acknowledged role as father of the small-parks movement has receded in historical significance compared with his contributions in journalism, photography, housing reform, and settlement work.[6] This selective approach overlooks Riis's increasing devotion to the cause in his reform activities throughout the 1890s and early 1900s.[7] Both unilaterally and through his work on government-appointed committees, Riis prodded city leaders to let sunlight and fresh air into tenement districts by replacing the most disease- and crime-ridden buildings with parks. When his fiery and emotional crusade led to the razing of Mulberry Bend, an infamous immigrant ghetto that formed the backdrop for many of his newspaper stories, the subsequent park provided Riis a dearly cherished personal victory over "deadly official inertia," individual property rights, and public apathy; it also provided the burgeoning small-parks and playgrounds movement with a strong precedent and a template for action.[8] Within ten years, park proponents were employing similar sources to craft similar arguments for replacing the "Lung Block" with a park—even adopting similar writing and photography styles, in Ernest Poole's case. Despite these multiple and obvious parallels, the two park campaigns arguably diverged in one key respect. Where Riis advocated destruction of tenement neighborhoods as a means of achieving small parks and playgrounds, Lung Block park proponents—as their proposals made clear—promoted small parks and playgrounds as a means of achieving the destruction of tenement neighborhoods.[9]

RIIS'S JOURNEY FROM RIBE TO REFORM

At first glance, Jacob Riis's formative influences made him an unlikely prospect for a career in American urban reform. Riis was born in 1849 in Ribe, a Danish coastal village situated far from railroads, telegraphs, and other technological innovations transforming the face of western Europe and the United States.[10] Once a flourishing medieval trading center, Ribe featured a largely preindustrial economy, strong traces of a feudal caste system, and a local culture centered upon its imposing twelfth-century church, "against whose strong walls," Riis recalled for American audiences, "the town leaned with its time-worn old houses and crooked streets as if seeking strength and comfort."[11] Against this quaint and rural backdrop, Riis distinguished himself further from his American reform colleagues through his lack of wealth, social connections, and academic credentials. As one of fifteen children subsisting on his father's modest schoolteacher salary, Riis grew up feeling the sting of material deprivation and hardship. He later became the only son to survive past the age of thirty, having lost one brother to drowning and six more to tuberculosis.[12] Never an enthusiastic student, Riis rejected a college education to apprentice as a carpenter; as a result, upon emigrating to New York in 1870, he found his occupational opportunities restricted to exploitative and often dangerous manual labor in harvest fields, coal mines, and factories. Too proud to beg or apply for relief, Riis endured years of hunger, homelessness, and rough treatment from law enforcement.[13]

While Riis's formative years in Denmark did not herald a career in social reform, they did shape the perspective he would later bring to American urban problems.[14] His faith in environmental influences gained traction among the "simple, honest, and good" people of Ribe, where "neighbor knew neighbor, and shared his grief and his joys."[15] Riis attributed their orderly, unhurried gentility to the stabilizing influences of family, religion, and tight-knit communities; these cultural traits, which he later portrayed as seamless extensions of the village's surrounding marshes and meadows, withered against the frenetic, temporal, and anonymous backdrop of the modern city.[16] Riis's fond memories of Ribe colored his impressions of American urban life throughout his literary career, "poking through his writing like a recurring dream."[17] Likewise, his humble beginnings and harsh introduction to America would set him apart from well-to-do reform colleagues who formed their impressions of the urban poor through abstract principles and statistics rather than direct experiences and emotions.[18]

By 1877, Riis had landed a reporting job at the *New-York Tribune*, where his office—directly across from police headquarters—provided an ideal vantage point for examining the city's geography, cultural groups, political rivalries, and social problems. Riis never lost his fascination with the deeper, universal "human element" lurking at the heart of the routine calamities he covered: "A petty tenement-house fire might hide a fire-bug, who always makes shuddering appeal to our fears," he later observed; "the finding of John Jones sick and destitute in the street meant, perhaps, a story full of the deepest pathos."[19] Over the next ten years, Riis cultivated a colorful style that encouraged his readers to see themselves in the unfortunate people he wrote about: prisoners who left heartfelt messages on their cell walls; a woman who awaited her husband's return, unaware that he had perished in a work-related accident; a two-year-old girl who wandered away from home, leaving her immigrant family in anguish; people who died alone in the city's hospitals, prisons, almshouses, and lunatic asylums, their meager personal effects unclaimed.[20] Although Riis's superiors cautioned him to discard his storytelling flourishes in favor of the plain facts, he came to relish the power of his subjective style to influence public opinion. If undertaken in the right spirit, he believed that a "murder story may easily come to speak more eloquently to the minds of thousands than the sermon preached to a hundred in the church on Sunday."[21]

Throughout the 1880s, Riis's police beat coverage expanded to include a broader array of social concerns such as street sanitation, housing conditions, food and water contamination, and infectious disease outbreaks.[22] He became a fixture at the city's health department, where he peered into microscopes alongside sanitary inspectors and acquired proficiency with mortality rates from statisticians.[23] Even as he incorporated these empirical methods into his work, Riis's perspective on urban issues remained firmly rooted in moral environmentalism. "I searched in vain for the real bacillus of the slum," he wrote; "it escaped science, to be identified by human sympathy and a conscience-stricken community with that of ordinary human selfishness."[24] Over time, he broadened his investigation to include the municipal inefficiency and corruption perpetuating slum conditions, and the reform efforts organizing in response.[25] Flash-lighting innovations from Germany enabled Riis to capture photographic images of dark tenement rooms and neighborhood alleyways and share them with his audiences in newspapers and public lectures.[26] As his reputation grew, so did demand for his work in national publications.[27]

In *How the Other Half Lives* (1890), Riis harnessed his signature literary style, his firsthand experiences as a police reporter, and his knowledge of emerging social-scientific and technological methods to educate Americans about the true conditions in New York slums. Drawing upon his own observations and a wide range of city-generated statistics, Riis took his readers on a guided tour of New York's tenement neighborhoods, highlighting the tightly interwoven relationships among immigration, low wages, high rents, over-crowding, saloons, high death rates, and arrests.[28] He then illustrated how these combinations of factors shaped the lives of individuals and families in heartwrenching descriptions and photographs. Central to his book was the conviction that "we are all creatures of the conditions that surround us, phys-ically and morally."[29] Riis felt that tenement children stood little chance of becoming decent citizens in homes resembling "a pigeon-hole in a coop along with so many other human animals." By the same token, he believed that nature redeemed "the child of common clay" by awakening "the instinct of beauty, of love for the ideal" that distinguished civilization from savagery. "I have seen an armful of daisies keep the peace of a block better than a police-man and his club," he argued, "seen instincts awaken under their gentle appeal, whose very existence the soil in which they grew made seem a mockery."[30]

How the Other Half Lives presented an alarming picture of tenement life to the middle and upper classes, placing Riis and New York's social prob-lems on a national stage.[31] Reviewers praised the book's authenticity: "Mr. Riis knows the East Side and its slums and alleys and tenements as perhaps no other man in this city knows them," crowed his new employer, the *Evening Sun*; "No writer has so minutely described the exact status of the wretched inhabitants of our tenement houses as Mr. Riis," agreed the *New York Press*. Critics also noted the book's broad appeal, filled as it was with "statistics for those who care for that sort of thing [and] suggestions for the charitable worker." It also contained engaging stories, photographs, and sketches "for those who are merely curious and who wish only to be entertained." During a time when "slumming" constituted an upper-class leisure activity and occu-pied its own genre in popular travel literature, the voyeuristic nature of Riis's work fueled sales. "He has written a plain, unvarnished tale, and yet the inci-dents are thrilling," the *Press* noted.[32]

The popularity of *How the Other Half Lives* supplied Riis with the creden-tials and public recognition he needed to issue calls for drastic action in the cities. As he continued writing and lecturing about working-class conditions throughout the 1890s, his efforts attracted interest and assistance from "men of sympathy, of learning, and of power": most notably Theodore Roosevelt, an up-and-coming politician who, upon reading *How the Other Half Lives*, imme-diately contacted Riis with offers to help.[33]

At the same time, Riis's growing success complicated as well as facilitated his mission of bringing rich and poor closer together. Because Riis under-stood that appealing to genteel audiences meant keeping them comfortable as well as engaged, his attitude toward the working classes in *How the Other Half Lives* often bore traces of the same condescension, exasperation, and dis-

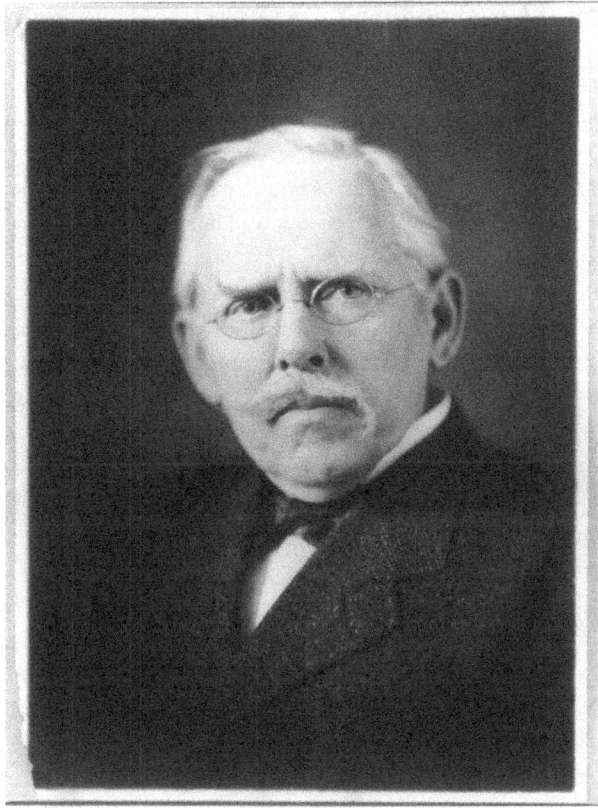

4.1. Jacob Riis. This portrait, taken by photographer Pirie MacDonald in 1904, is held in the Library of Congress, Washington, DC.

gust evident among other social commentators of his day.[34] For example, he confirmed his readers' image of tenement dwellers as "shiftless, destructive and stupid" before driving home his environmentalist argument that "they are what the tenements have made them."[35] Likewise, he helped his readers make sense of New York's diverse working-class population by relying upon racial and ethnic stereotypes already familiar to them.[36] Jews, he informed them, believed that "money was their God"; Italians learned "slowly, if at all"; both groups "carr[ied] their slum with them wherever they go." If both groups rose "only by compulsion," they still ranked ahead of the "Chinaman," who "[did] not rise at all."[37] In downplaying the significant social barriers that Italian, Jewish, and Chinese immigrants faced to advancement in urban America, Riis emulated the detached and critical perspectives of wealthier, "old-stock" Americans.[38] This conflicted approach to the poor—humanity and harshness, civility and condescension, brotherhood and bigotry—would set the tone for his subsequent battle with the slum.

THE PARKS AND PLAYGROUNDS MOVEMENT IN NEW YORK CITY

Riis joined the ranks of social reform at the precise moment when parks agitation acquired a fresh burst of momentum in New York City.[39] The movement for green spaces did not begin in earnest until the city's population began spiraling upward in the 1840s, compelling notable New Yorkers such as newspaper editor William Cullen Bryant and horticulturist Andrew Jackson Downing to recognize the importance of providing a refuge from the stresses of encroaching urban-industrial development—a "green oasis for the refreshment of the city's soul and body."[40] While their objectives reflected European trends in culture and urban planning, advocates argued that public parks also appealed to Americans' growing sense of nationalism by promoting their own natural resources and republican values.[41] If Old World empires had accepted the wisdom of redistributing aristocratic holdings to benefit ordinary citizens, how much more should Americans—a casteless people stirred by the westward ambitions of Manifest Destiny—feel entitled to lands reserved for their enjoyment?[42]

Central Park, carved out of the center of Manhattan in the late 1850s, boasted a carefully sculpted landscape of wooded pastures, open grasslands, and ponds connected by pedestrian and riding paths. Its designer, Frederick Law Olmsted, intended for the park to serve as not just an aesthetic marvel for its well-to-do neighbors but also a personal sanctuary for "hundreds of thousands of tired workers" who could not afford to leave the city.[43] In creating common spaces similar to the public parks and gardens of Europe, where citizens from all walks of life could "enjoy together the same music, breathe the same atmosphere of art, [and] enjoy the same scenery," Olmsted and likeminded contemporaries hoped that the park would stimulate a feeling of fellowship and community fast disappearing in American cities.[44] In keeping with the romanticism of the period, they also believed that mere exposure to the park's carefully maintained tranquility could refine "the most unfortunate and lawless classes" into adopting the middle-class values of "courtesy, self-control, and temperance."[45]

Central Park became a point of civic pride among genteel New Yorkers, inspiring other large-scale public recreation areas on the municipal, state, and national levels.[46] It "bears the stamp of a kindly and poetic genius," remarked William Dean Howells of Olmsted's work, "giving to the city-prisoned poor an image of what the free country still is, everywhere."[47] Yet the project undermined its founders' visions of class solidarity by placing the park at a substantial distance from working-class neighborhoods; by abruptly displacing more than a thousand immigrants and African Americans who had eked a living off the land; and by adopting a stratified layout that promoted what Roy Rosenzweig and Elizabeth Blackmar have described as an "elaborate class choreography of use."[48] On the carriage roads and promenades, upper-crust New Yorkers formed a "broad torrent of vehicular gentility" that drew barbs from cynical observers.[49] Parkgoers of more modest means visited the pedestrian areas on Sundays, where they encountered more than a hundred types of signs—and scores of vigilant "keepers"—cautioning them against rock climbing, flower picking, athletic games, and other activities that risked marring the pristine appearance of the grounds.[50] Despite its billing as "the people's park," New York's first large-scale public space proved over time to be more accessible and welcoming for people whose lifestyles and tastes reflected those of its designers.[51]

By the 1880s, as the effects of unregulated development grew more visible in working-class neighborhoods, urban park advocacy shifted from away from aesthetic boosterism and toward the sanitary and social concerns driving the public health and housing reform movements. Thirty years after Central Park's founding, bacteriological discoveries confirmed popular miasmatic associations between disease and dark, stuffy, overpopulated spaces; moreover, a new generation of social experts now agreed that sprawling landscape parks offered less prosperous New Yorkers little protection against the debilitating effects of city life.[52] "After a long day's work," protested Bureau of Labor Statistics employee Elgin Gould, "they do not feel disposed to go, as they usually must, a long distance to reach one, and then find nothing to do but take a short walk before darkness comes. To expect them to do it is absurd."[53] A series of smaller, streamlined "air holes" scattered throughout the city, Gould and others reasoned, could supply working-class New Yorkers with the fresh air and sunshine denied them in tenements, factories, and schools, enabling them to maintain stronger defenses against disease.[54]

Although small-parks supporters valued function and efficiency over aesthetics, they still shared their predecessors' conviction in the power of environment to mold human beings. Declaring that "foul air prompts to vice and oxygen to virtue," one Boston physician speculated that "if there was an attractive park convenient [the workman] would seek it as instinctively as the plant stretches towards the light." Likewise, Gould agreed that green and sunny urban spaces were valuable for "bring[ing] back hope as well as health to multitudes."[55] Growing labor unrest, such as the 1886 Haymarket bombing in Chicago, also highlighted the urgency of addressing promoting class harmony through uplifting recreational spaces.

All of these late nineteenth-century urban concerns intersected sharply in the growing child. Contemporary scholars of human development, most notably G. Stanley Hall, viewed the transitions from infancy to adulthood as mirroring the stages of human evolution from savagery to civilization.[56] Play, they believed, offered children a safety valve for channeling these primitive impulses in age-appropriate ways, enabling them to become healthy, productive, and orderly citizens. To that end, the lack of play opportunities for working-class city children worried many socially conscious Americans. "They are driven from their crowded homes in the morning," explained journalist-reformer Walter Vrooman, "chased from the street by the police when they attempt to play, and beaten . . . [by] the janitor's wife when found in the hallways or on the stairs."[57] Lillian Wald, of New York's Henry Street Settlement, recalled children's dogged attempts to play checkers in a crowded street market, their board "precariously perched on the top of a hydrant"; she also sympathized with the "fretful small boy" who complained when "the 'cop' had snatched his dice . . . nobody wanted him to chalk on the sidewalk, and he had been arrested for throwing a ball."[58] Hull House founder Jane Addams witnessed similar frustration among neighborhood children in Chicago. "Although they start over and over again," she lamented, "even the most vivacious become worn out . . . and take to that passive 'standing 'round' varied by rude horse-play, which in time becomes so characteristic of city children."[59] Denied appropriate outlets for their play instincts, such children learned to associate amusement with vice and authority with the enemy, growing up "into not healthy men and women, but into monsters."[60]

Based on their conception of childhood as a fleeting window "when character is plastic and can be molded for good or evil as clay in the potter's hands," playground advocates—Addams in Chicago, Wald and Charles Stover in New York, Joseph S. Lee in Boston, Stoyan Vasil Tsanoff in Philadelphia—demanded that cities set aside spaces for future citizens to indulge and master their "animal spirits."[61] In New York's densely populated tenement districts, this required clearing multiple 25-by-100-foot lots, each with an owner demanding compensation.[62] Recent housing agitation addressed this problem through the Small Parks Act of 1887, which allotted the city up to $1 million annually for acquiring land to convert into public parks. The city, led by reform-minded mayor Abram Hewitt, moved quickly to establish parks on vacant lots that it already owned; these first efforts lacked the sweeping views and aesthetic flourishes of Central Park, consisting of asphalt paths, a few trees and shrubs, rows of benches, and a fence.[63] They shared Central Park's tight restrictions, however, prompting Vrooman to complain that "our park officials [feel] that it is better for grass to grow green over children's graves than yellow under their feet."[64]

This municipal indifference toward working-class conditions led reform-minded New Yorkers to favor more drastic methods of intervention.[65] "If the houses are crowded," urged Felix Adler, founder of the Society for Ethical Culture, "the government must interfere"; Gould, using the analogy that "no cure for cancer [existed] except the knife," argued that the only solution for "irremediably insanitary" tenements was to tear them down.[66] As property condemnation emerged as a viable alternative to enforcing compliance with health and housing codes, reformers rallied around municipal small parks and playgrounds as a worthy goal. Soon, Riis would provide forward momentum for this burgeoning movement with his crusade against "the foul core of New York's slums": Mulberry Bend.

LETTING THE LIGHT INTO MULBERRY BEND

By the time Riis arrived in America, Mulberry Bend had long been associated in the popular imagination with immigrants, filthy and dilapidated housing, shady business dealings, violence, and frequent epidemics.[67] Pursuing police beat stories for the *Tribune* made Riis intimately familiar with the area's streets and narrow passageways, known to locals as "Bottle Alley," "Thieves' Alley," and "Bandits' Roost." Inside the houses, the squalor and hardship he witnessed while touring with health inspectors "gripped my heart until I felt that I must tell of them, or burst, or turn anarchist, or something."[68] Riis's desires for action found a catalyst in his coverage of Adler, who railed against Mulberry Bend in his public lectures as "one of the greatest plague-spots in New York . . . a sink of corruption and disease."[69]

In *How the Other Half Lives*, Riis devoted a full chapter to detailing how the dark haphazardness of Mulberry Bend's built environment revealed itself in the idleness of its tramps and thieves, the ignorance of unregulated street vendors and teenaged mothers, or the filth and illnesses of large families confined to a single room. In brief, picturesque swirls of local color—a flirtatious and pretty girl, spirited hagglers on the street, fluttering red bandannas—Riis also relayed hints of a diverse and struggling community whose vibrancy shone through "its household work, its bargaining, its love-making . . . or idling when it has nothing better to do." Basing his opinion on a combination of statistics and his personal impressions, however, Riis concluded that Mulberry Bend represented "a vast human pig-sty . . . swarming with unwholesome crowds" that defied municipal attempts to improve or control it.[70]

Riis's solution of "letting in the light" bridged older associations among nature, health, and morality with the recapitulation theory of contemporary play advocates. By replacing Mulberry Bend with a park, Riis hoped to enrich the lives of tenement children who amused themselves by scrawling "Keeb of te Grass" on fences, although "there was not . . . a green sod within a quarter of a mile."[71] On a broader scale, he also wanted to strike a blow against the public indifference and administrative neglect that enabled similar trouble spots to flourish.[72] "As long as [Mulberry Bend] stood," he later explained, "the slum had backing, as it were."[73] On a more personal note, the same dark alleys that fueled his literary rise also contained bitter memories from when he first walked them as a tramp himself, "long enough to taste of its poison." These painful memories amplified his conviction that "the blow must be struck there, to kill."[74]

Riis had reason to believe that his plan would succeed. Other American cities in the early 1890s, including Boston, Philadelphia, and Kansas City, were developing expansive park systems; moreover, the Small Parks Act now gave New York the legal grounds it needed to condemn private property for that purpose.[75] Even so, Riis's battle with Mulberry Bend dragged out across multiple city administrations, none of which demonstrated enthusiasm for the project.[76] For years, Riis applied steady pressure through newspapers, national magazines, and the lecture circuit, employing vivid language that characterized the Bend as morally and physically infected.[77] "[The Bend] taints whatever it touches," Riis declared; "wickedness and vice gravitate toward it and are tenfold aggravated, until crime is born spontaneously of its corruption." He promoted destruction as the only effective solution: "Recovery is impossible under its blight," he insisted; "Rescue and repression are alike powerless to reach it."[78]

Meanwhile, Riis expanded his efforts from publicity to participating directly in government. He served on the 1894 state Tenement House Commission, which prioritized small parks alongside its efforts to improve safety and building codes. After determining that one-third of New Yorkers lived below Fourteenth Street—where park acreage made up barely one-fortieth of the city total—commissioners secured passage of a law requiring the municipal government to provide two parks there within three years, along with open-air playgrounds for all subsequently built public schools. The commission also authorized the Department of Health (NYCDOH) to condemn unsanitary properties for the public good, a development that gave reformers a weapon against "every old ramshackle, disease-breeding tenement house" in New York.[79]

After expending $1.5 million in damage awards and assessments, the city finally took possession of Mulberry Bend in 1894, where "for a whole year," Riis fumed, "it complacently collected the rents and did nothing."[80] Razing the tenements and building the park involved three more years of public prodding, scandals, and changes in leadership.[81] When Mulberry Bend Park opened in June of 1897, during Mayor William Strong's reform-friendly administration, Riis described it in the glowing terms he usually reserved for his childhood memories of Ribe: "The sun shone upon flowers and the tender leaves of young shrubs. . . . Crowds of little Italian children shouted with delight over the 'garden,' while their elders sat upon the benches with a look of contentment such as I had not seen before in that place." The park, in giving working-class New Yorkers a space of their own, gave reformers a decisive, tangible victory for "decency and good government"; "It is as if the old bad days were gone with it," Riis remarked, "and a new reckoning begun."[82]

As had been the case with Central Park forty years earlier, Mulberry Bend Park's significance lay in what it lacked as well as in what it provided. Despite Riis's insistence on the importance of playgrounds, the park consisted solely of

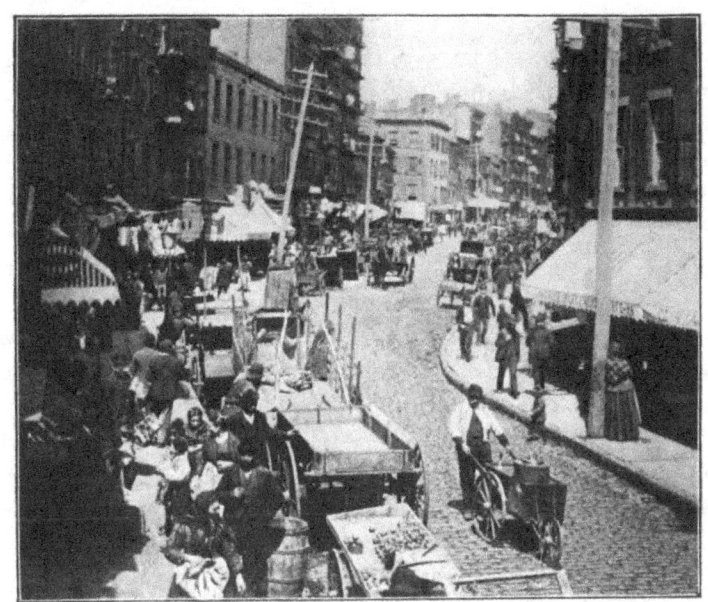

The Mulberry Bend.

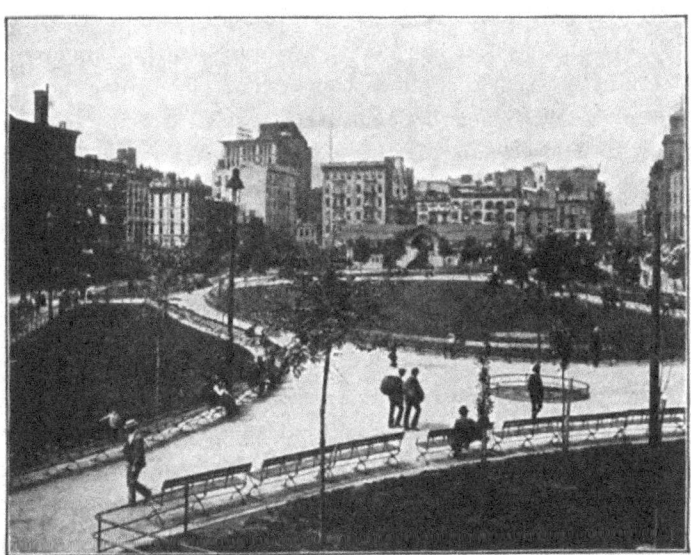

Mulberry Bend Park.

4.2A AND B. A photograph of the Mulberry Bend neighborhood from the late 1880s (top), originally published in Jacob Riis's *How the Other Half Lives* (1890). More than ten years later, Riis included this picture in *The Battle with the Slum* to showcase the before-and-after contrast with the recently opened Mulberry Bend Park, pictured above. Reprinted from Riis, *The Battle with the Slum* (New York: MacMillan, 1902), 277, 289.

asphalt paths, benches, and patches of grass bordered with wire to discourage pedestrians from walking on them. "Places of this sort are well called breathing spaces," Lee observed scornfully; "you can go there and breathe, but there is very little else you can do."[83] Also missing were 2,600 residents—young and old, lodgers and families, street vendors and tramps—who were abruptly displaced to make room for the park. Reflecting upon their departure, Riis speculated that the loss of people's homes now afforded them "a chance for their purely human qualities to expand," which the Bend had been "choking and smothering every hour."[84] Enough vacant apartments existed all over Manhattan to shelter them, he reasoned, provided they were willing to move.[85] "It is not where they shall go, but that *they shall not go there at any rate*," he concluded, "that is the important thing." While he did not include any reactions from the displaced residents themselves in his accounts of Mulberry Bend's transformation, Riis maintained that the permanent scattering of their community would work out for the best: "Something is gained in the mere shifting about," he wrote; "some of the dirt is lost on the way."[86]

Flush with his Mulberry Bend victory, Riis began outlining a broader vision for tenement district "breathing spaces" through the Committee on Small Parks, a citizens' advisory group that Mayor Strong appointed in June of 1897. Drawing on police and NYCDOH statistics, the committee compiled the number and density of people in each ward, including children less than fifteen years of age, and the death rates in each ward compared to the city as a whole. They then compared these numbers with a map they created of the city's parks, schools, and neighborhoods that featured the highest statistical incidence of crime, death, disease, and overcrowding. Based on these empirical findings, Riis, the committee's secretary, concluded that "the children seem to have been forgotten" in the city's rampant development.[87] Drawing upon the same European examples that Downing and Olmsted had used to justify Central Park's construction forty years earlier, Riis now downplayed their aesthetic marvels in favor of their recreational opportunities. "Amid all the wealth of shrubbery, flowers, statuary and fountains are spaces . . . devoted exclusively to games," he reported, "while in the very walks may be found . . . innumerable children digging holes and playing with the dirt heaps thus created." He then cited the new park at Mulberry Bend as proof that battling the slums "was not a question of moving an unruly population, but changing its environment"—a conclusion that overlooked the thousands of residents who were, in fact, compelled to move in order to enable the park's construction.[88]

The committee issued fourteen recommendations for small parks and playground sites throughout the city, which languished when Strong lost his bid for reelection. His successor, Robert A. Van Wyck—a "peppery Tammany mayor" who had won on the slogan "To Hell with Reform"—thereafter accorded Riis's committee "as much authority as a committee of bootblacks."[89]

Agitation for breathing spaces shifted once again to the private sector. There, Riis joined Stover, Wald, and other settlement workers in forming the Outdoor Recreation League, a citizens' pressure group that maintained their own playground equipment at several unimproved municipal sites in hopes of persuading park officials to assume the responsibility themselves.[90] Meanwhile, in his impassioned writings and public lectures, his ongoing pleas to "let in the light" suggested a powerful metaphor for civic reawakening. "For every slum block you tear down to make room for a playground," he told a Chicago audience in 1899, "you let the sunshine into the souls of 10,000 children who, in the next generation, will pull this great city out of the mire."[91] Pointing to Mulberry Bend's recent transformation, Riis imbued this light with self-governing, even mystical qualities. Averring that "scarce a knife has been drawn, or a shot fired" since the park opened two years earlier, he explained that "it is not that the murder has moved to another neighborhood. . . . It is that the light has come in and made crime hideous."[92]

Riis's parks advocacy throughout the 1890s, alongside members of the Outdoor Recreation League and other organizations, provided a template and a precedent for up-and-coming reformers to build upon. Veiller drew heavily on Riis's research for the Committee on Small Parks and the Mulberry Bend campaign for his 1900 Tenement House Commission report, which pointed out that Manhattan's tenement districts—which housed roughly two-thirds of its 1.6 million people—still contained only forty of the island's 1,141 acres set aside for parks.[93] Agreeing with Riis that sunlight and fresh air created "a total change in the character of the neighborhood," Veiller then listed sixteen "city wildernesses" that he recommended for future park sites—one being the block bounded by Cherry, Catherine, Hamilton, and Market Streets.[94] Riis's work also provided younger, more technically oriented activists such as Veiller a springboard to push against. While Veiller valued Riis's abilities as a writer and publicist, he dismissed Riis's approach to urban problems as "unscientific," unsystematic, and impractical. Replacing slums with parks "does not 'let in the light' as you seem to think," Veiller explained to Riis in 1900; "there are no rooms in any of the surrounding buildings that are any lighter for this park," other than "the front apartments . . . which already have ample light."[95] These criticisms, along with Veiller's reluctance to credit the 1894 tenement commission or Committee on Small Parks with meaningful changes, fueled Riis's resentment toward him.[96] While Veiller and Riis maintained an alliance going forward, their fundamental incompatibility in outlook mirrored a broader conflict between romantic and social-scientific waves of reform.

Fusion candidate Seth Low's mayoral victory in 1901 facilitated the revival of long-tabled municipal park projects, as well as new ones all over the city. Within the next two years, Lower East Siders had Corlears Hook Park, on the eastern tip of Manhattan; Seward Park, at East Broadway and Essex Street;

and Hamilton Fish Park at East Houston, Stanton, Pitt, and Sheriff Streets, among others.[97] As with Mulberry Bend, each of these three-to-four-acre parks replaced blocks of condemned tenements: Corlears Hook Park replaced the Hook, an area known for prostitution and gang violence, and Hamilton Fish Park replaced "Bone Alley," home to generations of ragpickers.[98] Through the efforts of the Outdoor Recreation League, many of these parks boasted playgrounds as well.[99] While reformers lauded new municipal parks and play-grounds as "proof what can be done with the waste spaces in the midst of tenement districts," those who lived in these "waste spaces" often viewed the situation differently.[100] "Is Bone Alley healthy?" Nicholas Balzer, unofficial mayor of the neighborhood, repeated incredulously to a reporter. "Look at me. I was born there, lived there until I grew up to be a strong, able-bodied man. . . . There are dozens of old men around here who were born and brought up in the alley."[101] Other locals pointed to "Frau Gurnurneger," a toothless, white-haired, and evidently vigorous woman who had lived in "Bone Alley" for sixty years.[102] These protests, while subjective and anecdotal, suggest that the mortality rates and lurid descriptions wielded by Riis and others did not support "Bone Alley" residents' lived experiences of health and community.[103]

As these "breathing spaces" sprouted throughout tenement districts in New York and other large cities, Riis hailed them as the long-anticipated culmination of seeds he had planted with his crusade to wipe out Mulberry Bend.[104] In *The Ten Years' War* (1900), *The Making of an American* (1901), and *The Battle with the Slum* (1902), he documented his early contributions to a movement he expected to continue, casting its light outward to illuminate and redeem all areas of urban society. When Seward Park in 1903 became the first municipal site in the country to include a permanent playground, Riis per-ceived the event as more than a victory for working-class city children; he saw it as "the dawn of a new day" in which the nature, close-knit communities, and enlightened civic awareness of Ribe could dispel the darkness of corruption, greed, and ethnic tensions. At the official opening, he asked the large crowd to "always remember this day and this meeting, for here a new citizenship is born today, a citizenship that shall look to the ideal, not always to the material; that shall carry in loving regard ever the city of its home . . . [that] shall wipe the word slum forever from its page."[105]

"WANTED: A BREATHING SPACE"

When Ernest Poole, Lilian Brandt, and Robert de Forest shared their respec-tive proposals for replacing the "Lung Block" neighborhood with a park in September of 1903, they had ample reason for viewing the project as one of a steady stream of municipally approved "breathing spaces." Their efforts unfolded in the favorable climate of Low's reform administration, and rested upon a sturdy scaffolding of precedents achieved over a decade of public health, housing, settlement, and park activism. While they traced the roots of the Lung Block campaign to Veiller's "city wildernesses," all of them drew upon Riis's work in some fashion. Where Poole adopted Riis's signature formula of statistics, photographs, and colorful prose, Brandt and de Forest stressed Riis's familiar themes of moral environmentalism and cited Mulberry Bend as the basis for their project. Their proposals, while differing in styles and approaches, overlapped on three main points: that dysfunctional working-class spaces posed a physical and moral threat to the city; that parks and playgrounds represented a more beneficial use of these spaces; and that the "city wilderness" of Cherry, Catherine, Hamilton, and Market Streets needed this transformation more than any other.

As statistician for the Charity Organization Society of the City of New York (COSCNY)'s Committee on the Prevention of Tuberculosis (CPT), Brandt built her case for a new park on the few tabulated numbers at her command; consistent with her previous work, she grounded these numbers with analysis containing a number of sweeping generalizations and class judgements. In "Wanted: A Breathing Space"—which immediately followed "The Lung Block" in the reform journal *Charities*—Brandt defined "city wildernesses" as "tracts of an unmitigated material hideousness that cannot but have its effect on the life of the people." She did not offer further clarification on these arbitrary terms, possibly because she presumed *Charities* readers to possess the same aesthetic filters she did.

Brandt then drew her readers' attention to one such "city wilderness": "a small, irregular polygon on the East River, bounded by the approach to Brooklyn Bridge, the New Bowery, East Broadway, and Pike street." Her accompanying map placed this irregular polygon at the center of a one-hundred-acre parcel of the Lower East Side estimated to contain forty-five thousand people.[106] Within a hand-drawn arrangement of lines and shapes denoting wards, major streets, and distances from existing parks, Brandt arrived at the proposed project site through a series of metaphorical abstractions. Automobiles on New Bowery and East Broadway posed "natural barriers as real as a navigable stream" for pedestrians, while Pike Street functioned as "a sort of watershed from which the streams of people will flow down east to Seward Park, and west to the new one." While Brandt appeared to take traffic patterns into account when sketching these parameters, her "natural" analogies conveyed an understanding of tenement dwellers as an unthinking, aggregate element rather than heavy concentrations of individuals, each moving in their own purposeful direction. This reflected park supporters' intent focus on how tenement spaces were occupied, rather than how they were being used. "It is evident," Brandt informed her audience, "that there are practically only two factors in the composition of this picture—the houses, and the people who live in them."[107]

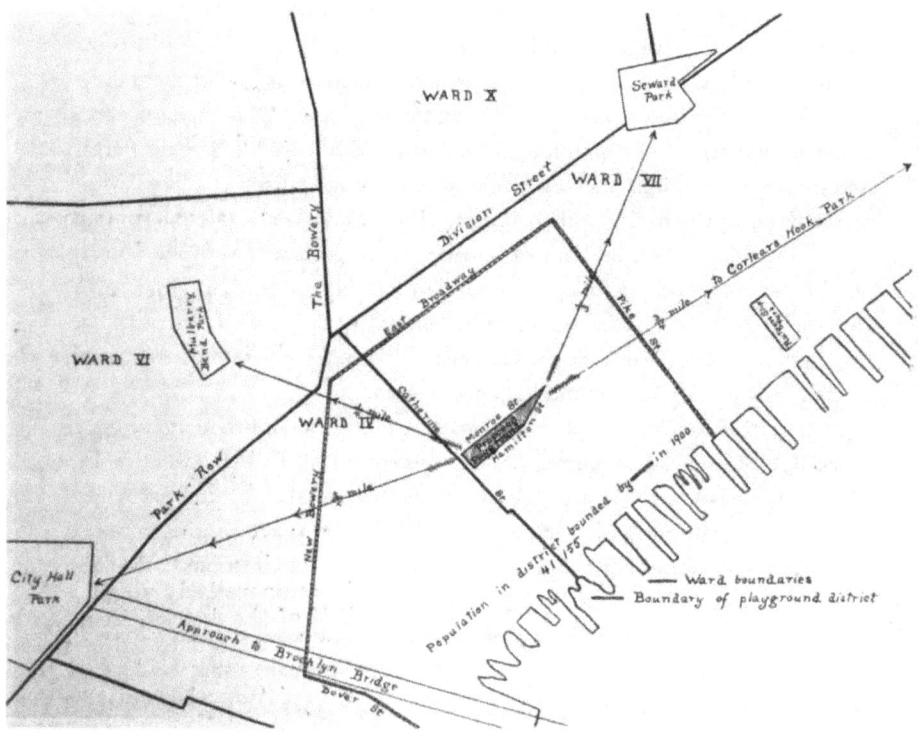

4.3. This hand-drawn map of the Lower East Side appeared in Lilian Brandt's "Wanted: a Breathing Space" in the September 1903 issue of the COSCNY journal *Charities*. The darkened shape at the center denotes the Lung Block park campaign's original proposed site, immediately adjacent to Cherry, Catherine, Hamilton, and Market Streets. Reprinted from Brandt, "Wanted: A Breathing Space," *Charities* 11, no. 10 (1903), 201.

Having isolated the key variables in the "city wildernesses" problem, Brandt outlined how each constituted a dangerous misuse of city space. She established the substandard, derelict nature of the houses by listing the extensive improvements that COSCNY colleagues de Forest and Veiller—now in charge of the brand-new Tenement House Department (THD)—deemed necessary for making them "halfway fit for human habitation." She then illuminated the hazards from thousands of working-class immigrant families, whom she characterized succinctly as "not a homogenous population," cramming into these dwellings at a rate far above the city average. Their problematic distribution in problematic spaces endangered health and values, Brandt argued, resulting in "a high death-rate and a low moral rate." "It is not going too far," she concluded, "to argue . . . that the population as a whole is degenerate."[108]

Having framed the area's problems in metaphorical and spatial terms, Brandt now presented the solution in medical terms. A "whole city of people crowded on one hundred acres of land," she declared, constituted ample proof "that a small park was, to use a physician's term, 'indicated.'" Clearing the space of houses and people would unleash its "latent regenerative forces," transforming it into "a strategic point for letting in sun and air to work the same miracles that they have worked in Mulberry Bend." Here, Brandt devoted considerably less attention to reimagining the space than she had to rationalizing its destruction. She offered tentative details of "a miniature Seward Park" with "a sand-pile for the small children and a corner, or a border, of grass and trees, where women may sit with their babies," along with a playground that had "apparatus for games and athletic exercises, presided over by an organizer of recreation." Under the watchful eyes of professionals, the park would provide residents with safe and appropriate outlets for physical energies, an "intellectual stimulus" for mental energies, and a sensory oasis "to relieve the prevailing hideousness of the crowded district."[109]

Notably, Brandt's proposal neglected to mention if these "city wilderness" inhabitants shared her assessments of their environment as "hideous," or whether they welcomed the idea of a park. In keeping with her previous research, the aggregate filters she used—population density, nationalities, death rates, arrests—suggest that Brandt viewed her working-class subjects through the lens of surveillance and enforcement agencies rather than through direct interactions. "One of the curious things about the tenement-dwellers of New York is the narrowness of their range," Brandt remarked when explaining the need for situating small parks within walking distance; "with the new world all before them their life is nevertheless generally contained within a few blocks." Dismissing this pattern as "curious" revealed not only a lack of familiarity with the factors limiting working-class New Yorkers' mobility but also an apparent lack of interest in exploring them further.[110] This detached, critical tone was not unique among social workers. When discussing the rate at which the Lower East Side population was increasing, Brandt included this comment from one of her colleagues: "It is a horrible thought . . . that *that population* is increasing at all."[111] If Brandt and her associates did not consult residents about the park project, such comments suggest that they did not value "that population's" opinions very highly.

Meanwhile, the park proposal was also working its way through the bureaucratic maze of New York City government. Appropriating land for a public park required approval from the Board of Estimate, a powerful central body that controlled, among other things, the city budget and the acquisition and disposal of public property.[112] Its approval in turn rested upon recommendations from the commissioner of parks for Manhattan, William R. Willcox; the Board of Local Improvement; and the Board of Aldermen, a body of elected representatives that voted on budgets and other financial matters. Once the proposal cleared those administrative hurdles, it would take months—possibly years—for the city to seize individual lots from private hands, raze the buildings, and begin laying out the park. Having observed this process in Mulberry Bend and other tenement neighborhoods, Lung Block park proponents felt optimistic about their prospects. With Willcox already offering his support, "it now seems probable that the Board of Aldermen also will favor the scheme," Brandt remarked in *Charities*, and "the approval of the Board of Local Improvement will then be assured."[113]

When de Forest appeared three weeks later before the Board of Estimate to formally propose a park for the block bordered by Cherry, Catherine, Hamilton, and Market Streets, he did so in his official capacity as THD commissioner. As longtime COSCNY president, however, he had monitored the plan's progress closely from the beginning. It was de Forest's respected position in the reform community, rather than in municipal government, that ensured a strong showing of supporters from COSCNY, the East Side Civic Club, the Outdoor Recreation League, and the Henry Street Settlement.[114] Before this group of lobbyists and city officials, de Forest deftly walked the line between public administrator and influential private citizen—coyly alluding to the proposal that fellow COSCNY members had submitted to the board, then claiming authority as an appointed city official to speak "on this subject which is of such vital importance to the tenement dwellers of that district."[115]

De Forest's objective, in keeping with Brandt's and Poole's, was to firmly establish Cherry, Catherine, Hamilton, and Market Streets as the boundaries for a dysfunctional space requiring immediate intervention. "I know of no tenement house block in this City," he informed the Board of Estimate, "which is so bad from a sanitary point of view, from a moral point of view, or from a criminal point of view." Disclosing the 197 code violations that his agency's inspectors had uncovered for the block that year, de Forest linked them with a local death rate nearly 75 percent greater than the city's. Then, drawing on testimony from the New York State Tenement House Commission that he had overseen with Veiller in 1900, de Forest repeated Hermann Biggs's charges of "permanent infection," boosting their significance with Biggs's unsubstantiated claim that only half of tuberculosis cases were reported to the proper authorities.[116] Segueing smoothly between physical and moral contamination, de Forest noted that "the block is occupied in large part by abandoned women, [and] criminal, vicious and disreputable people." He then speculated that police records, not cited in his report, would nevertheless "undoubtedly show an unusual number of arrests" for the area.[117]

More of a high-level administrator than a ringleader in this park project, de Forest drew on his professional skills as an attorney to remind Board of Estimate members that the city's power to acquire and destroy working-class neighborhoods rested on solid legal ground. "The establishing of small parks in tenement districts in this City," he declared, "has always gone hand in hand with the demolition of unsanitary slums"—a precedent that, while technically correct, only dated back to Riis's campaign against Mulberry Bend a decade earlier. As de Forest cited Mulberry Bend and other specific examples, he did not mention Riis by name, nor did he extol the benefits of sunlight, fresh air, and playgrounds. Instead, he boldly stated what Brandt's rudimentary playground sketches had only implied: that destruction, not creation, drove this latest park effort. "The reason for . . . Mulberry Bend Park was to destroy the notorious Mulberry Bend," de Forest argued, "which only a few years ago was the haunt of criminals and thieves, and a source of grave sanitary evils"; the same, he added, had been true for the areas now occupied by Seward, Hamilton Fish, and Thomas Jefferson Parks.[118]

In concluding that "every consideration of public health, morals and decency require that the buildings on this block be destroyed at an early date," de Forest purported to be speaking not just for himself or his colleagues but for "the many honest, decent and industrious working people" who could not afford to move to healthier surroundings. de Forest's confidence in speaking for tenement dwellers on this issue appeared to stem not from direct exchanges with them, but from his belief that serving as THD commissioner automatically qualified him to represent their interests: a mark of the noblesse oblige spirit that had long defined his approach to charity work.[119] Assuming that any reasonable person would agree with him, de Forest advised any skeptics to "personally inspect the district and the particular block" for themselves. Whether Lung Block park supporters declined to consult the people living there, as Brandt did, or claimed to speak for them, as de Forest did, one thing was clear: if they had not fully embraced Riis's vision of "letting in the light," they had accepted his uncompromising terms of victory in this latest "battle with the slum."

"AWAY WITH MANHATTAN'S 'LUNG BLOCK'"

When the park's publicity campaign began in earnest in September 1903, the city's major newspapers gave it the same encouraging coverage they had given other recent park efforts. Whether they summarized Brandt's work or reproduced it verbatim, at least four prominent dailies treated her appeal for "breathing spaces" as a legitimate news story requiring little additional verification or investigation by their own staffs.[120] The accompanying headlines— "City Wilderness Park," "New East Side Park," "More Breathing Space," "For a New Playground"—signaled these newspapers' stance toward the park idea as a vast improvement over what already filled those spaces. The *World* urged its readers to imagine "close to 100,000 persons crowded together [in] ancient tenements," with "thousands of children playing in the roadways, dirty and unkempt . . . whose only refuge from the sunless rooms, where they live in disease-breeding surroundings, is the street." Several newspapers noted that the proposed park area included the block bounded by Cherry, Catherine, Hamilton and Market Streets, which Brandt had described as "one of the worst tuberculosis-scourged neighborhoods in the city . . . notorious for three generations for the number and brutality of its crimes."[121] Calling the situation "a painful showing for a modern city," the *World* threw its support behind the project, declaring that a park in Cherry Hill would "clear a passage for pure air into diseased lungs."[122] One week later, the same newspapers published lengthy excerpts from Poole's *The Plague in Its Stronghold*, including enlarged disease maps and photographs of "plague rooms" where multiple deaths had transpired.

Notably, although these newspaper stories promoted park supporters' conceptualization of working-class spaces in terms of contaminated houses and people, they nevertheless continued to characterize the block as a vivid example of a larger tuberculosis problem. With headlines like "Lesson of the 'Lung Block,'" "Some Plague Spots in New York," and "Call to Combat the Mighty Plague of Consumption," city dailies called upon their readers to support the CPT's vbroader mission of building sanitariums and assisting poor consumptive families.[123] Once de Forest publicly targeted the neighborhood for demolition at the Board of Estimate hearing, however, newspaper coverage narrowed abruptly from New York's antituberculosis effort to sensational depictions of the medical and moral dangers radiating outward from one neighborhood.[124] "Malodorous, filthy, offensive to every sense," raged the *Evening Telegram*, "with no ray of cheering sunlight dispelling the awful gloom"; "an example of the most disgusting manner of living," agreed the *Herald*. Blown-up stock photographs from Veiller's tenement house reform campaign helped readers visually associate the "Lung Block" with "reeking stairways . . . filthy drains and sinks, cobwebbed ceilings and dust-covered floors." Reporters described their wary treks up dark, unventilated staircases into a world of "vile dens and foul apartments," where children ran naked and grownups drank and swore. Outside, the streets resembled a "garbage lot" where "the saloons . . . sell only the vilest spirits," and "not a day passes that the dread hearse does not pay a visit."[125]

In their zeal to convey the hopelessly contaminated state of the houses, these sensational "Lung Block" stories often revealed little, if any, direct contact with the inhabitants. Referring to them as "clannish" and "a people who live among themselves," the *Evening Telegram* shrugged off their lives as "a dark and unfathomable mystery." When residents did appear in these stories, they often assumed the roles of the anonymous "degenerates" in Brandt's and de Forest's appeals. "The evil men and women who make their lairs here

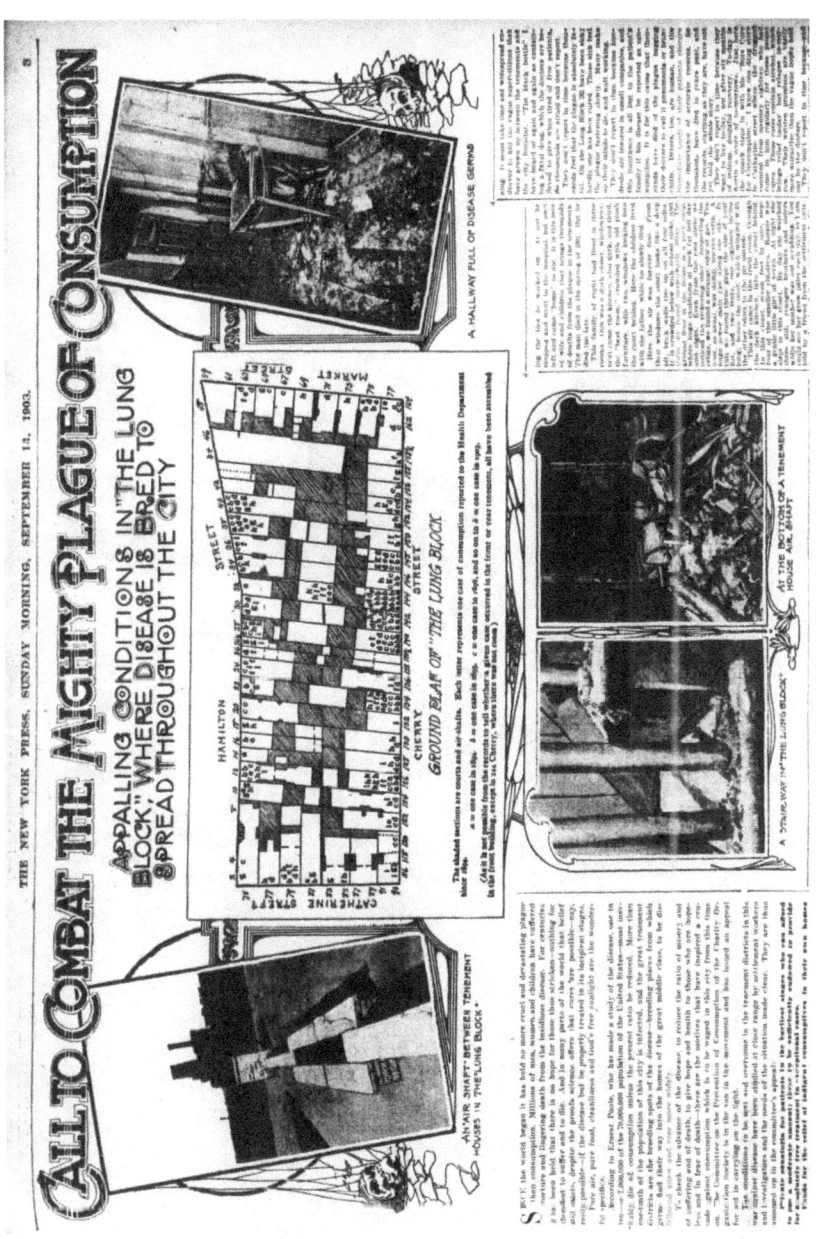

4.4A–C. Several notable examples of the sensational coverage that city newspapers gave the Lung Block park campaign. Note the central importance of the tuberculosis map in each instance, as well as penned illustrations in the margins embellishing already ghoulish portrayals of the health risks involved for residents (particularly children). "Call to Combat the Mighty Plague of Consumption," *New York Press*, September 13, 1903, 3; "City Block a Plague Hotbed," *New York Herald*, September 13, 1903, 5; "Horrors of 'Lung Block,' Where Consumption Holds Sway, Described by an Investigator," *Evening Telegram* (New York), October 17, 1903, 9.

Scenes in Tenement District Where Tuberculosis Claims Many Lives

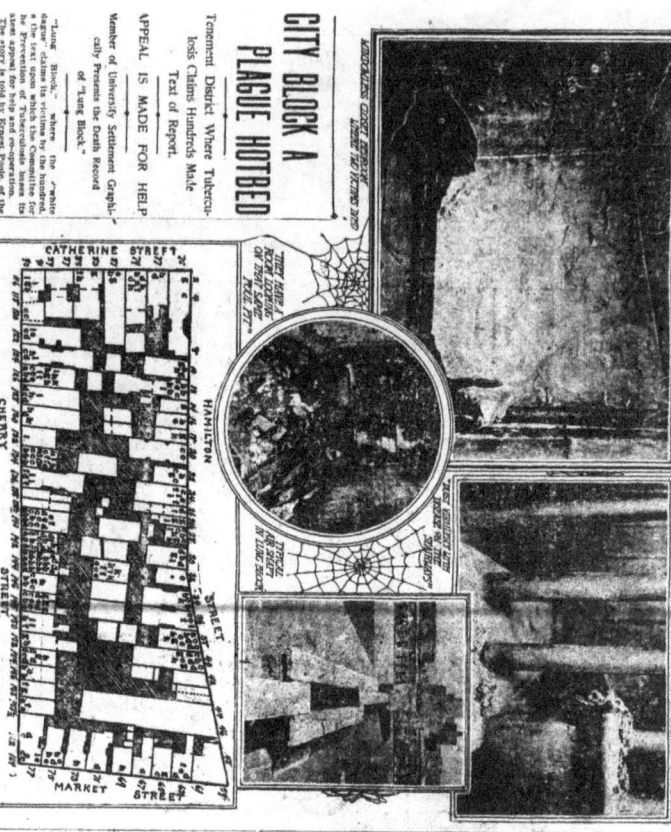

CITY BLOCK A PLAGUE HOTBED

Tenement District Where Tuberculosis Claims Hundreds Male Test of Report.

APPEAL IS MADE FOR HELP

Member of University Settlement Graphically Presents the Death Record of "Lung Block."

"Lung Block," where the tenement district claims its victims by the hundred, is the subject of an appeal for help and co-operation.

CUSTOMS RECORDS BROKEN

Duties for Three Days of Last Week Amount to $3,200,000, Indicating High Water Mark Since Establishment of New York House, in 1789.

Horrors of "Lung Block," Where Consumption Holds Sway, Described by an Investigator

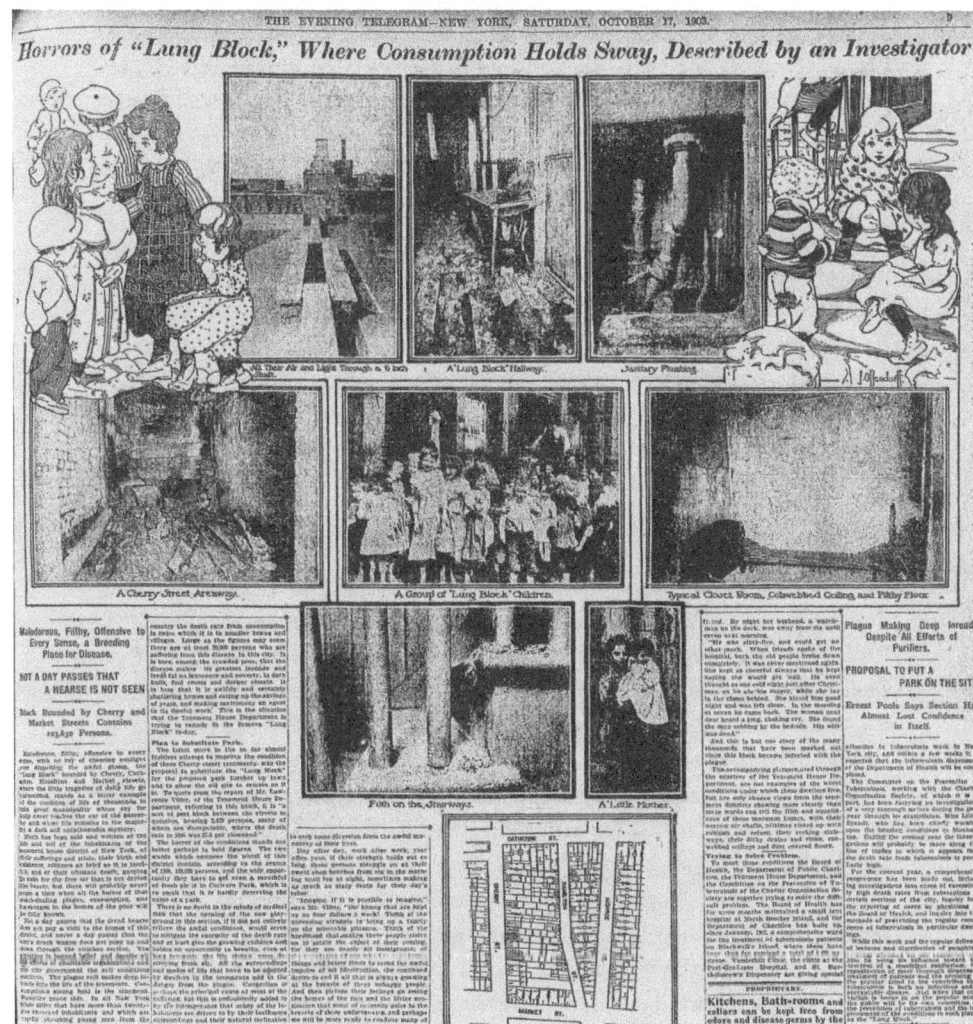

All Their Air and Light Through a 6 Inch — A "Lung Block" Railway. — Sanitary Plumbing.

A Cherry Street Areaway. — A Group of "Lung Block" Children. — Typical Closet Room, Cobwebbed Ceiling, and Filthy Floor.

Filth on the Stairways. — A Little Mother.

Malodorous, Filthy, Offensive to Every Sense, a Breeding Place for Disease.

NOT A DAY PASSES THAT A HEARSE IS NOT SEEN

Block Bounded by Cherry and Market Streets Contains 103,850 Persons.

Plague Making Deep Inroads Despite All Efforts of Purifiers.

PROPOSAL TO PUT A PARK ON THE SITE

Ernest Poole Says Section Has Almost Lost Confidence in Itself.

PROPERTY-OWNERS.

Kitchens, Bath-rooms and cellars can be kept free from others and disease germs by the occasional use of

CIGARS.   CIGARS.   CIGARS.

TO CELEBRATE ANNIVERSARY.

. . . hide from the police by day and prowl at night," the *Herald* informed its readers. "With the arrival of the bluecoats, feet patter swiftly over the uneven pavements . . . like rats running from a dog."

Portrayals of the block's noncriminals were only marginally less degrading, containing the same mixture of pity and disgust found in Riis's *How the Other Half Lives*. The *Herald* reporter, while interviewing a woman standing outside her apartment, assessed coolly that "she might have been fair once. Not over twenty-five years, she looks fifty. Her calico dress is tattered. Her hair hangs in a mass of snarls. Her face has not been washed this day." A brief exchange revealed that she shared a single room with four children and her husband, who "earns about $7 a week when he can work"; from the "hacking cough" accompanying her responses, the reporter speculated that "she ha[d] not long to live." He peered through her doorway at ill-clad children, "an apology for a stove," and a picture of Christ on the wall. These disjointed observations yielded to alarm as "coarse, discordant" voices from elsewhere in the building reached a crescendo of "wild shrieks [and] a volley of profanities." Amused by the reporter's reaction, the "faded woman" informed him that her neighbors were "at it again," an explanation that, when it appeared in print, likely raised more questions about her life than it answered.[126]

Some journalists did not try to hide their contempt. "To look upon the mode of life in this block," remarked the *Herald*, "is to wonder how these people can exist. It is an existence, nothing more." Living there, the writer speculated, "must make men desperate and women forget that even within their hardened lives there is some hope of getting away from such surroundings."[127] Prominently featured experts did little to alter the impenetrable gloom that such stories cast on the neighborhood. "Imagine, if it is possible to imagine, the homes that are kept up on four dollars a week!" Veiller was quoted as saying in the *Evening Telegram*. "Think of the unceasing struggle to bring up a family on the miserable pittance . . . of the temptation of one who has seen better things and better times to resist the awful impulse of self-destruction . . . that is always gnawing at the breasts of these unhappy people."[128]

Ironically, the photographs accompanying these descriptions often conveyed a less drastic scenario. In a *World* article from September, a barefoot child identified as a "typical Lower East Sider" beamed into the camera; a circle of young girls gazed up from the pavement with a mixture of curiosity and bemusement; mothers and their children gathered sociably on a front stoop; a large group of boys, attired in long-sleeved shirts, pants, and caps, stood stiffly at attention above the caption, "children in [nearby] Oliver Street want a park."[129] Reporters struggled to reconcile their own perceptions with the fact that "Lung Block" inhabitants evidently managed to enjoy themselves. One, when describing a room that sheltered three families as "distressing," observed with some puzzlement that "the occupants do not seem to think so.

They were happy, seemingly, when the photograph was made." Disavowing all knowledge of how these families managed to navigate their crowded living arrangements, he promptly abandoned the effort, pronouncing it "too great a puzzle to solve."[130]

Board of Estimate members tabled a final decision on the park for another hearing in mid-November, citing key changes in the proposal and Mayor Low's absence.[131] As the date for the next park proposal hearing approached, a sense of invincibility began to pervade the project's coverage. When *Charities* discussed the topic in October, its confident tone made clear that the headline—"Lung Block or Park-Playground—Which?"—did not seriously question the project's merits, nor its prospects for success. Noting that "little persuasion [was] required" for Board of Estimate members to accept the park idea for consideration, the journal buried details of the upcoming hearing amid lengthy excerpts from de Forest's proposal.[132] Similar optimism flashed in the city's daily newspapers. "The Lung Block," trumpeted the *Herald*, "with all its sad memories, will soon be a thing of the past." "That the movement . . . will be successful there is no doubt," agreed the *World*, declaring that "nowhere else In New York is a community so handicapped as this, nowhere else . . . is the proportion of crime and disease so great."[133]

As the block's destruction appeared imminent, people and organizations began stepping forward to claim a share of the credit. Noting that "the Lung Block . . . is to be razed," a *World* reporter added that "as advocated by the *Evening World*, a beautiful park is to mark the spot."[134] Two days before the scheduled hearing, Willcox publicly endorsed the project with an enthusiasm that betrayed his Johnny-come-lately role. "Nobody," he declared in the *World*, "knows better than [NYCDOH commissioner Ernst J.] Lederle, [tenement house] Commissioner De Forrest [*sic*] and myself of the awful conditions existing in the Lung Block." While Biggs, Veiller, or Poole might have bristled at Willcox's claim, they likely would have approved of his similarly enthusiastic, if exaggerated, assertion that "there is no place on the face of earth where the tubercular plant has such an opportunity to thrive in the systems of both young and old."[135]

Such forceful statements, born of expert knowledge and righteous indignation, granted no legitimacy to doubters or detractors. Yet they existed, their opposition growing more vocal as the hearing date approached. Roughly one-third of a *World* article from early November, ironically titled "All Agree the Lung Block Shall Go," dealt with strong objections from a local politician.[136] Alderman Isaac Marks, after "studying this question from every side," concluded that a small park at Cherry, Catherine, Hamilton, and Market Streets did not serve the best interest of his constituents, many of whom lived in the vicinity. Frankly acknowledging his own political interest in the matter, Marks nevertheless maintained that small-parks advocates had already introduced enough "breathing spaces" in the area, citing a public pier two blocks away and two other parks within walking distance.[137] "You cannot expect me to help wipe out the small storekeeper," he protested, "compel people to leave the homes they have occupied for years and years simply because of this agitation." He placed the block's tuberculosis problem at the threshold of the agency responsible for exposing it in the first place: the city health department. If Lederle "exercised the same sanitary vigilance [there] as he does in other parts of the city," Marks charged, he "could stamp out tuberculosis in the Lung Block and there would be no need of a park there."[138]

Park proponents chalked up Marks's opposition to shortsightedness: "Human life," declared Willcox scornfully, "is nothing compared to votes from the view of a politician."[139] Only ignorance or indifference, Willcox reasoned, could prevent people from realizing the advantages of replacing a tuberculosis-ridden slum with a restorative "breathing space." He echoed de Forest's challenge to "to walk through Hamilton street from Catharine to Market, and . . . see what a great good the razing of the tenements will do, and in their place a park of green grass and trees." Neither statement included alternative solutions that did not require destroying thousands of homes, nor entertained the possibility that Marks's constituents might not subscribe to the images of their neighborhood that Willcox and others promoted to disinterested outsiders. When Marks asked a reporter, "Why don't [park supporters] turn the whole east side into a park and be done with it?" he challenged their claims to higher moral ground by suggesting that they valued "breathing spaces" more than people—a charge that Willcox's rebuttal did little to dispel.[140]

When viewed against a larger backdrop of urban-park advocacy, the campaign to plant a "breathing space" at Cherry, Catherine, Hamilton, and Market Streets denoted one of a string of similar efforts taking place in New York and other cities at the turn of the century. This campaign grew directly out of the 1890s small parks and playgrounds movement, which promoted fresh air, sunshine, and greenery as essential for leading productive lives. Unlike their mid-nineteenth-century predecessors, small-parks advocates no longer accepted the passive landscape gazing of Central Park as sufficient for instilling health and civic virtue in its working classes. Instead, they argued, working-class people needed opportunities to use these natural elements actively and directly. This point resonated with greater urgency as the city swelled with working-class immigrants whose children lacked suitable places to play, and germ theory reinforced popular associations between crowded slums and deadly contagion. The impetus behind "breathing spaces," as with the parallel public health and housing movements, merged the moral environmentalism of earlier generations with modern demands for stronger municipal oversight to curb the excesses of unfettered urban development.

Born into the romantic age and propelled to national fame in the Progressive age, Jacob Riis bridged the aestheticism of Frederick Law Olmsted's generation with the social-scientific empiricism of his contemporaries. Within his own time period, his insistence on fresh air and sunshine over property and profits situated him within a broader, interrelated network of urban activism that included Hermann Biggs's push to control tuberculosis in the tenement districts, and Lawrence Veiller's crusade to outlaw dumbbell air shafts. Riis's reform work throughout the 1890s helped refashion eminent domain from a rhetorical concept into a weapon that reformers could use to reclaim and transform working-class spaces. His subsequent Committee on Small Parks recommendations informed Veiller's list of "city wildernesses," which then provided the opening for Lilian Brandt to promote the block bounded by Cherry, Catherine, Hamilton, and Market Streets as a future "breathing space." While historians have characterized Riis's small parks and playground advocacy as side ventures from his settlement or housing reform work, Riis viewed it as central to his reform agenda, at one point calling it "the logical sequel to 'How the Other Half Lives,' and the thing I have aimed at for years."[141] While his determination to "let in the light" met with skepticism among colleagues, none could dispute his talent for breathing life into their causes and instilling public awareness. "Though I'd like to reform almost every other reformer I ever knew," conceded Lincoln Steffens, "I shouldn't change Riis . . . in any particular, least of all in his roaring follies."[142]

Despite Lung Block park supporters' reluctance to publicly acknowledge Riis's influence and contributions, their reliance on his methods and the precedent he established made clear their indebtedness to his battle with Mulberry Bend. Both campaigns combined modern and authoritative maps, photographs, and statistics with older cries of irredeemable physical and moral contamination, courting sensational coverage that portrayed their target communities as both dangerous and doomed. Likewise, both campaigns incorporated the same top-down approach and class biases. Riis's work with Mulberry Bend, and later the Committee on Small Parks, reinforced the idea that public advocacy was a job for experts: people with the proper credentials for gathering the evidence needed to craft a successful proposal. This evidence typically resided with organizations that monitored as well as served the poor: private charities, settlements, and public agencies. Thus, it was not the poor themselves, but expert-driven impressions of the poor that ultimately determined which working-class neighborhoods remained and which were marked for destruction—something the former denizens of Central Park, Mulberry Bend, and "Bone Alley" understood all too well.

When Robert de Forest approached the Board of Estimate in September 1903—as COSCNY president *and* the city's Tenement House Commissioner—his case against the Lung Block bulged with Biggs's disease maps and Veiller's "city wilderness" designations, Brandt's statistics and Poole's alarming literary portraits, all intended to drive home the same points Riis had made in Mulberry Bend about how working-class spaces should be used. What de Forest did *not* include were Riis's impassioned and substantive arguments for the park and playground that would follow, a sign that at this point in the Lung Block park campaign, destruction took priority over creation.

As the proposal neared its final hearing before city leaders in November of 1903, increasingly heated exchanges between supporters and critics revealed not only competing visions of working-class needs but also traces of a much broader cultural conflict unfolding in New York political discourse. Alderman Isaac Marks, son of Jewish immigrants and a Democrat, dispensed Tammany power at the local level while Parks Commissioner William Willcox, an old-stock Republican and Ivy League graduate, served in Mayor Seth Low's cabinet.[143] However, in the wake of municipal elections occurring one week before, these men's backgrounds and government positions no longer reflected the true balance of power between them. While Marks looked forward to representing his constituents for a third consecutive term, Willcox—along with Veiller, de Forest, and other appointed officials in Low's two-year administration—prepared to make way for the mayoral victor, George B. McClellan Jr., and a return to Tammany rule. New Yorkers, it appeared, had decisively rejected reform." Low's failed reelection bid would occupy reform's disgruntled ranks for many months afterward. For the moment, however, with the Lung Block campaign's most powerful supporters having become lame ducks overnight, Willcox's shrillness signified both an awareness of the project's vulnerability and a fierce commitment to pushing it through before city administrations changed. Focused on these harsh political realities, park supporters redoubled their efforts, unaware that their most outspoken and unyielding opponent had yet to appear from within the "Lung Block" itself.

Chapter 5

"MY POOR PEOPLE NEED HOMES, NOT PARKS"

James Curry and Working-Class Counterperspectives on Reform

In the previous four chapters I charted the "Lung Block's" emergence as a public health threat through germ theory and disease maps, and its gradual transformation into a reform target through the moral environmentalism and muckraking idealism inspiring the settlement, urban housing, and park movements. Despite the resulting park campaign's weighty arsenal of evidence, widespread publicity and resounding support from key city officials, the block bordered by Cherry, Catherine, Hamilton, and Market Streets remained standing for the next thirty years. What force, or combination of forces, prevented this "breathing space" from becoming a reality?

Answering this question requires examining this campaign from the perspective of the working-class immigrant population for whom the park was intended. Hampering this approach is the reality that nearly all surviving sources from the park campaign—maps, statistics, photographs, publicity pamphlets, newspaper articles, municipal documents—originated with "outside" individuals and organizations bent upon the block's destruction.[1] This objective colored their perceptions and filtered their fact-gathering efforts, yielding depictions of the neighborhood as medically and morally contaminated. Whether park proponents surveyed these streets on foot with notebooks and cameras or on paper through abstracted renderings and numerical tabulations, they appeared to take little interest in how residents themselves perceived their immediate surroundings. Recovering the perspectives of "Lung Block" denizens involves applying against-the-grain interpretations to sources originally created for monitoring their poverty, crime, and contagion levels; using their voting patterns as rough proxies for their stances toward reform; and relying upon cultural mediators who lived among them and claimed to represent their interests.

One such cultural mediator, James Bernard Curry, stands in stark contrast to the urban reformers who have commanded the previous four chapters. He did not hail from old-stock Yankee wealth, nor did his career path include Ivy League universities, settlement houses, or city newsrooms. The son of Irish immigrants, Curry came up through public and religious institutions to serve Lower East Side tenement populations as a priest for more than thirty years. The perspectives he developed through these experiences led him to oppose the park project as unnecessary and even detrimental to families already occupying that space. When placed in the broader context of the 1903 municipal elections, Curry's outspoken opposition—and the bitter indignation it evoked from park supporters—highlighted fundamental class divisions regarding day-to-day priorities, expectations from government, and visions of how American cities should look and function. In the wake of the decisive Tammany victory that brought the park project to a halt, New York urban reformers lashed out against what they perceived to be their opponents' corruption and self-interest. However, the evidence suggests that their political and park campaigns foundered on dwindling popular support—a direct result of reform's failure to bridge these class divisions.

THE EVOLUTION OF JAMES CURRY'S WORLDVIEW

James Curry's working-class perspective took shape through the poverty, instability, and loss permeating his early years. His parents, Peter and Ellen, emigrated to America along with nearly two million others during the Irish potato famine of the 1840s and 1850s. Upon disembarking in New York, they joined the swelling ranks of the foreign-born working class.[2] By 1853 they had married and taken up residence on East 28th Street between Second and Third Avenues, one of many emerging Irish enclaves scattered throughout New York.[3] Here, Peter Curry and his brother-in-law, Cornelius Horgan, worked as butchers, a demanding but lucrative occupation into which relatively few Irish immigrants had ventured by the 1850s.[4] Horgan had moved uptown before James was born in 1857, leaving Peter and Ellen Curry to raise six children amid the din and stenches of slaughterhouses, stables, iron works, and masonries.[5] A sanitary report from the mid-1860s blamed the area's overcrowding, filth, and ventilation deficiencies for turning the houses into "prolific fever-nests"; it also singled out slaughterhouses for the health risks associated with "decaying animal matter . . . and offensive effluvia," as well as their potentially demoralizing effects on children, "who are often curious witnesses of these disgusting scenes of blood and slaughter." While the report focused on environmental contributors such as outdoor plumbing and poorly maintained streets, it also condemned the tenants themselves as "the lowest grade of [laborers] . . . almost entirely Irish and of Irish descent . . . degraded, filthy in their habits and improvident."[6] By this point, health and social workers in New York had been making similar conflations between Irish backgrounds, illness, and immorality for thirty years.[7]

James Curry was among the local children whose moral development was in jeopardy, according to the sanitary inspector. The sounds and smells of animal death accompanied him daily to the nearby school, to church, and back home to the multistory brick house containing his family's butcher shop and at least a dozen other tenants.[8] Death also assumed a human specter for Curry, claiming four of his siblings before he reached the age of ten.[9] All the while, his father's health declined—a common pattern among Irishmen whose long hours of manual labor increased their vulnerability to opportunistic infections like tuberculosis and pneumonia.[10] By the time Peter Curry died in 1869, his family had left their house and butcher business for a nearby tenement that his brother-in-law owned. Ellen Curry, the first tenant listed for the house in the 1870 census, may have acted as housekeeper.[11] The oldest daughter, Margaret, then died a year later, leaving fourteen-year-old James with the daunting prospect of supporting his mother and two younger siblings.[12]

James Curry found himself at this difficult crossroads at a time when Irish immigrants and their children still encountered formidable obstacles to economic and social advancement in American cities.[13] Although Irish-born New Yorkers numbered two hundred thousand—or one out of four residents—by 1860, and constituted the largest ethnic group of shopkeepers, lack of education and marketable skills still relegated many of them to the city's docks, warehouses, construction sites, and factories.[14] They were also disproportionately represented in the city's courts and prisons, constituting 80 percent of the fifty-eight thousand persons convicted of criminal offenses in 1860.[15] However, they had achieved more headway in the public sector. Having arrived in New York during political suffrage's expansion to include nearly all white male adult citizens, Irish immigrants responded to the Democratic Party's overtures enthusiastically—in part because their nativist detractors tended to align with the rival Whigs.[16] As their votes strengthened the Democrats' grip on city government, Irish-born supporters benefited through employment opportunities within the municipal ranks.[17] By the mid-1850s, 27 percent of New York City's police force and one-tenth of its elected representatives were Irish or of Irish descent; by 1860, they made up more than a third of the police force, nearly a quarter of elected representatives, and 40 to 50 percent of the city's public school employees.[10] This trend paralleled those of other large northern and midwestern cities, where the proportion of public employees with Irish backgrounds increased from 11 percent in 1870 to 30 percent in 1900, while the proportion of the labor force with Irish backgrounds remained stable at 20 percent.[19] While a substantial number of Irish Americans had attained middle-class status by 1870, approximately 40 percent still toiled as manual laborers or domestic servants; wealth and prestige would elude most of them for decades to come.[20]

Beyond their poverty and lack of marketable skills upon arrival in urban

America, Irish immigrants toiled against nativists' perceptions of them as a threat to American economic, political, and cultural freedoms. In an age of rapid industrialization, their increasing numbers drove wages further downward and accelerated the deskilling of manufacturing and artisanal trades; this ensured their place in a fixed caste of replaceable wage earners, undermining the egalitarianism of American free labor ideology.[21] Likewise, their pragmatic willingness to exchange their political loyalty for direct material assistance fueled the urban political machine, which threatened democracy through fraudulent and occasionally violent methods of suppression.[22] Finally, their overwhelming adherence to Catholicism challenged mainstream Americans' self-image as Anglo-Puritans, raising questions about the extent to which immigrant loyalties were divided between Old World and New.[23] "We are fast losing our identity as Americans," the Presbyterian newspaper *Evangelist* warned its readers in 1849, "and shall soon fall into a meager and powerless minority. The reins of power and influence are passing from the hands of Americans to those of foreigners."[24] Nearly forty years later, this nativist attitude still flourished in elite Protestant circles. "This country is not Ireland or Germany," declared the Reverend Howard Crosby, who led the city's Society for the Prevention of Crime during the 1880s; "[our institutions] are American . . . and we do not intend to surrender them to arrogant and impudent foreigners who abuse our hospitality by their insulting effrontery."[25] This anxiety permeated all levels of native-born society. "The Yankee hod-carrier, or Yankee wood-sawyer, looks down with ineffable contempt upon his brother Irish hod-carrier or Irish wood-sawyer," observed New England intellectual Orestes Brownson in 1845; "in his estimation, 'Paddy' hardly belongs to the human family."[26] In the privacy of their diaries, patrician New Yorkers George Templeton Strong and Theodore Roosevelt, respectively, reviled the Irish as being as "remote from us in temperament and constitution as the Chinese . . . brutal, base, cruel, cowards, and as insolent as base" and "a stupid, sodden, vicious lot . . . equally deficient in brains and virtue."[27] Aspiring Irish Americans thus contended with discrimination on the job, political groups seeking to curtail their naturalization and voting opportunities, and popular caricatures depicting them as violent, drunk, or lazy—all variations of the intolerance they had experienced from the ruling Anglo-Protestant class in Ireland.[28]

James Curry forsook the butcher's apron, the factory, and the political machine in favor of another avenue of Irish American upward mobility: the Roman Catholic Church. Across the Atlantic, this institution had provided impoverished Irish tenants with sanctuaries from British colonial oppression; in urban America, it now provided impoverished Irish immigrants with sanctuaries from nativist hostility, as well as vehicles for cultural assimilation.[29] Between 1840 and 1865, immigration from Ireland and Germany swelled

New York's Catholic population to more than 300,000, or nearly half of the city's total. As this sudden influx boosted the church's visibility and clout, it also strained the church's resources. On average, each priest in 1850s Manhattan served 4,500 Catholic New Yorkers across twenty-one parishes; by 1870 the number of parishes had doubled, with more than half of them sponsoring their own schools. Even so, one priest judged this exponential growth to be "entirely inadequate to the wants of the Catholic population."[30] Between 1870 and 1900, the number of priests in America continued climbing from 3,780 to 12,000; this trend unfolded most dramatically in cities, where demand was greatest.[31]

Living in a city where most of the church's leading figures were Irish born, Curry may have also felt drawn to the priesthood for its insulation from direct competition with US-born Protestants.[32] A priest's salary stretched considerably further than that of a butcher in nineteenth-century New York, taking into account the room and board provided and additional stipends for special masses, weddings, and funerals.[33] Likewise, the priesthood conveyed an air of prestige and authority that elevated Curry's social standing.[34] For working-class Catholic families, the clerical collar signified "a magical key" that unlocked the privileges of upper-class life.[35] Several blocks from the Currys' home, the sprawling sanctuary of Saint Stephen's—one of New York's fastest-growing churches, with twenty-five thousand parishioners—boasted elaborately carved marble, fine Italian paintings, and soaring sculpted angels. "The blue vaulted and fretted ceiling is sustained by graceful pillars and studded with stars," marveled a contemporary guidebook; "light pours in through beautiful stained-glass windows, casting their multicolored hues on pew and marble aisle."[36] Such handcrafted opulence offered Curry and other Irish Americans a coveted glimpse of paradise—a refuge from the hardship, tragedy, and indignities that formed the contours of their lives outside church walls.[37]

Here, Curry heard the sermons of Edward McGlynn, an Irish American who distinguished himself from other Catholic priests with his outspoken social activism regarding poverty and labor conditions. His "zeal, self-sacrifice and eloquence" secured him a reputation for being, according to one close associate, "'easily the chief' . . . among the priests of the metropolis."[38] Like Curry, McGlynn had grown up in a large family and lost his father early; timely intercession from his parish priest and archbishop enabled him to attend a Catholic university in Rome, where he earned multiple degrees.[39] Through a Latin school he established in the basement of Saint Stephen's, McGlynn extended the same vocational opportunities to "poor but worthy young men of the parish" who displayed aptitude and interest in an ecclesiastical career.[40] Curry's first steps toward the priesthood likely started here. He also attended the College of Saint Francis Xavier, a Jesuit day school providing low-cost education for Catholics who could not afford to attend nearby Fordham University.[41] Curry then traveled to Rome, where the church continued to provide him with opportunities and experiences denied him at home: rigorous academics, picturesque scenery, and interactions with students of different cultural backgrounds from all over America and Europe.[42] When the Irish immigrant butcher's son returned to New York, he did so with a college degree and a profession; the methods by which he attained them would ensure his ongoing allegiance to Irish Catholic, rather than American secular, institutions.

CURRY'S EARLY CAREER IN SAINT JAMES PARISH

Curry embarked upon his clerical career during a volatile period in which Catholic leaders debated the church's identity and direction in America. Liberal Catholics wanted to preserve the essentials of church doctrine while embracing the progressive, optimistic spirit of the age; conservatives maintained that the church's integrity and survival rested upon its ability to withstand rather than accommodate the forces of change.[43] Throughout the 1880s and 1890s, these factions clashed repeatedly over a host of contemporary issues. How to accommodate the growing wave of Catholic immigrants from Italy and Poland without rendering the church an ethnic and ghettoized fortress against nativism? Alternately, how to combat popular anti-Catholic stereotypes that aligned the church with Old World despotism and ignorance without compromising traditional principles? As labor-capital relations worsened, should the church respond by defending the rights of the workers who filled its pews on Sundays, or by condemning them for challenging higher authority? Should Catholics assert their rights as American citizens by enrolling their children in public schools, or should the church pour its resources into a parochial system that preserved traditional values at the risk of walling their followers off further from the mainstream?[44] For New York, a city at the forefront of large-scale national developments, a prominent seat of American Catholic power, and home to prominent leaders on each side of these issues, these questions held special significance. McGlynn, Curry's childhood priest from Saint Stephen's, served as a lightning rod for these differences with his increasingly radical stances against capitalism. His public campaigning for Henry George, a socialist mayoral challenger who attracted significant Irish support in 1886, posed a direct challenge to the insular, top-down approach of New York's conservative Catholics—the most powerful being Archbishop Michael Corrigan. The conflict culminated in McGlynn's temporary excommunication, polarizing Catholics on both sides of the Atlantic.[45]

When Curry arrived at Saint James Catholic Church as a curate in the 1880s, the Lower East Side parish served approximately twenty-five thousand people, many of them working-class Irish immigrants and their children.[46]

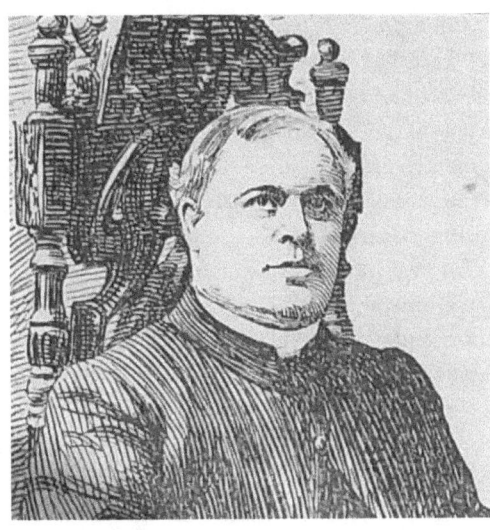

5.1. A sketch of the Rev. James B. Curry, published on the front page of the *Catholic News*, April 18, 1908.

Depending on their proximity to East River docks, parish neighborhoods ranged in character from quiet, family-oriented enclaves to rougher areas featuring saloons, brothels, and sailors' boardinghouses.[47] Against this variable backdrop, Saint James's pastor, John Kean, exemplified a delicate balance between power and obedience. A "powerful and magnetic personality" who exercised authority over most aspects of his parishioners' lives, Kean supervised the 1,500 children who attended the city's largest parochial school, organized many of their social activities, and ordered them home every night at nine o'clock from his rectory window. Kean also closely supervised the conduct of parish adults: when a local saloonkeeper persisted in the frowned-upon practice of serving women, Kean fought him for five years until the saloon went out of business.[48] Between 1880 and 1900, Saint James's growth mirrored that of other New York Catholic churches as Kean expanded the parish's offerings beyond the school to include an orphanage and fifteen social clubs, with an army of volunteers to sustain their funding and labor.[49] These developments underscored Saint James's important role in the community. It "was the heart and center of the parish," recalled one of Smith's children, "an intimate part of our daily lives."[50] Meanwhile, throughout this period of expansion on the parish level, Kean presented himself as a loyal and devoted subject to higher church authorities—"a source," recalled one colleague, "from which they could always find support."[51]

At the time Curry assumed leadership of Saint James in the early 1900s, one reporter described him as a "wholesome, solidly built man of kindly visage, keen eyes and a square jaw," armed with "an agile wit and determination of the bulldog type."[52] He fielded outsiders with vigilance: "We know every man, woman and child about here," he later boasted, "and when a new face shows up we ask to whom it belongs."[53] Among insiders, Curry was "ardent yet amiable [with] a noble, generous nature"; "a lover of truth and justice . . . [whose] word was gospel."[54] As he fulfilled his customary duties of preaching, hearing confessions, fundraising, visiting the sick, and officiating at milestone events, he worked to uplift his parishioners by promoting the mainstream middle-class values of modesty, temperance, industry, and thrift.[55] Referring to the parish's children as "my boys and girls," he followed Kean's example of overseeing their education by day and enforcing strict curfews by night.[56] Curry provided a clubhouse to keep older working boys off the streets during their leisure hours, and threatened schoolgirls with expulsion if he found them socializing on the nearby pier after dark.[57] Curry did not shrink from disciplining neglectful parents either, with one newspaper likening the sting of his rebukes to "a whip of scorpions."[58] As he monitored his parishioners' activities, he defended them fiercely against the class and ethnic biases hounding them in mainstream publications. Describing his Working Boys Club members to reporters as "good boys [who] come from good parents," he insisted that "while they have not got the money nor the good clothes of Fifth Avenue youths, their moral stamina is equally good."[59] Despite all these efforts, Curry still despaired over the gap he perceived between the number of children in his parish and the resources to care for them. "I see around me a field weighty with ripened wheat," he confided to Archbishop Corrigan in 1901, "and whilst we reap, the field seems to grow thicker and heavier. I always feel that much more is to be done."[60]

At first glance, such concerns would appear to align Curry with progressive urban reformers. So would his advocacy methods, which moved up conventional chains of command while courting publicity pressure. For example, when Curry aimed in 1901 to curb illicit activities featuring a rowdy dance hall and prostitutes in a nearby square, his escalating complaints to the police commissioner, and then journalists, brought about a stronger law enforcement presence there.[61] The following year, Curry issued calls to close a brothel operating near a clubhouse he had organized for working boys in his parish. When the boys then faced retribution from policemen who had collected bribes for protecting the brothel, Curry notified city officials; when his complaints had little effect, he launched a public counteroffensive that resonated through newspapers all over the city.[62] "If the police want work to do," Curry thundered from his pulpit, "they can get it by closing up the disorderly houses that dot this district"; if not, he volunteered to lead the men of the parish in carrying out the work themselves.[63] The resulting publicity triggered a shake-up at the precinct, bringing about an increased responsiveness from the police.[64] "Let [Curry] hear of anything wrong in the parish," remarked one sergeant afterward, "and up those steps he comes, and it's not 'If you please, Mr. Captain,' or 'You'd oblige me, Mr. Sergeant' . . . but 'Now then, boys, what's the meaning of these happenings. Get out there and put an end to them.' . . . [W]hen we see him coming, we know there's work ahead."[65]

Despite these overlaps with urban reformers in objectives and methods, Curry perceived no common cause with them—quite the opposite. "I don't want anybody to class me as a crusader," the priest cautioned reporters when detailing his battles with vice and police corruption; "I am not starting to reform New York or the East Side, but I am going to take a hand in protecting the boys."[66] Unlike Jacob Riis, Curry harbored no desire to effect change beyond Saint James Parish, which he patrolled as its spiritual and moral protector.[67] Unlike Lawrence Veiller, Curry saw his activism flowing not from visions of impartial and professionally administered government but from the moral authority bequeathed to him through God and the church. This parish-bound perspective encouraged Curry to view social problems as isolated matters to be addressed and resolved within local power networks. These networks, in which he played a central role, sometimes functioned along lines that reformers rejected as shady and undemocratic. For example, when Curry encountered police resistance in shutting down the brothel near his boys' club, he approached Paddy Divver and "Big Tom" Foley, immigrant saloonkeepers, fellow parishioners, and Tammany power brokers capable of pulling strings in high places.[68] Living in an assembly district firmly in the grip of the political machine, Curry did not share reformers' image of Tammany leaders as corrupt and shifty; he related to them as fellow Irish Catholics with businesses, families, and the resources to help when needed. By contrast, Curry regarded urban reformers as outsiders whose motives toward the poor could not be trusted. Most of them hailed from Yankee-Protestant backgrounds that he and other Irish Catholics had learned to associate with discrimination, proselytization, or both. Because Protestants dominated the staff of social settlements as well as church missions, Curry often made little distinction between them, placing both efforts in the same class as brothels and saloons in terms of the risk they posed to his parishioners' souls.[69]

In the months before the Lung Block park campaign began, Curry registered his disregard for reformers when rejecting an overture from the nearby settlement that Riis had founded several years earlier. Describing himself as "perfectly indifferent" to the settlement's aims, Curry informed the head worker that "the responsibilities of my parish . . . need my constant and undivided attention. My sympathies run in distinctly religious lines." Underscoring the divisions he perceived between them, he continued, "To workers in fields outside of mine I wish success, but I beg to be left alone in my own . . . I trust to please the Divine Master, if not with extraordinary success, at least with the heart and will that I devote to my work. All-absorbed in that work, I cannot attend to any other."[70] With these remarks, Curry asserted his departure from reformers in placing God and the needs of his parishioners above broader social agendas, and in favoring parish-centered solutions to working-class immigrant problems.

"MY POOR PEOPLE NEED HOMES, NOT PARKS"

The Board of Estimate and Apportionment, consisting of the mayor, comptroller, president of the Board of Aldermen, and all five borough presidents, held their regular meetings upstairs in the west wing of City Hall. Their room, a former council chamber reputed to be among "the finest in the building," boasted several fine portraits; renovations undertaken during the summer had revealed a secret stairway from the Boss-Tweed era leading down to the basement, away from angry constituents.[71] On this Friday morning, mild for mid-November, the meeting drew the usual combination of city officials, petitioners, and journalists. Yet the balance of power in the room had shifted dramatically since the board's previous meeting in late October. Three board members—Mayor Seth Low, Manhattan president Jacob A. Cantor, and Brooklyn president J. Edward Swanstrom, all elected in 1901 on the Fusion ticket—now anticipated being replaced in two months. Their successors, all Tammany Democrats, would join the five board members who had won reelection eleven days earlier. Of these, four were Tammany Democrats, two of them having abandoned the Fusion ticket for Tammany's only weeks before the election. These two men—Comptroller Edward Grout and Board of Aldermen president Charles Fornes—were absent this morning, having sent surrogates in their place.[72]

When the park project for Cherry, Catherine, Hamilton, and Market Streets came up for review, a notable cross-section of public health experts, housing reformers, and settlement house activists stood up to briefly restate the points that Robert de Forest, Lilian Brandt, and others had raised before the same board in September. "I have never seen such filth and disease-breeding conditions as exist [there]," physician Sigard Adolphus Knopf testified, claiming that the neighborhood contained "hundreds of pale-faced children" at risk for tuberculosis. Veiller, speaking for the Tenement House Department (THD), condemned the block's houses as "filthy places of habitation . . . [where] neither light nor fresh air ever penetrate." These structures "could not be put in a sanitary condition by fumigation or disinfection," assured James Graham Phelps Stokes, a young settlement worker and millionaire philanthropist.[73] Representing the Outdoor Recreation League, Henry Street Settlement founder Lillian Wald called for replacing this "danger spot" with a "breathing space" and playground, a point upon which her fellow proponents predictably agreed. "If these children are to be saved," insisted

Knopf, "it must be by means of pure air and sunlight, of which they . . . have been deprived since birth." Veiller reminded other city officials that replacing crowded tenement blocks with parks had become "established policy."[74] To this, Manhattan parks commissioner William R. Willcox added his bold declaration that "the day for discussion on the necessity for small parks in the tenement districts is past."[75]

As Curry awaited his turn to speak, the preceding events of his life and career ensured that he would evaluate such arguments warily, critically, and personally. What park advocates presented as rows of dot-filled rectangles on disease maps, he knew to be streets of brick-and-mortar homes filled with human beings. Streamed through the filters of his working-class, Irish American upbringing, the public-spirited tones of this proposal for disease prevention and community improvement fairly crackled with nativist, highbrow contempt. As his parish's sworn spiritual guardian—as a man representing a people who still carried bitterness from their forced eviction and dispossession in Ireland—Curry embraced vocal opposition to the park as the only honorable course of action.[76] Seth Low's stinging defeat had already rendered the project vulnerable to public criticism. Representing his constituents at the meeting, Alderman Isaac Marks delivered the same points he had made to newspapers several days earlier: his district had enough parks, and unsanitary conditions reflected upon the THD and Board of Health.[77] For the park's opponents, success would hinge upon their ability to discredit campaigners' arguments and evidence while maintaining the credibility of their well-heeled, professionally oriented listeners.

Curry presented his counterarguments with diplomacy and charm. While he did not dispute the campaign's central premise—assuring board members that he "underst[ood] perfectly how to appreciate the oasis of parks in the midst of a thickly populated district"—he agreed with Marks that the block bordered by Cherry, Catherine, Hamilton, and Market had reached a saturation point with breathing spaces. To the east, Curry observed, the block already featured two slips "as wide and as spacious as squares in parks"; beyond that stretched "the broad expanse of the river, and the day-enduring smile of the sun, all untaxed and rent free." To the north, south, and west lay eleven parks, many of which he credited "the worthy City Fathers" with providing in the past decade: Corlears Hook Park, Grand Street Park, Hamilton Fish Park, Rutgers Park, and Seward Park, "not to say anything at all of Battery Park, Bowling Green Park, City Hall Park, Jeannette Park, Mulberry Bend and Paradise Parks." With most of these sites situated well within a mile of the block, Curry assured the board—perhaps lightly, perhaps sarcastically— that "if our people need the warm life-giving rays of the sun, or desire to draw into their lungs long, deep draughts of pure ozone, they can be had at the small expense of a slight exertion in a short walk."[78]

Curry then moved from assessing the project's merits to questioning its motives. He used park supporters' descriptions of overcrowding as a launching point for acquainting his audience with the needs of "our people": the working-class tenants who packed into these houses to be "close to their work, [which] gives the poor man a warm dinner and saves car fare and lunch bills." Knocking down tenements in congested neighborhoods "betokens more the desire of getting rid of the poor rather than of helping them," Curry argued, calling upon the "honorable Board" to acknowledge "the truth that it is a thousand times better to improve the dwellings of the poor than to raze their homes to the ground." Having claimed the high moral ground, Curry joined Marks in holding the city's health and housing departments partly accountable for the sanitary violations that park supporters condemned so vehemently. "Why not enforce the Tenement House Laws," Curry demanded, "see to it that landlords pay fair wages to honest and sober janitors and housekeepers . . . [to] cleanse the halls and areaways and keep clean the sidewalks and streets?" Noting that more than a hundred of the tuberculosis deaths reported over the past nine years came from six houses, he suggested tearing those down and erecting model tenements in their place. "My poor people need homes," he insisted, "not parks."[79]

Having undermined the project's merits and motives, Curry then turned his attention to the charges of contamination that inspired it in the first place. He began with the public health statistics associated with the block, deftly employing language that undermined their legitimacy even as he professed to uphold it. "I have never questioned the genuineness of the *alleged* reports of the Board of Health," he stated; "nor have I inquired into the *real* causes of death in the district," which, he speculated, could be "cholera infantum, senility, or some other disease with a sesquipedalian name." The large turnover of families in tenement apartments could just as easily indicate that infected humans were contaminating the houses, rather than the other way around, he argued; this would mean that "the seeds of consumption which proved fatal in these surroundings did not originate in Cherry street, but in some other portion of the city, even in some other country of the world." Curry then introduced letters from local physicians confirming the general health of the block's residents—physicians who "understand thoroughly the sanitary conditions of this neighborhood, and appreciate most intimately the needs of our people." While these physicians visited the block frequently, Curry maintained that they came to deliver babies, "healthy, country-loving, newborn citizens for our great metropolis." These infants would eventually grow into a "swarm of healthy children that gather around the humble but honest fireside, despite the theories and speculations of our twentieth-century reformers."[80]

With the project's merits, motives, and supporting evidence now on shaky ground, Curry now moved to redeem the block's tarnished image. Citing twenty years of living and working in the area, Curry pointed out that the "Lung Block" designation had not existed "until these petitioners wished to grab it for a park . . . [it is] a term used to further this grabbing scheme, that is all." Curry then cited specific passages from Ernest Poole's *The Plague in Its Stronghold* that exhibited a strong nativist bias. "'So come hundreds of others in this neighborhood,'" Curry read aloud, "'men and women, young and old, drunk, bestial, vile, forever steadily sinking. Hard drinking triples suscepti-bility to consumption. This is seen most of all in the Irish.'" He continued, "'The body of the block is packed with Irish and Italians and a sprinkling of twelve other peoples. All these image best the dissipation, the shattered vitality which eats into savings, starves the home, then gives the plague easy entrance, and makes it a constant danger to all the family.'" Refuting these statements as "slanderous falsehoods," Curry deplored their dissemination far and wide through "villainous articles . . . written by reporters who could be bought for any price from a glass of beer to a dollar." As a result, parishioners from Cherry, Catherine, Hamilton, and Market Streets were "grossly misrep-resent[ed] . . . to our fellow-citizens as a district of thugs, cadets, fallen women and brawling, drunken, foul creatures," Curry fumed, "guilty of every crime against Sinai's laws."[81]

Knopf, Veiller, Stokes, Wald, and Willcox sat in silence as a clergy-man flatly contradicted their medical and social-scientific expertise, then denounced their publicity campaign as insulting and inaccurate. The worst was still to come, however. No longer content with defensive tactics, Curry now launched into a fiery counteroffensive that laid bare his contempt for urban reformers. The park's masterminds, he alleged, were "a few idealists who come from palatial homes to tell the poor how to live." Their underlying motive was "to decimate the democratic proletariat" by razing tenement neighborhoods. Their evidence was incomplete and firmly slanted against the ethnic poor, its fixation on tenement districts obscuring the fact that alcoholism and tubercu-losis affected all classes of people. "The drink might be cheap whisky, it might be champagne," he pointed out; "the sick man may be the poor man of Cherry Hill, or it may be the rich man in his Fifth-Avenue mansion."[82] If tuberculosis favored the tenements, Curry insisted it was because of the constant clouds of germ-laden dust filtering in from poorly maintained streets. This dust, which harbored "the death-dealing sputa" of tuberculosis sufferers, met diminished resistance in "the condition of our people, who, healthy or delicate, sick or well, are forced . . . to toil day after day, [from] the very early morn long before our theorists have arisen from their comfortable beds, [until] long after the setting of the sun . . . when their more blest fellow-men have already had some hours of sleep." Drawing from the experiences of an immigrant butcher's son as well as those of a parish priest, Curry continued: "Toil they must, toil for themselves, toil for the[ir] large families . . . toil until they drop exhausted by the effort, drop into their coffins and their graves, victims of disregarded theories, say these petitioners; martyrs of most heroic self-sacrifice, say I." With that, Curry asked board members to reject the park "for our people's sake, for a good name and reputation are of much more value to our people, poor as they are, than the realization of reform dreams and . . . the fancies of faddists."[83]

In the short span of ten minutes, James Curry had challenged park proponents' claims to superior and objective knowledge across multiple fronts. Pitting lived experience and firsthand observations against the reformers' detached expertise, he recast the project as an unnecessary hardship to residents; its creators as wealthy, impractical meddlers who had their own agendas; its evidence as flawed or fabricated; and its publicity as a smear campaign fueled by sensationalism, class snobbery, and xenophobia. In the process, Curry elevated the residents from a degenerate rabble of "foul creatures" into "our people": a struggling community of human beings who were "decent and respectable," "humble but honest," deserving of warm dinners, agreeable lodging options, and dignity. As board members mulled the project's future, Curry intended for them to see this park proposal the way he did: not as a benign community improvement venture but as a professionally polished act of class aggression.

THE REFORM REACTION TO "NEIGHBORHOOD INERTIA"

When Board of Estimate members moved to table further discussion of the park until the next meeting, newspaper coverage deviated sharply from the park project to its critics. Calling Curry's statement a "sensation," the New York Herald acknowledged that it "had evidently been prepared with great care," inferring strong parallels with his defense of the parish against police harassment the previous year.[84] The Times and the Press noted Curry's "vehemen[ce] in resenting the imputation that the block was a 'lung' block," while Sun readers were treated to lengthy direct quotations, delivered "in plain terms."[85] While these accounts included his inflammatory remarks about reformers and reporters, only the Tribune characterized them as "vicious." Rather than engaging Curry's accusations directly, the city's news outlets merely reproduced them, savoring the colorful copy he provided.[86]

Park supporters and their allies reacted to Curry's testimony with quizzical bemusement. "There may be minds so skeptical as still to find," Charities editors observed caustically, "in the death-rates, the number of contagious diseases, and other figures presented at the previous hearing, evidence that the writers . . . must be in some degree blinded to the real sanitary conditions."[87] The same withering dismissiveness pervaded newspaper editorials, one holding Curry accountable for "the almost-universal regret in civilized lands that . . . the advice of the clergy is not quite so often asked and somewhat less frequently followed."[88] Another notable pattern among these reactions was their marked detachment from the displacement-related hardships the park would impose upon thousands. At the hearing, Veiller countered Curry's displacement concerns with a list of recent civic improvements in which "large numbers . . . had been displaced with little apparent inconvenience to anyone." Rather than clarify what, if any, efforts proponents had made to determine the park's impact to residents, *Charities* faithfully reiterated Riis's Mulberry Bend dictum that "the displaced population . . . [would be] quickly absorbed in the surrounding blocks." Citing a large number of new law tenements under construction with no clear timetables for completion, it concluded that the park's impact on local residents was "negligible."[89] The evening *World* likewise remained focused on long-term objectives, arguing that a new park meant "a healthier life for those babies on the block, whose presence there it is expected to prolong." This rosy prediction overlooked how the park, in actuality, would scatter those babies in every direction.[90] While a second *Times* editorial conceded "some force in [Curry's] assertions" regarding the humanitarian implications of proceeding, to hesitate on those grounds "would prevent the removal of practically every evil of long standing."[91]

Moreover, park champions refused to recognize critics' firsthand knowledge of the block and its residents as a legitimate claim to authority; on the contrary, they regarded it as a liability disqualifying their opponents from any serious consideration. When reviewing Isaac Marks's objections from the Board of Estimate hearing, *Charities* remarked cynically that "not all the forensic elaboration employed served to conceal the underlying reason for opposition, which was the unwillingness to see [his] constituents scattered."[92] Likewise, they maintained that Curry's decades of direct involvement had damaged his credibility by rendering him too close to the problem. He was "misled by a view too close and a knowledge too personal and intimate of the people who live in the 'lung block' and its vicinity," the *Times* suggested. "Their virtues, heroically maintained in the face of enormous obstacles, appeal to him more than do the cold mathematics of the Health Department, and he sees the terrors and horrors incidental to every wholesale eviction too clearly to appreciate its ultimate benefits." Secure in their conviction that these "terrors and horrors" served a worthwhile purpose, *Times* editors adopted a charitable, even patronizing tone toward the priest's fiery attacks. "He need not worry about a lack of homes for the very poor," they assured their readers soothingly. "The demand for them will certainly create them, and so much better than the old ones will they be that the number of the very poor will tend to decrease." Viewed through the long-range lens of progress, destroying tenement neighborhoods would vanquish not only the diseases of poverty, but poverty itself: an idea ushering nineteenth-century moral environmentalism seamlessly into the twentieth. "Homes make people," the *Times* declared confidently, "almost as much as people make homes."[93]

When the Board of Estimate tabled the park issue indefinitely three weeks later, pending the upcoming transition between mayoral administrations, the same city dailies that had filled their front pages and editorials with the Lung Block crusade buried the news item deep in their back pages. The *Evening Telegram* referred to the move as a "temporary setback," while other newspapers forecast grimmer odds for a reform-aligned project left to "the tender mercies of the Tammany Tiger."[94] Alarmed by the prospect of their own "Mulberry Bend" triumph slipping away, park supporters adopted a more militant approach. An unsigned editorial subsequently appeared in the *New York American*, which deftly captured how the campaign's detachment toward park-site residents had hardened into indifference, its smug indulgence toward critics had sharpened into impatience, and its zeal had boiled over into impotent rage.[95] The editorial charged several unnamed city officials with thwarting efforts of "the Board of Health, the Tenement-house Department, the Department of Parks and of numerous societies, settlements and physicians" to turn the neighborhood into a park and playground.[96] Citing statistical evidence from "eminent experts," the editorial reviewed the campaign's main talking points: that the tenements harbored deadly bacteria; they "[could not] be made fit for human habitation by any known method of disinfection"; and "that nothing short of razing the infected buildings w[ould] adequately protect the community." It jolted readers' fears by associating plague with place: "In the darkness and dirt of the 'Lung Block' the germs of tuberculosis live for years," it stated unequivocally.[97] Declaring "no need of multiplying illustrations," the editorial branded the neighborhood "a menace to the public welfare" whose only chance at redemption lay in its eradication. It rejected even more forcefully the logistic and ethical problems of displacement, countering that "almost any public improvement could be opposed with equal reason and equal folly." This indifference toward the park's evictees degenerated into outright hostility toward its critics: "The notion that the immediate and short-lived comfort of a few is of more consequence than the future and permanent welfare of the many is antiquated, and needs burial, badly," the editorial barked; "public servants who, actuated by such notions, thwart the public interests, need burial, similarly."[98]

The voice behind this unsigned editorial almost certainly belonged to Ernest Poole, who had pitched a piece fitting this description to the reform-friendly *American* one day after the park's tabling.[99] In defending the project, Poole framed the issues at stake as a binary power struggle between corrupt politicians and "eminent experts"; antiquated notions and scientifically proven facts; short-term upheaval and long-term urban planning; the "comfort of a few" and the "welfare of the many"; evil and good; wrong and right. This intractable mindset left park supporters with few alternatives for regarding their opposition as anything other than ignorant, self-serving, and irrelevant; it also conveyed their inability or unwillingness to address underlying weaknesses in their approach. After all, if the need for a "breathing space" at Cherry, Catherine, Hamilton, and Market Streets was so solidly and expertly established as to be immediately self-evident to anybody of intelligence, how could a few uninformed obstructionists bring it to a halt?

One possible answer is that the park's opposition was not uninformed. Both Curry and Marks were university-educated professionals who made a living serving their communities. While neither possessed formal training in public health or the social sciences, their firsthand familiarity with the proposed park site would have acquainted them with the environmental hazards there. For example, in a letter he wrote two years earlier to Archbishop Corrigan, Curry described the poor facilities where Saint James children attended school. Noting the church basement's lack of access to light and air, he worried that the "heavy, greasy, damp atmosphere" violated city health codes, in addition to hampering children's education. "Already vitiated before the children have assembled in it," Curry complained, "what must be the unhealthy condition of that same air after it has been inhaled and exhaled by our little ones?"[100] Curry's letter demonstrates that he not only accepted the connection between environment and disease but shared park proponents' concerns about its effects on his "little ones."[101]

Meanwhile, Poole's shrill defense of "the public interests" raises the question of just how far support for the park extended beyond reform circles. Park proponents appeared to derive their understanding of the public interest through germ theory, moral environmentalism, and citywide data generated by public and private institutions. Based on Veiller's breezy assurances and Poole's callous disregard for "the short-lived comfort of a few," the public whose interests they claimed to represent clearly excluded those living in the proposed park site. Opponents, by contrast, derived their understanding of the public interest from direct interactions with individuals and families who relied upon their leadership. Maintaining their positions as political and spiritual leaders rested upon their ability to advocate for and safeguard the priorities of their working-class constituents, making their own interests and those of their constituents indelibly linked. When park proponents attributed Marks's opposition to political self-interest, they did not consider that he might be defending a different set of "public interests." Having determined the public interests for themselves, they perceived Marks's opposition not as a reflection of his constituents' priorities but as an obstruction of their own.

When the park issue appeared in the city's opinion pages, it became even clearer that the "public interest" represented different things to different groups of New Yorkers. While top-brass editorials consistently promoted the park as a means of health and civic advancement, opposing arguments struck a more sympathetic chord with rank-and-file readers. "Parks are well enough," wrote George Trebor, a Brooklyn undertaker, to the *New York Times*, "but I agree with the Rev. Father Curry that we cannot drive these people out and into the river, for we hold out a practical invitation for them to come here. . . . We must give them consideration on Cherry Hill, notwithstanding the objections of Murray Hill, or any other hill."[102] Other readers suggested that the city adopt less drastic methods. "Acquire this property," advised Manhattan stockbroker Harry A. Groesbeck. "Raze the buildings, destroy by fire the germs which are supposed to exist there, and sanction the erection, even by private means, of a model tenement. . . . Father Curry is right: what these people need [are] homes, not parks."[103]

THE LUNG BLOCK CAMPAIGN IN POLITICAL PERSPECTIVE

When investigating whether Curry's objections reflected larger patterns of public dissatisfaction in New York, it is helpful to view the park plan and its critics within a broader context of reform setbacks in New York City during the fall of 1903. The failed reelection bid of Fusion mayor Seth Low, which unfolded along the same timeline as the doomed park campaign, had a simple enough explanation on the surface: the coalition of Republicans, Democrats, and independents who had supported his reform agenda in 1901 eventually disintegrated along traditional party lines. More specifically, Low's determination to govern efficiently and impartially had embittered his allies across the political spectrum, and antagonized merchants and wage workers with bureaucratic interference they had not experienced under Tammany rule.[104] As a result, the Fusion reelection campaign drew the same critiques that dogged the Lung Block park project: the proponents' reputation as idealistic "outsiders," their inability to relate to working-class needs and desires, and their hostile imperviousness to criticism.[105]

Critics from inside and outside the Fusion camp saw many of these weaknesses personified in Low himself. Born into a wealthy mercantile family and educated at Harvard, he "was of the old stock," his nephew recalled; "original America bred him."[106] Low honed his administrative skills as mayor of Brooklyn in the 1880s, and later as president of Columbia University. Swept into office on a wave of bipartisan fury following the corruption scandals of Robert Van Wyck's Tammany administration, Low interpreted his victory as a public mandate for fiscal responsibility, transparency, and principled leadership.[107] Within two years, however, his aloof bearing and rigid adherence to doing things by the book had eroded his support base.[108] One journal's lukewarm profile in May 1903 praised Low's "remarkable self-control" and "choice words chosen with academic precision" before conceding that despite his cordiality, close associates regarded him as "a cold man."[109] The weekly reform magazine *Independent* attempted to counterbalance the "glacial" aspects of

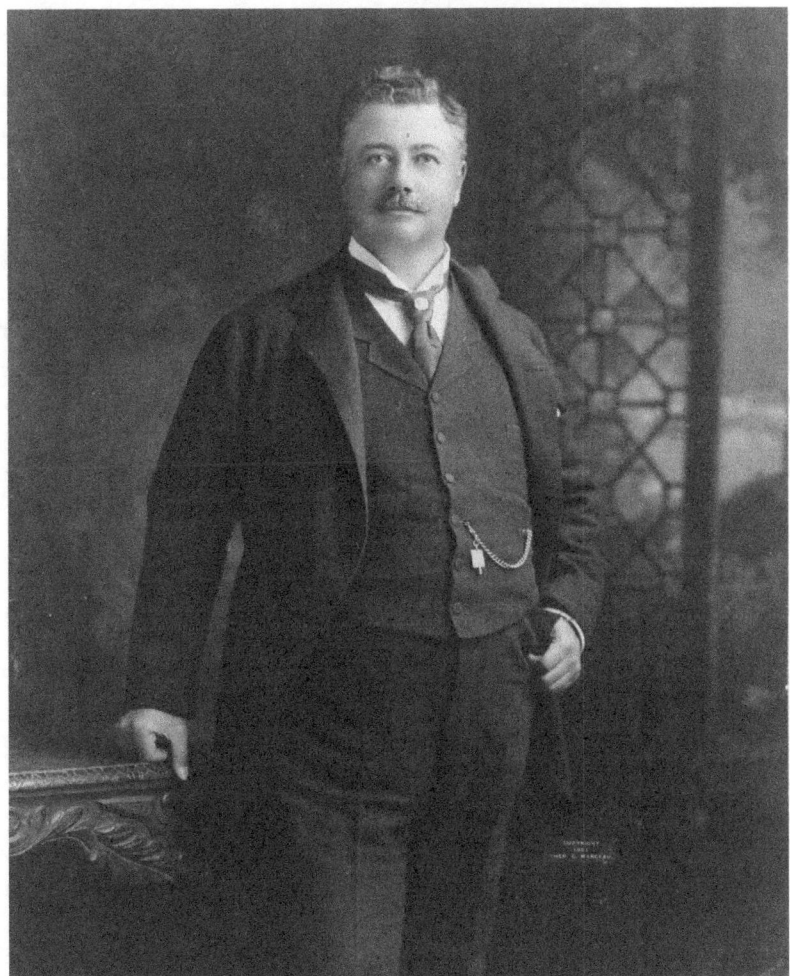

5.2. Seth Low, 1900s. This portrait, taken by Theodore C. Morceau in 1901, is held in the Library of Congress Prints and Photographs Division, Washington, DC.

Low's personality with glowing accounts of his kindness toward former servants, including "a very pretty story about an old nurse" that only reinforced his silk-stocking image.[110] The pro-business *World's Work* agreed that while Low was not "a mixer," "not brilliant nor imaginative," it still endorsed him for reelection as "eminently sane, safe, and conservative."[111]

As election day approached, Low's austerity and lack of charm had worn thin even among his staunch allies. His own district attorney spoke publicly against his renomination, arguing that "egotism, self-complacency and constitutional timidity are not the elements to make a leader, nor do they attract the love and support of an American electorate."[112] Muckraking journalist Lincoln

Steffens, when describing Low's smile, noted that "there is no laughter back of it. . . . The appealing human element is lacking all through." Steffens classified these deficiencies as symptoms of a larger public relations problem. Low's "good abilities are self-sufficient," he wrote; "his dignity is smug; his courtesy seems not kind; his self-reliance is called obstinacy because, though he listens, he seems not to care; though he understands, he shows no sympathy . . . Mr. Low," Steffens concluded, "is the bourgeois reformer type."[113] This searing judgment, issued bluntly from one bourgeois reformer to another, closely paralleled Curry's accusations of high-minded, hardhearted indifference.

Low's air of cold, superior aloofness carried over into his policies. His cabinet selections disproportionately favored professional experts and civic-minded gentlemen from his own social rank, stirring up early public concerns about his "los[ing] touch with the masses."[114] These concerns grew with his enforcement of state laws limiting public recreation and liquor sales on Sundays, which imposed Yankee-Protestant standards of behavior on working-class New Yorkers—many of them Irish and German immigrants who were liquor dealers, or saloon patrons who resented being denied opportunities to socialize on their one day off from work.[115] Meanwhile, Low's replacing patronage with civil service examinations imposed limits on working-class opportunities to participate directly in government.[116] People seeking to air their grievances about these and other issues encountered a related problem: Low's lack of accessibility. "You could see the Tammany Mayor if you had any complaints to make," a local union representative fumed; "now, you can get no nearer the Mayor than his secretary."[117] Low's supporters expressed similar frustrations. One letter, published anonymously in the New York Herald, argued for replacing Low on the 1903 Fusion ticket, citing his "slow-moving mind that rejoices in its own obstinacy" and his existence on "an altitude far removed from [the people]." He "does not and cannot understand their life and their real, personal civic aspirations," the writer asserted.[118] These complaints, levied against Low from inside and outside his administration, mirror the complaints Curry levied against park advocates and their indifference toward poor people's immediate material needs.

Tammany's new boss, Charles F. Murphy, used such missteps to his advantage. A saloonkeeper and son of Irish immigrants, Murphy had earned a "shrewd, silent, and aggressive" reputation among Fusionists."[119] "He looks dense," observed Steffens, "but he acts with force, decision, and skill."[120] Murphy had worked on healing internal rifts during the previous two years, culminating in Grout and Fornes—key Fusion Democrats in Low's administration—returning to the party fold. For Low's challenger in 1903, Murphy settled on George B. McClellan Jr.: son of a famed Civil War general, a Princeton graduate who studied law at Columbia, and a United States congressman with a reputation for being in but not of the urban political machine.

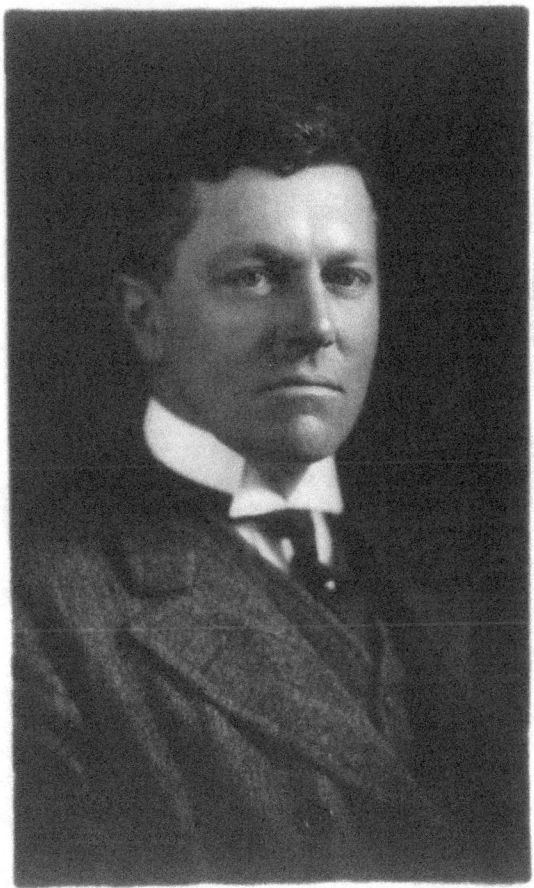

5.3. George B. McClellan Jr., circa 1905. Photo by Pirie McDonald, held in the Library of Congress Prints and Photographs Division.

Moreover, unlike Low, McClellan was personable.[121] While McClellan gave stump speeches throughout the city in three foreign languages from his open motor car, Low continued relying heavily on well-spoken surrogates, posters, and increasingly militant newspaper endorsements.[122]

With internal and external discontentment toward Low mounting—culminating in two of Low's top Democratic officials, Grout and Fornes, accepting Tammany's nomination for reelection—Fusion supporters fired back with the same defensiveness evident among the Lung Block campaigners. They stressed Low's accomplishments: fairer assessment and collection of taxes; streamlined city payrolls and budgets; improved and expanded services; new public schools, parks, bridges, and subways begun; a corrupt police force brought to heel.[123] While Low's administration "may not have been perfect ... not expert,

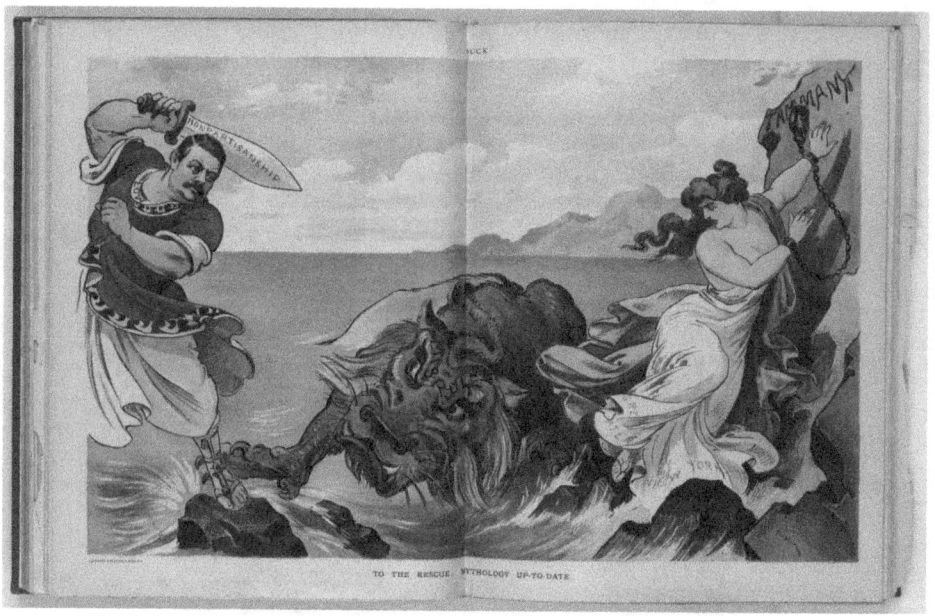

5.4. In this 1901 *Puck* illustration by Udo Keppler, titled "To the Rescue: Mythology Up-to-Date," then mayoral challenger Seth Low is depicted as Perseus defending Andromeda, representing the city of New York, from the ravages of a sea beast. This symbolism is intended to suggest a city being terrorized by the tiger (here, a hybridized sea-tiger) of Tammany, as indicated by the label on the rock to which New York is chained. Low wields a sword representing "nonpartisanship"; the beast's forehead bears the word *misrule*. Published in *Puck*, October 30, 1901, centerfold. Held in the Library of Congress Prints and Photographs Division. I am indebted to Elizabeth Richey, classicist and Head of Technical Services at the University of California, Irvine, Libraries, for her interpretive contributions.

not coordinated, certainly not wise," Steffens judged that by contemporary American standards, it was "not only honest but able, undeniably one of the best in the whole country." Fusionists pleaded for more time. "Two years," complained the *Independent*, "was hardly enough for a fair beginning."[124] In their desperation to convince readers that an imperfect nonpartisan administration was still superior to Tammany's, pro-Fusion analogies grew starker and more polarized. Tammany stood for bloated corruption, shortsighted selfishness, vice-ridden evil; Fusion represented honest efficiency, farsighted nonpartisanship, virtuous good.[125] The fact that these diametrically opposed sets of terms could be—and often were—collapsed further into "Celtic" and "Anglo-Saxon," or "American" and "un-American," revealed the ethnic undercurrents shaping the ethical chasms Fusionists perceived between their brand of public service and Tammany's.[126]

Throughout the fall of 1903, these loaded terms not only framed the issues for both the Fusion and Lung Block park campaigns, but also revealed the same intolerance toward dissenting viewpoints. Insisting that reform had already "made good," Fusionists viewed the upcoming municipal election as a test of New Yorkers' fitness for self-rule. "The great question is this: Are the people of the metropolis of the Western world capable of maintaining a government of the people, by the people, for the people?" posed the *New York Press*.[127] "Do we Americans really want good government?" Steffens asked his readers. "Do we know it when we see it? Are we capable of that sustained good citizenship which alone can make democracy a success?"[128] After listing a series of sharp contrasts between New Yorkers' quality of life under Tammany and reform administrations, Riis placed responsibility for the city's future squarely on his readers' shoulders. "You who believe in decency, in honesty, in good government . . . stand up and be counted," Riis demanded. "Sit and shake your head," he chided skeptics, "wait to see how the cat will jump. . . . Too late you will find that the cat is a [Tammany] tiger, and that it was you who let it in."[129] Should the city's electorate permit that to happen, the *Tribune* concluded harshly that "it deserves again to suffer at the hands of criminals."[130]

The park and political campaigns also manifested similar degrees of polarization in the city's opinion sections, prominently displaying editorials endorsing reform leadership as the only sensible course while confining objections to the margins. "[Low's] platform told us of a liberal Sunday law," one such reader complained to the *New York Times*, "which [now] seems to be only a dream." This unrealized promise confirmed the writer's belief that the Low administration "placed men in positions that do not know the city or its people, and . . . do not care to be instructed by others, who at least have the city's interest at heart."[131] Likewise, a self-professed Democrat rejected Low's policies as "too much government and too little liberty." "The small shopkeepers have been bullied and harassed by the [mayor's] underlings," he fumed to the Brooklyn *Daily Eagle*; working-class New Yorkers "have been governed as if by divine right . . . deprived of their legitimate and accustomed pleasures . . . their protests unheeded. If you think, or Mr. Low thinks, that they have accepted all this . . . you are both in error."[132] Anti-Fusionists particularly resented their political views being portrayed as counter to intelligence, morality, and good citizenship. Inferring that the newspaper denied Tammany supporters "the right to be called a good citizen," the *Times* writer accused its editors of losing touch with the common people. "Go out among the people that cast their votes on election day," the writer urged, "and do not take the cue among those that prefer to play golf rather than to accept the rights of citizenship."[133]

These dissenting opinions illuminate another characteristic common to both political and park campaigns: while proponents viewed the contest as a struggle between opposing ideas, such as honesty and corruption, opponents portrayed it as a struggle between opposing groups, more specifically commoners and elites. In challenging Low's reform agenda, Tammany supporters defined themselves as enemies not of good government but of unpopular and oppressive elitism. "Government of the masses by the classes . . . that is what Mayor Low typifies," argued the *Evening Journal*. "He is the reverse of a Democrat—an aristocrat."[134] Low's comptroller, shortly after accepting Tammany's nomination for reelection, defined the race as "a question whether a majority of the people is to rule the city or . . . a select few."[135] This characterization of the conflict followed the party line exactly. "Mayor Low is narrow-minded and bigoted," declared the *Tammany Times*; "by birth and training he is incapable of sympathy with the common people . . . believes the Declaration of Independence was written for only swell club members . . . plays golf on Sunday, and has boys and men arrested for playing baseball on the same day . . . won't meet [with] committees of reputable citizens . . . promised liberal enforcement of the excise law and broke his pledge . . . is a pliable tool in the hands of [the Republican] Governor."[136]

Based on this broad sampling of published criticisms, issued from inside and outside the Fusion camp during the fall of 1903, Curry's and Marks's opposition to the park paralleled larger patterns of dissatisfaction with reform. Election results likewise confirm this. On November 3, Tammany Democrats swept every major race in every borough but Staten Island, with their mayoral challenger, McClellan, defeating Low by more than sixty thousand votes.[137] The *Herald* cited a "complete breakdown" of Fusion, with thousands of disgruntled Republicans withdrawing their support while Democrats unified around the Tammany banner once more. Prominently placed editorials to the contrary, "the tide was simply strongly in favor of the democracy and a wide-open town," the newspaper concluded—an observation that evoked Tammany's overthrow of William Strong's administration six years earlier with the campaign slogan "To Hell with Reform."[138]

Out in the streets, wildly cheering crowds celebrated the Tammany victory with noisemakers, cannon and fireworks, creating an "ear-splitting din that ran the length of Manhattan and over the bridge to Brooklyn."[139] Years later, Low's nephew could still recall "boys and girls running up and down the streets, and hear them crying between prodigious blasts down their tin horns, 'The lid is off!—The lid is off!'"[140] In the Bowery, Fusion banners were set ablaze.[141] Despite chaotic traffic snarls and heavy police presence, newspaper reporters marveled at the peaceful jubilation permeating the event. "Young women of good breeding locked arms with men they never saw before and whom they would fail to recognize today," the *Herald* reported, "and . . . paraded up or down the street, all rejoicing in their liberty."[142] "There were no Low murmurs on Broadway," quipped the *Morning Telegraph*; they were all

Table 5.1: Selected municipal election results from November 1903 (grouped by office, party, assembly and election district)

Office	Candidate	Assembly District 4	Election Districts 1 and 2
Mayor (citywide)	George B. McClellan (Tammany)	3,565 (52%)	429 (74%)
	Seth Low (Fusion)	2,297 (33%)	105 (18%)
Comptroller (citywide)	Edward M. Grout (Tammany)	3,564 (52%)	420 (72%)
	Frederic W. Hinrichs (Fusion)	2,237 (32%)	113 (19%)
President, Board of Aldermen (citywide)	Charles V. Fornes (Tammany)	3,550 (52%)	418 (72%)
	Edward McGuire (Fusion)	2,237 (33%)	114 (20%)
Borough President, Manhattan (citywide)	John F. Ahearn (Tammany)	3,687 (53%)	438 (75%)
	Cyrus L. Sulzberger (Fusion)	2,200 (32%)	97 (17%)
Alderman (District 4)	Isaac Marks	3,342 (49%)	401 (69%)

Source: Official Canvas of the Votes Cast in the Counties of New York, Kings, Queens and Richmond, City Record, December 31, 1903, supplement.

loud, and spelled 'McClellan.'"[143] Meanwhile Fusionists, having watched the cat jump, accepted defeat philosophically. "Well, we were licked, weren't we?" Riis remarked to his longtime colleague and friend, Elgin Gould. But, he said, "I would rather go under a hundred times with the record of the Low administration than with . . . Tammany."[144] Other Fusionists' reactions ranged from Riis's stoicism to the dejection of his friend, Theodore Roosevelt, who concluded disgustedly that "the dog has returned to its vomit."[145]

If Curry's and Marks's park opposition paralleled broader patterns of discontentment with New York reform, what might 1903 voting patterns from the "Lung Block" area reveal about locals' stance toward the park? Inside the Fourth Assembly District, where the neighborhood straddled the first and second election districts, Tammany candidates received just over half (51 to 53 percent) of the approximately 6,900 votes cast for mayor, comptroller, president of the Board of Aldermen, and Manhattan borough president, with Marks receiving just under 50 percent of the vote for district alderman (table 5.1).[146] By contrast, only 33 percent of Fourth Assembly District voters supported Low and his Fusion candidates in the same races.[147] When narrowing the focus to a smaller portion of the assembly district that included the proposed park site, this disparity becomes even more dramatic. In the first and second election districts, Tammany candidates received between 72 and 75 percent of the vote, with Marks receiving 69 percent of the vote for district alderman; Fusion fared even more dismally, with 17 to 20 percent supporting Low and his candidates for the same offices.[148] While these voting patterns cannot be used as direct proxies for locals' stances on the park issue, the results are nevertheless suggestive. In a list of registered city voters published two years later, 61 percent of those with "Lung Block" addresses identified as Democrat, 18 percent as Republican, and 20 percent as unaffiliated. These patterns, when compared with those from 1903, indicate locals' remarkably consistent tendency to vote along party lines, and Tammany lines in particular.[149] The fact that local Tammany representatives Marks and John F. Ahearn carried the district in 1903 with decisive majorities suggests that their park opposition reflected not just their own views but those of their working-class immigrant constituents—their public. Fusion's crushing defeat among the same population only reinforces this idea.

In the aftermath of the failed park project, the eleventh-hour public opposition mounted by people claiming to represent the residents of Cherry, Catherine, Hamilton, and Market Streets was often attributed to shallow, self-serving motives. For example, the New York Evening Post conflated Curry's stance with those of Tammany district leaders who "have always opposed the razing of tenements for park purposes, simply because it disperses the people and endangers the political status quo."[150] Pinning the park's failure entirely on these last-minute detractors, however, overlooks the extent to which political timing altered the project's fortunes. If proponents had launched their Lung Block campaign in the 1890s, while Hermann Biggs compiled his disease maps and Jacob Riis battled with Mulberry Bend—or during the optimistic early days of Seth Low's administration, when the brand-new Tenement House Department began issuing violation orders—the block might have vanished along with other tenement neighborhoods into a string of Lower East Side "breathing spaces." By the time the Committee on the Prevention of Tuberculosis had settled on a brick-and-mortar target for their activism, however, a significant number of New Yorkers had soured on reform rule. As a result, the park campaign's most active phase unfolded amid a larger political contest that placed Low's Fusion administration—and reformers in general—under harsh public scrutiny. Throughout the fall of 1903, both park and political campaigns drew criticism for their tone-deaf approach to working-class problems and their high-handed superiority regarding their methods. When Tammany's decisive victory revoked reformers' public mandate to govern, it also obliterated the administrative backing that park proponents relied upon. In this new and inhospitable climate, their indifference toward the fate of displaced families left them vulnerable to the same charges of coldhearted elitism ascribed to Low and his allies. When Board of Estimate members tabled the park project, their decision could be read not only as an endorsement of Curry's and Marks's arguments, but also as a frank acknowledgment of the bleak terrain confronting reformers in the wake of their municipal losses.

While Fusionists and park advocates blamed their defeats on oppositional ignorance and selfishness, the evidence suggests that their campaigns foundered on the gulf dividing them from their opponents regarding how they interpreted "the public interest." Reformers envisioned the public interest as a series of long-range, citywide improvements, and embraced an impartial, business-oriented administration as the best means of achieving them. Their opponents viewed the public interest in more local and personalized terms, structuring it around working-class constituents' immediate priorities. Reformers faulted this parish- and district-centered approach as shortsighted and inefficient; if left unchecked, they feared that it would keep the city's immigrants forever cloistered in squalid and dilapidated ethnic ghettos, subsisting on papist decrees and shady power brokers' handouts. Opponents countercharged that reformers cared more about ideas than people, their wealth and privilege having blinded them to the working-class struggle to carve out opportunities and resources from systems of exploitation and neglect. The central question driving the 1903 municipal and park campaigns involved the kind of city that twentieth-century New Yorkers wanted. Whose public would prevail, and whose interest?

The block bordered by Cherry, Catherine, Hamilton, and Market Streets formed a crucial battleground where urban reformers and working-class intermediaries projected these competing visions of the public interest onto the same point in space. Park proponents perceived the public interest as a wide green expanse where tenement children could grow healthy and strong in body and morals; they arrived at this perception through maps, statistics, and their own unfavorable impressions of the neighborhood. Curry and Marks believed that they were protecting the public interest by preventing the evictions of thousands of people already occupying that space; they based their belief on firsthand familiarity with residents' living and working patterns. When Ernest Poole accused the park's detractors of self-interest, he took the position that impartial expertise equipped urban reformers with the ability to perceive the needs of the block's tenants more accurately than the priest and politician who dealt with them directly. This position, stated outright on many of the city's editorial pages, echoed Robert de Forest's claim that his role as Tenement House Commissioner automatically qualified him to represent the interests of tenement dwellers. By contrast, park opponents' frequent references to "my people" and "my constituents" suggested that they perceived little distinction between their own interest and their public's—a perception that the 1903 election results appeared to confirm. Interpreting the Tammany victory as proof of New Yorkers' civic unfitness, as many reformers did, overlooked the Fusion missteps that had repelled Republican and Democratic supporters alike. Moreover, the city's exuberant postelection celebrations suggested that working-class New Yorkers did not share reformers' view of Tammany as a threat to democracy, nor did they view an impartial business administration as sympathetic to their needs. By contrast, George W. Plunkitt, a prominent Tammany district leader in the early 1900s, attributed his party's following to its accessibility and pragmatism in a crisis. "Everybody in the district knows him," Plunkitt said of the typical district leader; "everybody knows where to find him." He celebrated alongside constituents at weddings, parades, and religious festivals, and helped them over rough patches with jobs, material goods, and bureaucratic leverage.[151] "If a family is burned out I don't ask whether they are Republicans or Democrats," Plunkitt explained; "I just get quarters for them . . . and fix them up till they get things runnin' again. It's philanthropy, but it's politics too—mighty good politics."

When reformers dismissed this good-neighbor policy as pandering for votes, Tammany leaders did not deny it; for them, that was the point. The district leader's "heart is in his work," Plunkitt argued, "for his subsistence depends on its results."[152] They encouraged naysayers to judge Tammany's good works not by the underlying motives but by the outcomes. "Think of the hundreds of thousands of foreigners dumped into our city," urged Tammany boss Richard Croker in 1898, asserting that "there is not a [reformer] in the city who would shake hands with them." He argued that his party's "helpful" overtures—however calculatingly extended—"grafts them upon the Republic, makes citizens of them in short; and although you may not like our motives or our methods, what other agency is there by which so long a row could have been hoed so quickly or so well? If we go down into the gutter," Croker declared, "it is because there are men in the gutter, and you have got to go down where they are if you are to do anything with them."[153]

Occasionally, urban reformers stepped back from denigrating the urban political machine long enough to acknowledge the truth behind Plunkitt's and Croker's arguments. On the eve of the 1903 election, Steffens conceded that Tammany's strength lay in its inherent humanity. "Tammany kindness is real kindness," he observed, "and will go far, remember long, and take infinite trouble for a friend."[154] Decades of living among Chicago's poor had convinced Jane Addams that "protection and kindness" easily outranked a "sense of just dealing" in their hierarchy of desires, placing reformers at a distinct disadvantage. "What headway can the notion of civic purity, of honest administration, make against this . . . human friendliness, this stalking survival of village kindness?" she asked. "Compared with Tammany's hearty handshake and a pail of coal, or help with the rent, [reformers'] goodness is not dramatic; it is not even concrete and human."[155] Even as Riis railed publicly against Tammany methods, he grasped that the boss's appeal lay in his ability to transcend social boundaries as "a friend in need," and "one of them." While "the reformer comes to them from another world" to offer unsolicited instruction on the finer points of citizenship, Riis noted that the boss "lives among them," and "does not want to reform them; far from it." Instead, the boss "helped John to a job on the pipes in their hard winter, and got Mike on the force." Timely, relevant assistance, compassionately given, ensured working-class immigrants' allegiance to the urban machine because "they know him as a good neighbor, and trust him to their harm."[156]

Forging closer connections with working-class immigrants, these reformers acknowledged, required borrowing from Tammany's strategies. "If," Addams proposed, "we discover that men of low ideals and corrupt practice are forming popular political standards simply because such men stand by and for and with the people, then nothing remains but to obtain a like sense of identification before we can hope to modify ethical standards."[157] Written nearly twenty-five years after she founded Hull House, Addams's remark suggests her dissatisfaction with the settlement house experiment in creating the common ground she sought. Riis, who had long promoted settlements as a means of bridging the classes, called on reformers to abandon social theories and moral high ground in favor of the "humane touch." "A vigorous optimism," he argued, "a stout belief in one's fellow-man, is better equipment in a campaign for civic virtue than stacks of tracts and arguments, economic and moral. . . . When we have learned to smile and weep with the poor, the slum will have lost its grip and the boss his job."[158] Addams's and Riis's statements, published one year before the ill-fated Fusion and Lung Block campaigns, proved prophetic in both cases.

Curry needed no such primers for empathizing with the poor, for he started out as "one of them." He still considered himself one of them, as his abundant references to "my people" attest. While the Lung Block campaign's failure scattered its proponents in radical and conservative directions, it set Curry even more firmly on a course of social activism. As his targets expanded to include the unlawful sale of alcohol to minors and the unregulated distribution of cocaine, he continued presenting his public objections as those of a concerned citizen and parish priest—nothing more. "I am not conducting any crusade or instituting any new reform," he insisted during one of his publicized, self-administered saloon inspections in 1905; "I am simply reporting such violations of a certain law as I see in my own parish, where I have my home."[159] In reality, public interest in Curry's crackdowns extended well beyond the tightly defined parameters of his parish.[160] So did their ramifications, such as when his efforts to prevent a local druggist from selling cocaine to Saint James boys led to tighter state regulations, making him one of the earliest antidrug advocates in the United States.[161] Through it all, Curry continued to look back on his role in the Lung Block park project with satisfaction. "I did oppose the wiping out of this block and of my people," he declared years later, "and had I not done so vigorously, I would have been man and priest unworthy of the name." Alluding to the park's champions as "fake philanthropists and pseudo-humanitarians," Curry viewed their residual bitterness toward him as a badge of honor that validated the "righteousness and justice" of his cause, adding, "I am proud beyond all measure of that one action of my life."[162]

Conclusion

REDEMPTION(?) OF THE LUNG BLOCK

Despite their political setbacks in 1903, New York City reformers' hopes of putting a park on Cherry, Catherine, Hamilton, and Market Streets flickered intermittently until 1908, when the Tenement House Department—now part of George B. McClellan Jr.'s mayoral administration—implemented renovations bringing the block's dwellings into full compliance with the 1901 code regulations championed by Lawrence Veiller and others.[1] These renovations included eliminating outdoor privies, adding or enlarging hall skylights, replacing saturated woodwork around hallway sinks, waterproofing cellars, and adding additional fire escapes. "In so far as the houses can be made to comply with the law," the department concluded in its annual report, they were now "in as good condition as [those of] any other ordinary block in the city"; therefore, "the term Lung Block can . . . be regarded henceforth only as a misnomer."[2]

After years of maintaining pressure on the Tammany-controlled Tenement House Department through independently monitoring the block's housing conditions, the Charity Organization Society appeared to hail these developments as an acceptable alternative to a park. In a *Charities* article titled "Redemption of Lung Block," settlement worker Emily Dinwiddie reviewed the renovation measures with enthusiasm: "The casual visitor now is astonished to learn that this is the once famous 'Lung Block,'" she remarked, "and that these are the tenements of former ill fame brought to their present condition through the work of the Tenement House Department."[3] In reality, these structural changes offered only modest improvements. Skylights and interior windows transformed dark rooms and hallways into semidark rooms and hallways; notoriously foul air shafts remained unchanged; and more people than ever were packing into these houses. No one understood the compromised nature of this "redemption" better than park proponents who had demanded nothing short of complete obliteration five years earlier. Noting that the block now contained "458 more people to the acre . . . than in the days when the city was excited over it and the whole country was hearing of it," leading reformer-journalist Harold M. Finley concluded skeptically that "a prevailing idea that the 'lung' block and others of like gruesome reputation have been transformed into *model* blocks is a myth."[4]

In some respects, the timing of the this "redemption" reflected additional etiological shifts as tuberculosis experts began focusing more intently on sick people, rather than the inanimate structures housing them, as the reservoirs of infection.[5] Subsequently, New York antituberculosis activists turned from tenements to overcrowding as the root problem, culminating in a public exhibit on urban congestion in 1908 that involved the Tenement House Department, the Charity Organization Society, and dozens of public and private social agencies.[6] Arguably, park proponents' warming toward less drastic alternatives also signaled awareness of their narrowing prospects for securing victory on their original terms. In the five years since the 1903 park campaign, the Committee on the Prevention of Tuberculosis and the fledgling Metropolitan Parks Association—both offshoots of the Charity Organization Society—lobbied city leaders to revive the park project, eventually settling upon an adjacent block they hoped would attract less opposition.[7] "We believe that if this [adjacent] block be secured," Metropolitan Parks Association member and Henry Street Settlement founder Lillian Wald stated in a report of proposed sites she compiled for comptroller Edward Grout in 1905, "many of the evils of the Lung Block will automatically right themselves": a notable retrenchment from her colleagues' unyielding condemnation of the houses located one block south.[8]

Meanwhile, the settlement workers who had supplied much of the footwork for the 1903 park campaign—increasingly frustrated by their attempts to improve urban living conditions through conventional power mechanisms—had begun opting for more radical paths of activism.[9] Instead of fighting reluctant government officials and indignant landlords to redeem "lung blocks" one tenement at a time, Ernest Poole and James Graham Phelps Stokes argued, urban reformers should channel their efforts toward dismantling the capitalist system that created working-class poverty, sickness, and despair in the first place. "Who makes and maintains the slums?" Stokes asked in his public lectures. "Who is responsible for the deaths in the lung block?" Urging his listeners to look beyond sick buildings and demoralized tenants, he asked, "Is it not rather those who perpetuate the conditions . . . the landlords and the public? . . . In our blindness we say, 'It can't be helped.' Can't it?"[10]

Over time, these scientific and social trends narrowed the ideological gap between park supporters and critics. By 1906 the evening *World*—once among the Lung Block campaign's most ardent supporters—called on the city to replace the buildings on Cherry, Catherine, Hamilton, and Market Streets with model tenements, stating flatly that "the city can't turn every plague spot into a park."[11] Conceding that the city was "now fairly well supplied" with breathing spaces, the University Settlement shifted toward crediting James Curry with "sound logic" in rejecting parks as a weapon against the slum. Citing the cost to taxpayers of securing and clearing the lots needed for a park, and the increased housing demand that would affect adjacent neighborhoods with overcrowding and higher rents, the worker concluded that future park sites "must be chosen with sole reference to the . . . needs of the community . . . the remedy must fit the disease."[12]

Despite this growing consensus on the limitations of small parks in alleviating urban social problems, residual bitterness from the failed 1903 campaign continued festering among supporters and critics alike. When Curry publicly accused Jacob Riis's settlement of proselytizing among Saint James Parish children in 1908, Riis used the park's defeat as evidence that Curry posed a far bigger threat to local Catholics than settlement houses did. Settlement workers "would long since have made a playground and a breathing-place out of the infamous 'Lung Block' . . . but for the opposition of the very priest who today accuses them of giving the East Side a bad name," Riis fumed. "The lung block is in his parish, and he alone kept it there. If any relief has since been afforded its tenants by action of the authorities, that is due directly to the agitation kept up by its 'defamers.'"[13] Riis's tone of resentful indignation suggests that not all small-park proponents equated the recent renovations with redemption.

Predictably, Curry refuted Riis's countercharges with his own impressions from 1903, "that year when the settlement crowd demanded the razing of the entire block for a park" while he "stood alone for homes for my poor people, and . . . enforcement of the Tenement House laws." Curry savored the structural improvements as a personal victory, his terms having been met. "Surely the credit [for improvements] is due to the man who alone stood for homes against a park," the priest argued, "and not to the settlement people who so vigorously fought against my people and their homes in favor of a park . . . I fought for homes, not parks, for my poor people, and I won out."[14]

Riis's and Curry's heated exchange—encapsulated within their larger debate concerning the role of settlements in working-class immigrant neighborhoods—confirmed that both men perceived the stakes of the Lung Block park campaign to extend well beyond tuberculosis, dirt, or morality. In addressing how urban spaces should be reconfigured to further broader social aims, the campaign's central question—"Lung Block or Park-Playground— Which?"—raised still-larger questions. Who possessed the credentials for determining how working-class neighborhoods should look and function, and on what basis were these matters decided? If instilling fitness for American citizenship was the ultimate goal of small parks and playgrounds, as advocates often stated, whose ideas of fitness did these projects reflect?

Answers to these questions abound in Riis's reform writings from the 1900s, which move seamlessly back and forth between exerting his claims to American citizenship and promoting his vision for urban spaces. "I hate darkness and dirt anywhere, and naturally want to let in the light," Riis remarked in his 1901 autobiography, aptly titled *The Making of an American*. "I love to mend and make crooked things straight."[15] Using germ theory, moral environmentalism, social science, and eminent domain, he and other Progressive Era activists worked to make American cities lighter, cleaner, and straighter. Their efforts concentrated on the "breathing spaces" that parks and settlements provided for children of different backgrounds to forge a new, collective identity. "When James of Madison Avenue and Jimmy of Battle Row, or of Cherry Hill, lie groping in the dirt together for the same ball," Riis postulated in his rebuttal to Curry's accusations, "James will know that Jimmy is not a tough, though he hails from the East Side, and Jimmy that James is not necessarily a dude because he wears good clothes; but that they are just two good, square American boys together. And then the day will break when we shall pull together at the polls, too, being no longer strangers."[16] Riis did not elaborate upon how he pictured this transition being accomplished; having linked citizenship fitness with the appropriate use of space, he then devoted himself to creating spaces that he felt would support the natural working out of this process. He regarded his settlement house and others like it as crucial footholds in this battle, offering "the pledge of a better day, of the defeat of the slum with its helpless heredity of despair."[17]

From Riis's standpoint, Curry's opposition represented much more than a missed opportunity for another Mulberry Bend. It represented the deliberate obstruction of what parks and settlements meant: public health, social cohesion, and civic advancement. In Riis's view, Curry's opposition to the park campaign aligned with Old World ignorance, corruption, and ghettoization; dark rooms, disease, and death. In standing for his "poor people," Curry stood against the progress of civilization.

Curry challenged Riis's spatialized vision of citizenship in that he, too, was an American. A native-born son of Irish immigrants, he had spent most of his clerical career forging a church, school, and community from Riis's "helpless heredity of despair." In defending the rights of working-class immigrants to occupy and use urban spaces in ways that benefited them, he promoted his vision of America as a pluralistic society of equals who worked, studied, voted, and otherwise forged their own paths to citizenship without intervention from disapproving patricians. Curry perceived parks and settlements not as vehicles for promoting wellbeing and citizenship but as upper-class assaults on the dignity and autonomy of those already living there.

By revealing how these clashing visions of citizenship unfolded in space, the events of the Lung Block park campaign of 1903 reinforce historians' portrayals of Progressive social activists as fundamentally disconnected from the populations they claimed to be helping. Not surprisingly, these disconnects turned on class and culture. Having hailed from similar Yankee-Protestant backgrounds, attended the same prestigious schools, moved in the same elite social circles, and read and written for the same publications, they developed insulated, closed-circuit mindsets that allowed little room for reflection or compromise. In dismissing the intelligence and morality of their detractors they revealed their difficulties empathizing fully with the working-class, hand-to-mouth realities Lower East Side religious and political leaders experienced from a much closer vantage point.[18]

Moreover, the events of the Lung Block campaign confirm that Progressive Era social activists did not always perceive these disconnects as problematic; in certain times and places, they leaned into these disconnects consciously, deliberately, even militantly. Those relying upon social-scientific approaches, like Hermann Biggs, Lawrence Veiller, Robert Weeks de Forest, and Lilian Brandt, believed that maps and statistics yielded more impartial, objective, and accurate depictions of tenement life than direct observation and lived experience did. Aligning detachment with professionalism and expertise not only obviated the need for seeking out residents' perspectives; it offered grounds for dismissing residents' perspectives as shortsighted, misleading, and irrelevant. Ironically, this detachment did not prevent park proponents from claiming to speak for potentially affected residents anyway. Among wealthy philanthropists like de Forest, this pattern stemmed from a deeply ingrained sense of noblesse oblige; among middle-class professionals like Biggs, Veiller, and Brandt, it stemmed from contempt for tenement dwellers' "degenerate" values; among muckraking journalists like Riis and Poole, it stemmed from romantic notions of Christian uplift and brotherhood. All of these patterns rested on the same idea: native-born, old-stock, Protestant Americans—by birth, upbringing, and education—held the highest qualifications for transforming multicultural urban ghettoes into suitable incubators for future citizens.

Placing these disconnects under fire, as this failed park campaign does, reveals multiple cracks in the longstanding popular image of Progressive Era social activists as noble, high-minded humanitarians. Park supporters' insistence on viewing the neighborhood through an abstracted, aggregate lens, their frank and unapologetic lack of concern for the thousands of people their park would displace, and their increasing shrillness in the face of growing resistance, all belie urban reformers' pledge to bridge the social classes. Moreover, these characteristics give weight to their critics' charges of class aggression masquerading as social activism. To Poole and his CPT colleagues, "the public interest" was *their* interest; what was right and good from their perspective was right and good for everyone else, and they had scientific principles and reams of carefully tabulated data to prove it. Choosing germ theory, moral environmentalism, and eminent domain for their weapons, they set out on a determined crusade to remake New York's tenement districts in their own image—and failed, their lofty civic ideals weakened by the same strains of indifference and contempt that undermined the city's political reform movement.

The class and cultural disconnects revealed in the Lung Block campaign also encourage us to examine Progressive Era social activism's opponents more closely. Public opposition to reform did not lodge exclusively with wealthy capitalists; it also issued forth from ethnic community leaders like Curry and Isaac Marks, whose close identification with working-class immigrants led them to reject reform-friendly policies as biased and detrimental to "their people." That these cultural mediators also pursued their own interests in these conflicts did not invalidate their opposition; instead, it underscored the reality that park supporters—far from being the impartial civic advocates that they claimed to be—were pursuing their own interests as well. This last insight, which informed many of the reactionary Progressive Era histories of the 1960s and 1970s, was common knowledge to Curry and other critics of reform in the 1900s.

Today, the block bounded by Cherry, Catherine, Hamilton, and Market Streets is altogether unrecognizable from its "Lung Block" days. Saint James Catholic Church offered its last mass in 2014, its generations of Irish and Italian parishioners gradually replaced by a dwindling number of Latinx and Asian Americans. Now part of the Two Bridges neighborhood bordering Chinatown, the block features a number of sprawling housing projects, schools, parks, and playgrounds, many of them named for the early twentieth-century politicians and reformers populating this study: the Jacob A. Riis School (Public School 26); the Lillian D. Wald Playground; the Alfred E. Smith Housing Project. If Lung Block park proponents could walk through the area today, they would find it cleaner, greener, and more orderly. To the twenty-first-century historian straining to pick up the last faded remnants of bygone spatial and cultural battles, it feels sterile, colorless, and eerily quiet.

Two blocks away, the East River flows across the splintered, shattered remains of the "permanently infected" houses that once gave these streets notoriety.[19] Now occupying the former "Lung Block" site are the dozen thirteen-story apartment buildings of Knickerbocker Village. The housing project—a New Deal collaboration between large-scale developer Fred F. French and the Reconstruction Finance Corporation (RFC), a government agency created to stimulate the ailing economy through loans from the federal treasury—elicited cheers from the *New York Times* as a "vast improvement over the squalid tenements which it displaced." Some critics felt that these improvements came at the expense of character: a writer from the Works Progress Administration panned the buildings as "an overcrowded group whose essential monotony is barely relieved by the sparse planting which differentiates it from hundreds of equally undistinguished apartments farther uptown."[20]

By the time Al Smith's sledgehammer came down on the "Lung Block" in 1933, Hermann Biggs, Jacob Riis, and Robert Weeks de Forest were long dead; James Curry, who had left Saint James fifteen years earlier for a more prosperous Catholic congregation uptown, had died the year before.[21] Lawrence Veiller, by this time founder of the National Housing Association and a self-described "conservative reactionary," registered his strong disapproval of direct federal involvement in what he felt should remain a private business venture.[22] Ernest Poole, who had since become a Pulitzer-winning novelist, mentioned Knickerbocker Village only briefly in his memoir several years later.[23] Lilian Brandt, still working as a social statistician in New York City, did not speak publicly on the project.[24]

Surviving Lung Block campaigners' muted response to Knickerbocker Village stemmed at least partly from the reality that it had not been their direct public appeals thirty years earlier, but fundamental changes in supply and demand that brought the "Lung Block" crashing down. Following the First World War, stricter national quotas sharply curtailed the flow of immigrants into New York's Lower East Side. During the same period, a postwar boom in housing and public transit improvements lured more than half the area's population—at least two hundred thousand people—to "new law" apartment dwellings in outlying boroughs and beyond. By the early 1930s the block bordered by Cherry, Catherine, Hamilton, and Market Streets contained one thousand fewer people than it had in its "Lung Block" days; Depression-era unemployment rendered many of them unable to afford the plummeting rents.[25] Therefore, when French began buying up hundreds of buildings through various dummy corporations, most landowners were ready to cut a deal.[26] French succeeded where the 1903 park campaign had failed because he had the federal government for a business partner and because slums no longer paid in Depression-era New York; slum clearance did. Under these new conditions, the space bordered by Cherry, Catherine, Hamilton, and Market Streets yielded quickly to one of Manhattan's first public-housing experiments.[27]

When promoting the project, French harnessed the newfound profitability of destruction to decades-old, permanently infected claims from the Lung Block campaign. Replacing "old law" tenement neighborhoods with modern multifamily housing would rid the city of "disgraceful and disgusting sores ... [which] for more than a century, have been festering in our very midst, festering with disease and ... crime."[28] Accompanying French's formal proposal were dozens of contemporary photographs from the area surrounding Cherry,

Catherine, Hamilton, and Market Streets, their subjects consistent with the moral environmentalism of bygone muckrakers. Back yards abounded with trash; outdoor privies leaned precariously; a "destitute" family sat on broken chairs in an otherwise sparsely furnished room. Notably, these squalid conditions were recorded from properties immediately adjacent to the proposed site, rather than the site itself.[29] Other photographs linked unhealthy spaces with unhealthy activities: A multiage group of boys playing craps would be "provided with more wholesome recreation when Knickerbocker Village is completed," the accompanying caption promised, while images of weary, downcast men standing in bread lines or passed out on the sidewalk appeared calculated to convey the unlikelihood of collecting rents from the block's current population.[30]

By contrast, some of the messages that French intended to convey in these photographs appeared to be more successfully argued than proved. One such example features a small group of children sitting quietly at the curb of an intersection devoid of vehicle traffic, while a steady trickle of residents appear to be going about their daily business in the background. The caption transformed what could have passed for a quaint and leisurely street scene in any travel guidebook into documentable evidence of the "danger of street play for children." Likewise, a beaming family of seven gathered on a sunny stoop were "making the best of filthy rear yard," and young boys gathered around an imaginary pavement campfire were "making the best of squalor, as children will."[31] Stripped of such pessimistic commentary, some of the images tasked with representing spatial misuses could just as effectively—if not *more* effectively—have supported sympathetic descriptions of the neighborhood, such as one appearing in the *New Yorker* shortly after Knickerbocker Village opened. Despite many locals being out of work, the reporter observed, "You wouldn't know it to see them. They all look well fed and reasonably happy." Likening the surrounding neighborhood to "a small town," she noted local leaders' responsiveness and residents' determined pooling of resources. "There is a sort of community pride in not letting people go hungry or be evicted," she remarked. Five years into the worst economic depression the country had ever experienced, the local support networks of Curry's time were still recognizable.[32]

Completed in 1934, Knickerbocker Village offered the new law housing options that Curry and Marks had called for decades earlier. Each of the 1,600 apartments had adequate lighting and ventilation, along with the latest amenities: "No such thing exists here as the well-known inside room," an early promotional brochure boasted. Moreover, the project incorporated the "breathing spaces" that Brandt and Riis had argued were vital to poor city children. "More than half of the entire five acres is devoted to lawns, flowers, [and] trees," the brochure reported, along with "an enormous playground

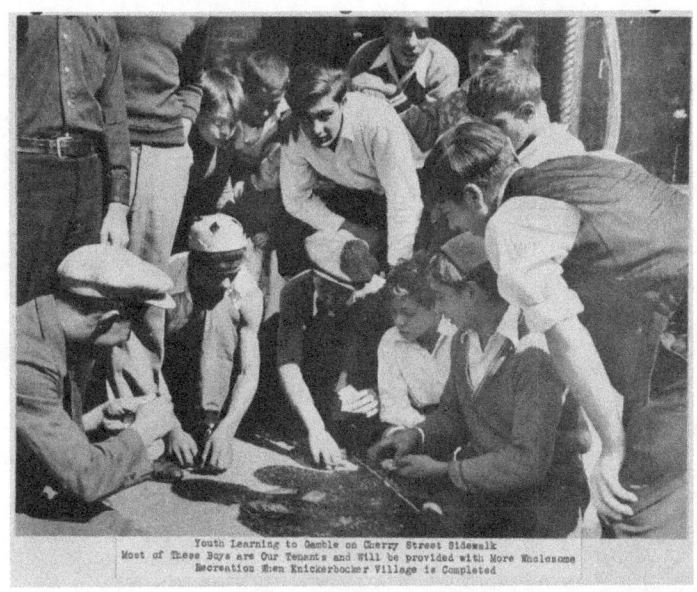

Youth Learning to Gamble on Cherry Street Sidewalk
Most of These Boys are Our Tenants and Will be provided with More Wholesome
Recreation When Knickerbocker Village is Completed

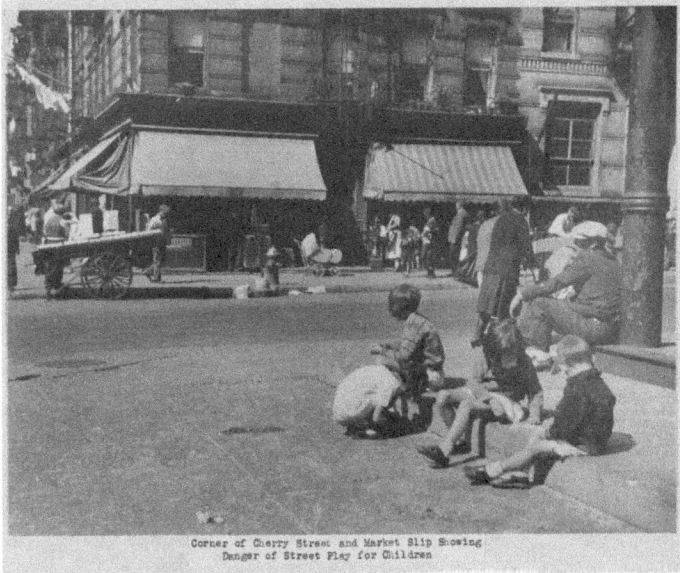

Corner of Cherry Street and Market Slip Showing
Danger of Street Play for Children

C.1A–D. These photographs, taken of the "Lung Block" neighborhood during the early 1930s, accompanied New York developer Fred F. French's formal proposal to build Knickerbocker Village on the site with federal funding. These images of Depression-era street life, bolstered by the grim interpretations set forth in the original captions, were intended to promote the same links between environmental and moral dangers that Ernest Poole and Jacob Riis had decades earlier. Photographs held in the Fred F. French Companies Records, Manuscripts and Archives Division, New York Public Library.

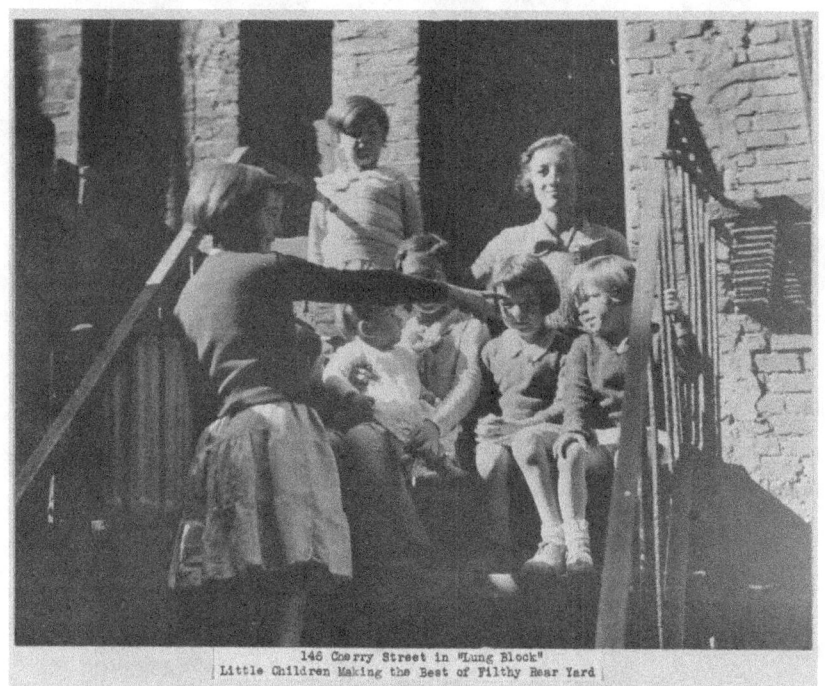

146 Cherry Street in "Lung Block"
Little Children Making the Best of Filthy Rear Yard

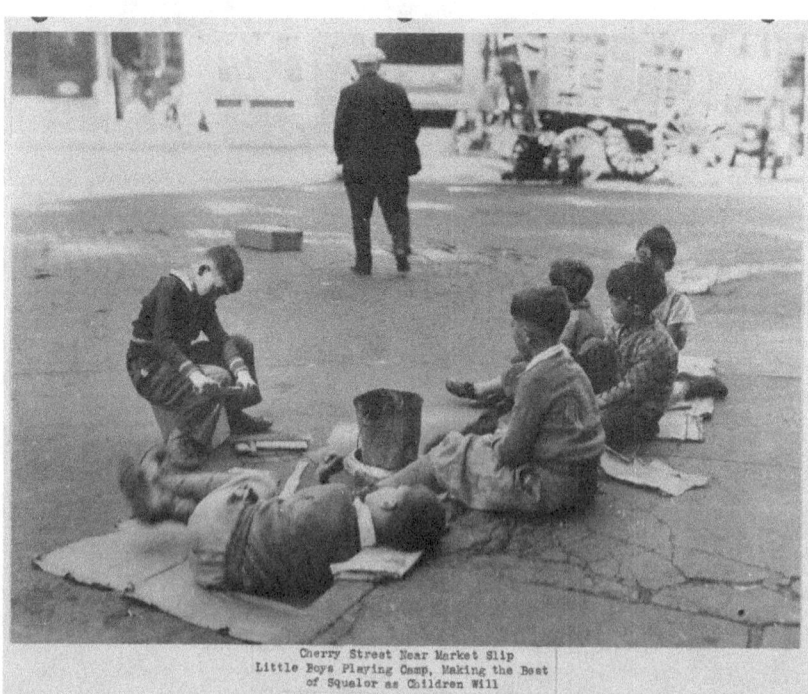

Cherry Street Near Market Slip
Little Boys Playing Camp, Making the Best
of Squalor as Children Will

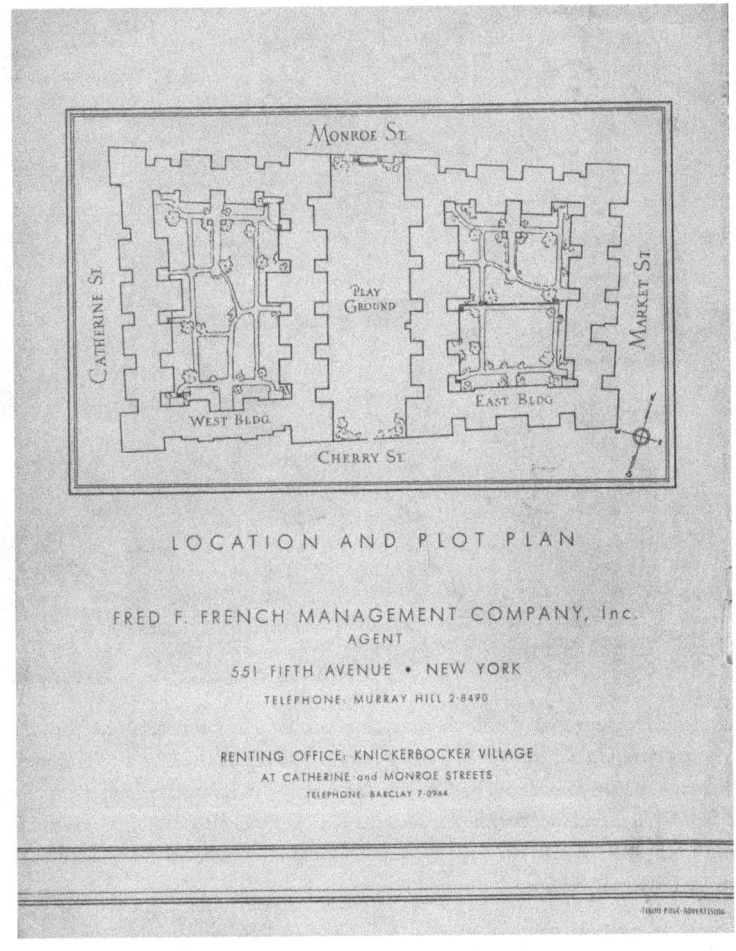

C.2. The balance struck between multifamily dwellings and "breathing spaces" in Knickerbocker Village appeared to satisfy the demands of bygone Lung Block campaigners. Original held in the Fred F. French Companies Records, Manuscripts and Archives Division, New York Public Library.

. . . equipped with sandboxes, swings, etc." As was the case thirty years earlier, supporters hailed the project not only for what it provided but for what it would replace. In an official statement, the RFC promoted Knickerbocker Village as "a modern, clean, light, apartment community" that would eliminate the hazards and dispel the evils of previous generations. "Filth and disease are bred in the buildings and in the narrow slot-like streets and courts," it asserted; "children, in many cases undernourished, are forced to play in streets in an environment which encourages waywardness and crime."[33] In tones reminiscent of Riis, French likewise assured potential supporters that the parks

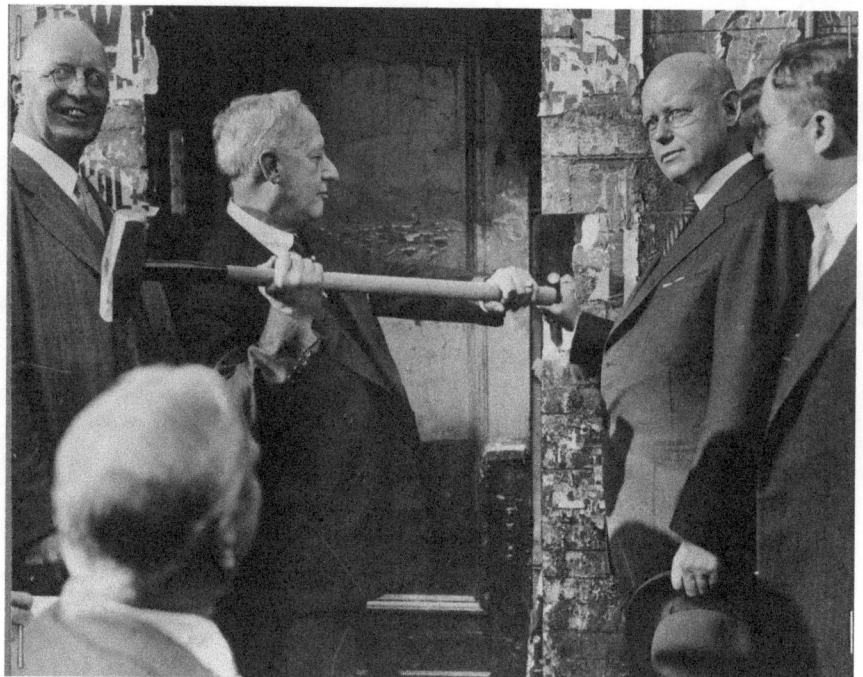

C.3. Before a large crowd of onlookers on October 10, 1933, former New York Governor Alfred E. Smith wields a sledgehammer to strike the first demolition blow in the neighborhood bordered by Cherry, Catherine, Hamilton, and Market Streets. Fred F. French, developer for the subsequent Knickerbocker Village, stands to his right. Photograph held in the Fred F. French Companies Records, Manuscripts and Archives Division, New York Public Library.

and playground at Knickerbocker Village would "assure a higher grade of citizenship" while eliminating longtime reservoirs of infection.[34]

One additional feature Knickerbocker Village had in common with the 1903 park campaign is that in the end, both failed to provide better housing for working-class New Yorkers. Despite Veiller's optimistic predictions that working-class demand would keep new law tenements at full occupancy, placing pressure on landlords to stay competitive through making improvements, this did not prove to be the case. As housing-reform skeptics had forecast years earlier, the additional costs of building to a higher standard carried over into higher rents, thus placing new law housing beyond the reach of most working-class tenants. Knickerbocker Village, with its rent prices being three to four times the local average, proved no exception. Only several displaced families relocated there, leaving the rest of the 1,600 apartments to be filled by junior attorneys, secretaries, clerks, city employees, journalists, and other young professionals who worked downtown.[35]

The irony of low-cost public housing neglecting the city's poorest did not escape public notice. Chiding the government for not taking on the job themselves, the *Nation* argued that "a nation that builds battleships from taxes can afford to build homes from taxes. . . . Public funds for housing should first be used to provide decent homes for workers at rentals they can afford to pay."[36] RFC chairman Jesse H. Jones, who was affiliated closely with the project, likewise conceded before a crowd of five thousand at Knickerbocker Village's grand opening that "it is people who are unable to pay the rents that even this project requires who most need consideration."[37]

These concerns aside, the federal government's role in creating Knickerbocker Village opened up new possibilities for fulfilling the missions of bygone park crusaders. Within a year, the Public Works Administration provided $25 million for New York City to continue replacing old law dwellings with modern multifamily housing units.[38] Under the city's new parks commissioner, Robert Moses, slum demolition would continue to transform New York City's skyline—and neighborhoods, and lives—for the next several decades under the banner of "urban renewal." Speaking to the crowd assembled for Knickerbocker Village's opening in 1934, Moses shrugged off the project's critics with the glib observation, "You can't be a perfectionist in New York and get anywhere."[39]

As for the block's former residents, they did not merely scatter. A social-settlement study conducted among 386 families displaced by French's project found 86 percent of them still living nearby. Noting that "a great majority of tenants expressed a desire to remain in the neighborhood," the study indicated that "most of the families have been residing [there] for a long period of time and many of the wage workers live within walking distance."[40] Over time, it became clear that the much-touted advantages of living in Knickerbocker Village would not extend to its working-class neighbors. "A special . . . police force guards at all times the entrances to the courtyards and the children's playground," the *New Yorker* reported; this was in response to Knickerbocker tenants complaining about "slum kids" heaving bricks and rocks at them, attempting to roller-skate in the complex's smoothly paved interior, and scaling fences to peer into apartment windows. Although such incidents eventually subsided, the two populations remained distinctly separate, with Knickerbocker Village providing working-class locals merely "a curiosity to stare at."[41]

When Al Smith hailed the Lung Block's demolition as "the further extension of the well-known theory of economic justice working out to the ultimate good of us all," it is not clear how he saw that justice working in the lives of the displaced immigrants and children of immigrants who had quietly shifted into old-law housing nearby, their living conditions roughly comparable to what they had left behind. But the tenants of the block bounded by Cherry,

REDEMPTION(?) OF THE LUNG BLOCK

Catherine, Hamilton and Market Streets had long lived apart from their fellow New Yorkers, hemmed in by barriers of language, geography and class. Only by dying in large enough numbers, from causes that posed a potential threat to others, were they once capable of commanding attention from society at large.

NOTES

INTRODUCTION

1. "Slum Work Begun by Smith's Sledge," *New York Times*, October 11, 1933, 25; Al Smith's entry found in Manuscript Census Returns, Tenth Census of the United States, 1880, New York County, NY, Enumeration District 32, National Archives and Records Administration microfilm publication T9, roll 868, page 16, records of the Bureau of the Census, Record Group 29, National Archives, Washington, DC, accessed through Ancestry.com.

2. Scholars occasionally mention the "Lung Block" as a dramatic example of urban tuberculosis prevalence or Progressive Era medical surveillance; see Ott, *Fevered Lives*, or Roberts, *Infectious Fear*. Recent histories of early twentieth-century social activism tend to remain rooted in the movement's achievements, even while attempting to redefine it from a variety of perspectives. Prominent examples include globally oriented works such as Rodgers, *Atlantic Crossings*, and Dawley, *Changing the World*; nationally oriented works such as McGerr, *Fierce Discontent*; and works centered around a single city, such as Recchiuti, *Civic Engagement*. This is also true for works addressing the darker aspects of Progressivism, such as Fronc, *New York Undercover*.

3. For example, Davis, *Spearheads for Reform*; Hofstadter, *Age of Reform*; and Lubove, *Progressives and the Slums* allude briefly to the ideological or cultural gulfs they perceived between reformers and working-class immigrants. Other twentieth-century historians who adopted a more critical perspective of the movement, most notably Sproat, *"The Best Men"*; and Boyer, *Urban Masses and Moral Order*; remained focused on activists' objectives of social control rather than the reaction their agendas elicited from working-class immigrant communities. By contrast, Nasaw, *Children of the City*, includes multiple instances of passive and active resistance that activists sometimes encountered in working-class immigrant neighborhoods. More recently, Fronc, *New York Undercover*—which explores the coercive, even extralegal nature of Progressive Era activists' attempts to regulate behavior—carries on this critical tradition, but goes further to address this gap in perspective between activists and the prostitutes, saloon owners, and ethnic community leaders who regarded the activists' efforts as restrictive and damaging to their livelihoods. Among other things, this study seeks to build

upon Fronc's quest for "a new understanding of the importance of the intersections of local knowledge, ethnic geographies, and the trade-offs made between ethnic and elite power brokers" in early twentieth-century New York City (62).

4. Kraut, *Silent Travelers*; Leavitt, *Typhoid Mary*; Shah, *Contagious Divides*; Markel, *Quarantine!*; Roberts, *Infectious Fear*; Abel, *Tuberculosis and the Politics of Exclusion*.

5. Notable examples of works that emphasize the role of mapping in the construction of knowledge about working-class urban areas include Shah, *Contagious Divides*; Roberts, *Infectious Fear*; Craddock, *City of Plagues*; and Blake, *How New York Became American*.

6. Stephanie Camp used this spatial approach to excellent effect when examining power dynamics between plantation owners and enslaved populations in *Closer to Freedom*.

7. Prominent examples include LeFebvre, *Production of Space*; Soja, *Postmodern Geographies*; and Harvey, *Justice, Nature, and the Geography of Difference*.

CHAPTER 1: "TO ROB CONSUMPTION OF ITS TERRORS"

1. See Duffy, *Public Health in New York City, 1866–1966*, particularly chapters 5 and 11.

2. Chapin, "Tribute to Dr. Biggs," 178.

3. Fee and Hammonds, "Science, Politics, and the Art of Persuasion."

4. Biggs's longstanding image as a white-coated demigod is directly traceable to Charles-Edward Winslow's exhaustive hagiography of the 1920s, which allegedly drew upon an extensive collection of Biggs's schoolwork, diaries, letters, and other sources. This material then vanished from the historical record, rendering Winslow the authoritative source on Biggs's life for at least the next fifty years. See Winslow, *Life of Hermann M. Biggs*. For examples of scholarship emphasizing Biggs's political acumen, see Fox, "Social Policy and City Politics"; Blancher, "Workshops of the Bacterial Revolution"; Fee and Hammonds, "Science, Politics, and the Art of Persuasion."

5. Ott, *Fevered Lives*, 22–26.

6. Kraut, *Silent Travelers*, 155.

7. Prudden, *Dust and Its Dangers*, 61.

8. Prudden, *Dust and Its Dangers*, 62.

9. Roberts, *Theory and Practice of Medicine*, 302. These descriptions supported a white, middle-class construction of tuberculosis. As Katherine Ott observes in *Fevered Lives*, "Other 'races' were excluded from participation in an illness that resulted in refinement of the body and ennoblement of the soul" (28).

10. The work of Koch and Pasteur had its predecessors, most notably J. A. Villemin, a French physician whose 1860s experiments suggested that consumption could be transmitted from one animal species to another via inoculation. Bates, *Bargaining for Life*, 16.

11. Ott, *Fevered Lives*, 70–71. This change developed even more gradually outside the medical and scientific communities. As late as 1939, only 18 percent of Americans believed that germs caused tuberculosis; by contrast, 52 percent still believed it was inherited, and 64 percent believed it developed from a rundown or malnourished condition, exposure to inclement weather, or hereditary factors. Gallup, *Gallup Poll*, 1:162.

12. For a concise overview of the bacterial revolution in America, see Duffy, *Sanitarians*, chapter 13. For a more extensive overview of technological advances in diagnosing and treating tuberculosis, see Ott, *Fevered Lives*, chapter 5.

13. Starr, *Social Transformation of American Medicine*, 79–144. See also Bonner, *Becoming a Physician*; Ludmerer, *Learning to Heal*; Kaufman, *American Medical Education*; and Rothstein, *American Physicians in the Nineteenth Century*.

14. Sedgwick, "Modern Medicine," 109.

15. Jordan, Whipple, and Winslow, *Pioneer of Public Health*, 57.

16. Gorham, "History of Bacteriology," 71–72.

17. Prudden, *Story of the Bacteria*, 136; Prudden, "Tuberculosis and Its Prevention," 631.

18. Hutchinson, *Preventable Diseases*, 126.

19. Winslow, *Life of Hermann Biggs*, 24.

20. Winslow, *Life of Hermann Biggs*, 31–32.

21. Winslow, *Life of Hermann Biggs*, 43.

22. Bonner, *American Doctors and German Universities*, 110–15.

23. Flexner, *William Henry Welch*, 119, cited in Markel, "Extraordinary Dr. Biggs," 2473.

24. For an example of how this professional skepticism worked, see Formad, "Bacillus Tuberculosis," 141.

25. Jacobi, "Inaugural Address," 163–64.

26. Examples of contemporary critiques include Draper, "Scientific and Practical Medicine," 7. See also Shattuck, "Specialism, the Laboratory, and Practical Medicine," 614. For a look at earlier critiques of germ theory, see Tomes, *Gospel of Germs*, 34–38.

27. "Bacteriology in Medical Colleges," 210; Gaertner, "Microscope," 615–16.

28. Notably, within only a few months of publicly rejecting germ theory in his classroom, Loomis implored Welch to stay on at Bellevue as his successor. Oshinsky, *Bellevue*, 161.

29. "Life of Service," 161. This eagerness on the part of recent American medical graduates to partake of European knowledge showcases another important aspect of the "transatlantic moment" Daniel Rodgers has described with respect to social reform movements during the late nineteenth century. See Rodgers, *Atlantic Crossings*.

30. Winslow, *Life of Hermann Biggs*, 65. As late as 1892, germ theory enthusiasts complained about bacteriology's slow and uneven dissemination into the medical community: while top medical schools included germ theory in their curricula, "there are schools in America so behind the age as to teach that bacteriology is nonsense." "Bacteriology in Medical Colleges," *Medicine*, 210.

31. Fox, "Social Policy and City Politics," 169.

32. Biggs, "History of the Recent Outbreak," 71. As subsequent historians have pointed out, Biggs's triumphant interpretation disregarded other factors that limited the cholera epidemic's spread: unseasonably cool weather, cleaner water sources, and inflexible quarantine policies that protected New Yorkers as a whole, even as they elevated the risk of illness and death for Jewish immigrants quarantined at Ellis Island. See Markel, *Quarantine!*

33. When Biggs joined the department in 1892 it had acquired a reputation among critics for being "a refuge for political place hunters." See Duffy, *Public Health in New York City, 1866–1966*, 92–93. See also testimony before the Mazet Committee, a group of state legislators investigating the extent of municipal corruption in 1899. *Report of the Special Committee of the Assembly*, 917, 3807–14, 4012, 5198; Fox, "Social Policy and City Politics," 184n58.

34. See Fox, "Social Policy and City Politics"; Fee and Hammonds, "Science, Politics, and the Art of Persuasion."

35. For an extensive account of Biggs's diphtheria campaign, see Hammonds, *Childhood's Deadly Scourge*.

36. Biggs, "Preventive Medicine," 630.

37. Biggs, "Preventive Medicine," 630.

38. Park, "Tribute to Dr. Biggs," 165. Notably, many of Biggs's public health innovations took place while Tammany was in power, even as some of his colleagues resigned in the wake of what they felt to be patronage appointments. Daniel Fox argued that this pattern calls into question contemporary (usually reform-based) critiques of Tammany as enemies to progress; it also renders suspect previous historians' portrayals of Biggs as a noble hero who suffered under the yoke of Tammany leadership, rather than a shrewd negotiator who successfully manipulated power structures to his advantage. Fox, "Social Policy and City Politics," 182–83, 185.

39. Nicoli, "Foreword," 159.

40. Blancher, "Workshops of the Bacterial Revolution," 109–10. Fee and Hammonds present the *Herald*'s antitoxin campaign as "the first time a public health department had tried to raise money directly from the public through a newspaper appeal; it was one of the most successful efforts ever recorded of raising money indirectly by bringing public pressure to bear on city officials." Fee and Hammonds, "Science, Politics, and the Art of Persuasion," 169. Other city publications also gave Biggs's diphtheria campaign favorable coverage: examples include the following articles from the *New York Times*: "Antitoxine in New York," December 2, 1894, 16; "Will Make Antitoxine," December 21, 1894; "A Home Supply of Antitoxine," January 5, 1895; "The Diphtheria Antitoxine," February 23, 1895, 4; "Value of Antitoxine," April 5, 1895, 5; "Marvels of Antitoxine," September 4, 1895, 2. Other major cities took notice of his diphtheria campaign as well: see "Explains the New Diphtheria Cure," *Chicago Daily Tribune*, August 26, 1894, 7; "Biggs on Anti-toxin," *Chicago Daily Tribune*, January 8, 1896, 12.

41. Howard Markel, "Long Ago against Diphtheria, the Heroes Were Horses," *New York Times*, July 10, 2007, F7. Ironically, Biggs's diphtheria program faced significant challenges from reform administrations, which saw the department's antitoxin production as competing unfairly with private enterprise. See Fee and Hammonds, "Science, Politics, and the Art of Persuasion," 180–81.

42. Evelynn Maxine Hammonds credits the antitoxin campaign with "explicitly providing Biggs with a public platform from which to promote bacteriological research and to defuse potential critics of his new disease-control program." Hammonds, *Childhood's Deadly Scourge*, 90.

43. Shrady, "Health Board and Its Official Diagnosis," 270.

44. Flick, "Contagiousness of Phthisis," 165–66. Nineteenth- and early twentieth-century Americans often used the term *phthisis* (taken from the Greek, meaning "to waste away") interchangeably with consumption and tuberculosis. Dunglison, *Dictionary of Medical Science*, 250.

45. In the years immediately prior to Koch's discovery, standard medical textbooks still attributed tuberculosis to an unfavorable combination of predisposing factors: family history, unfavorable climate, sedentary indoor life, "want of exercise, defective ventilation, deficiency of light, and the depressing emotions." Flint, *Principles and Practice of Medicine*, 206.

46. Davis, "Report of the Committee," 409; Formad, "Second Communication," 463; Formad, "Bacillus Tuberculosis," 141–42.

47. Public health officials had noted Americans' reluctance to put germ theory to practical use as early as 1888, when Chapin called for a systematic approach involving public education, disinfection, and isolation of tuberculosis patients—all of which Biggs adopted as crucial elements in his own public health campaigns. Chapin, *What Changes*, 44.

48. Biggs, "To Rob Consumption of Its Terrors," 758.

49. Biggs to Charles Wilson, health commissioner, in Department of Health of the City of New York (NYCDOH), *Annual Report* [. . .] *1893*, 24–26.

50. For a more detailed account, see NYCDOH, *Action of the Health Department*.

51. Germ theory's lack of immediate practical application proved to be a stumbling block for many clinical physicians, with one writer complaining that discovery of the tubercle bacillus had "added little to our actual knowledge of the causation of this most insidious disease." "Causation of Pulmonary Consumption," 86.

52. This trend to deromanticize tuberculosis only accelerated with time: physician H. de Carle Woodcock described the disease in 1912 as "coarse, common, vulgar . . . bred in foul breath, in dirt and squalor . . . the beautiful and the rich receive it from the unbeautiful poor. . . . Tuberculosis attacks failures." Woodcock, *Doctor and the People*, 185.

53. Knopf, "Plea for Justice to the Consumptive," 6. For a variety of specific examples of phthisiophobia, see Ott, *Fevered Lives*, chapter 7.

54. "Report of the Committee on Hygiene," 462.

55. Biggs and Huddleston, "Sanitary Supervision of Tuberculosis," 109.

56. Taylor, "Duty of a Physician," 18–19. During 1894, 1895, and 1896, physicians supplied 6, 9, and 13 percent of all tuberculosis cases reported to the health department, respectively—a modest rate of increase that Biggs attributed chiefly to informational pamphlets his department issued to physicians all over the city. NYCDOH, *Annual Report* [. . .] *1896*, 26–27.

57. Biggs, "To Rob Consumption of Its Terrors," 757; Biggs, Prudden, and Loomis, "Communications to the Board of Health and Circulars Issued by the Board in Relation to Pulmonary Tuberculosis," in NYCDOH, *Action of the Health Department*, 11, 12, 15, 32, 51, 58, 62, 65.

58. Flick, "Contagiousness of Phthisis," 175–76.

59. Jacob Riis described a tenement as "generally a brick building from four to six stories high on the street, frequently with a store on the first floor . . . four families occupy each floor, and a set of rooms consists of one or two dark closets, used as bedrooms, with a living room twelve feet by ten feet. The staircase is too often a dark well in the center of the house, and no direct through ventilation is possible, each family being separated from the other by partitions." Riis, *How the Other Half Lives*, 18. For more specific details, see de Forest and Veiller, *Tenement House Problem*.

60. Experiments conducted by Georg Cornet, a pupil of Koch, revealed the presence of tuberculosis bacilli on common surfaces inside the houses of people with tuberculosis; moreover, he found through inoculating guinea pigs that these bacilli were still capable of transmitting disease. Cornet, "Uber das Verhalten der Tuberkelbazillen"; Cornet, *Ueber Tuberculose*.

61. Biggs and Huddleston, "Sanitary Supervision of Tuberculosis," 25. Tenement districts were also canvassed by a growing network of city inspectors, visiting nurses, and "friendly visitors" from philanthropic organizations, all of whom complied with referring suspected tuberculosis cases to the health department. See Abel, "Medicine and Morality," 643–48.

62. Biggs and Huddleston, "Sanitary Supervision of Tuberculosis," 23.

63. Biggs, "Registration of Tuberculosis," 307.

64. Flick, *Control of Tuberculosis*, 7.

65. In the fourth ward, which had the largest reported tuberculosis prevalence in the city, four-fifths of the cases were confined to nine streets; moreover, 55 percent of the cases occupied ten percent of the ward's houses. The sixth ward revealed strongly similar patterns. NYCDOH, *Annual Report* [. . .] *1896*, 245–46, 249–50.

66. NYCDOH, *Annual Report* [. . .] *1896*, 252. In his unpublished dissertation, Blancher issues a strong critique of Biggs's maps as fundamentally biased. "No experimentation was involved, no inductive reasoning was employed, no controls were sought; its purpose was to justify a preconceived belief—the 'study' was, quite simply, a polemic." Blancher, "Workshops of the Bacterial Revolution," 197. Ott later concurred, arguing that these maps "created a false picture of the disease." Ott, *Fevered Lives*, 130–31.

67. Biggs and Prudden to Charles G. Wilson, president of the Board of Health, in NYCDOH, *Action of the Health Department*, 28, 30.

68. "Report of the Committee on Hygiene," 462. Daniel Fox discusses this link between etiology and public policy in his 1975 article "Social Policy and City Politics."

69. "Health Board and Compulsory Reports," 126–27.

70. New York was one of several large American cities debating compulsory notification of tuberculosis during the 1890s. Philadelphia physicians' objections centered on similar concerns, most notably patients' rights to privacy and physicians' rights to attend to their patients without state oversight. Flick rejected these concerns, arguing that since surveillance, education, disinfection, and isolation measures protected the public, public institutions should carry them out. "It is not proper to place upon the physician's shoulders duties which belong to the government." See Flick, *Control of Tuberculosis*, 6. Baltimore, which enacted the nation's first universally compulsory tuberculosis reporting legislation in 1896, encountered less resistance from its physicians; this may have stemmed from the measure's selective application among poor and racially segregated populations, who were less likely to receive physicians' services. By 1908, eighty-four cities with populations of forty-eight thousand or more had similar regulations on the books; Roberts, *Infectious Fear*, 92–94.

71. Biggs, "Preventive Medicine," 631, 634.

72. T. Mitchell Prudden, Biggs's longtime ally and president of the Academy of Medicine, and his successor, Edward G. Janeway, helped broker this compromise between Biggs and medical practitioners. Fox, "Social Policy and City Politics," 189–90.

73. NYCDOH, *Annual Report [. . .] 1896*, 254.

74. Knopf, *Pulmonary Tuberculosis*, 57.

75. Flick, "House Infection of Tuberculosis," 349–50.

76. Prudden, *Story of the Bacteria*, 75.

77. Lawrence Flick, T. Mitchell Prudden, Sigard Adolphus Knopf, and Hermann Biggs cite these experiments, conducted by Koch pupil Georg Cornet when declaring the tuberculosis bacillus to be capable of living indefinitely in dried sputa on common surfaces. Examples include Flick's remarks in "Discussion on the Advisability of the Registration of Tuberculosis," 4; Prudden, *Dust and Its Dangers*, 66; Biggs, "To Rob Consumption of Its Terrors," 761; Biggs, "Registration of Tuberculosis," 301. References to dust theory also appear in official health department reports, such as NYCDOH, *Action of the Health Department*, 12. References to other laboratory experiments and anecdotal evidence appear in Otis, "Causes and Conditions of Pulmonary Tuberculosis," 536–39.

78. Otis, "Causes and Conditions of Pulmonary Tuberculosis," 535.

79. Prudden, "Tuberculosis and Its Prevention," 632.

80. As late-nineteenth-century laboratory experiments favored direct-droplet transmission rather than dust as a more likely avenue for tuberculosis, experts developed a sharper appreciation of the conditions that needed to be in place for exposure

to the bacillus to result in active disease. Flügge, "Die Verbreitung der Phthise durch-staubtörmiges Sputum," 107–24.

81. See Tomes, *Gospel of Germs*, chapter 2.

82. Biggs, "To Rob Consumption of Its Terrors," 767. Within five years of New York's antispitting ordinance going into effect, 21 American cities had outlawed spitting; by 1916, 195 of 213 American cities with populations over twenty-five thousand had followed suit. See Abrams, "Spitting Is Dangerous," 430, 433.

83. Abrams, "Spitting Is Dangerous," 431.

84. See Tomes, *Gospel of Germs*, chapter 8.

85. Duffy, *Sanitarians*, 142.

86. Guerard, "Report on the Distribution of Tuberculosis," 36, anecdotal examples on 50–51.

87. Biggs alludes to these concerns in his letter to Wilson. Biggs and Prudden to Charles G. Wilson, president of the Board of Health, in NYCDOH, *Action of the Health Department*, 29. It would not be until 1905 that the first municipally owned sanatorium for tuberculosis care in the United States, Otisville, opened its doors in the Shawangunk Mountains northwest of New York City. There, Biggs implemented a "work cure" for impoverished people with consumption, convinced that the regimen of complete rest and abundant food provided at Saranac Lake and other upper-class sanitariums would turn "a working tuberculous person . . . into a fairly healthy loafer." Biggs, "Municipal Sanatorium at Otisville," 266.

88. Rosner, *Hives of Sickness*, 13. Ott discusses this point in *Fevered Lives*: "Middle-class consumptives, who lived and died in better neighborhoods, were not subject to such scrutiny. No one suggested destroying an infected brownstone or a suburban bungalow" (133).

89. Chapin, "End of the Filth Theory," 236; Chapin, "Fetich of Disinfection," 577. Notably, house infection did not disappear completely from the etiological landscape after the early 1900s; one 1910s study of tuberculosis in Philadelphia endeavored "to show *to what extent* house infection may be considered a factor in the spread of the disease," regarding the concept itself as "clearly established" based on a variety of anecdotal examples. Ward, "Study of the Deaths from Tuberculosis," 24–33.

90. See Wiebe, *Search for Order*.

91. Biggs, "Preventive Medicine," 637.

92. Winslow, *Life of Hermann M. Biggs*, 217.

93. Holt, "Tribute to Dr. Biggs," 170.

94. Winslow, *Life of Hermann M. Biggs*, 133–34, 136.

95. A number of scholars have explored the role of scientific mapping in asserting power, most notably Harley, "Deconstructing the Map." As Ott states in *Fevered Lives*, "Spatialization of disease as dots on a map distanced officials and reformers from the reality of the disease by making it less possible to think about the people involved. Dots carried no information about family, name, age, or how frightening a hemorrhage could be" (131).

96. "Wicked Streets Are Scarce in New York of Today," *New York Times*, September 20, 1925, X20.

CHAPTER 2: "CITY OF THE LIVING DEATH"

1. Lubove, *Progressives and the Slums*, 257–64.

2. Tolman, "Tenement House Curse," 659–60. This trend was established as early as the 1870s, when a guidebook referred to New York's tenements as "habitations, not homes." See McCabe, *Lights and Shadows*, 696–97.

3. Bocock, "Tenement Houses and Their Tenants," 112; Howells, *Impressions and Experiences*, 251; Riis, *Peril and Preservation of the Home*, 35; Morgenthau, "National Constructive Programme," 59.

4. This trend may have originated with Veiller himself when he selected housing reform as the starting point of his life story during an interview conducted in the late 1940s. See "Reminiscences of Lawrence Veiller," Oral History Collection, Columbia Rare Book and Manuscript Library (hereafter cited as Columbia RBML), 2–3. Subsequent portrayals reflect this orientation, based on an informal survey of following monographs dealing with housing reform in New York City: Lubove, *Progressives and the Slums*, chapter 5; Carson, *Settlement Folk*, 71; Plunz, *History of Housing*, 44–45; Rodgers, *Atlantic Crossings*, 194; Page, *Creative Destruction of Manhattan*, 94; Day, *Urban Castles*, 64; Fairbanks, "From Better Dwellings to Better Neighborhoods," 23; Blake, *How New York Became American*, 39; Barbuto, *American Settlement Houses*, 218–19.

5. This popular interpretation draws strength from the fact that Veiller's associates tended to recall him with respect rather than affection. Veiller's brother, playwright and screenwriter Bayard Veiller, included this curious (and solitary) reference to Lawrence in his autobiography: "a fine, upstanding, round-shouldered, bald exponent of law and order and justice and right living and right thinking." Veiller, *Fun I've Had*, 6. Even Roy Lubove, Veiller's most sympathetic biographer, characterized him in *Progressives and the Slums* as "abrupt and aggressive," lacking "the bubbling optimism and winsome personal warmth" of Jacob Riis (127–28). Since the early 1960s, historians have not ventured far from Lubove's assessment. In *Spearheads for Reform*, Allen Davis describes Veiller as "principally a technician and scientific reformer who believed that the housing problem could be solved by passing restrictive legislation and housing codes" (68). In more recent decades, historians have focused more on Veiller's "pragmatic realism" and shrewdness in politics. See Day, *Urban Castles*, 64; Fairbanks, "From Better Dwellings to Better Neighborhoods," 23; Blake, *How New York Became American*, 39; Barbuto, *American Settlement Houses*, 218–19.

6. Census and city-directory entries for Philip Veiller list him as a Wall Street broker in the early 1870s, a sugar refiner in Chicago in 1880, and an upper West Side banker in New York by 1889. *Trow's New York City Directory* (1872), 1179; Manuscript Census Returns, Tenth Census of the United States, 1880, Chicago, Cook County,

Ill., Enumeration District 185, National Archives and Records Administration microfilm publication T9, Roll 199, p. 321B, accessed through Ancestry.com; *Trow's New York City Directory* (1889), 2034. According to Lawrence's brother, Bayard, their father was an ambitious, class-conscious businessman who accumulated and lost several fortunes while he and Lawrence were growing up. Veiller, *Fun I've Had*, 30.

7. University of the State of New York, *101st Annual Report of the Regents*, 560; University of the State of New York, *104th Annual Report of the Regents*, 2:721; New York Board of Education, *49th Annual Report*, 245; New York Board of Education, *46th Annual Report*, 298.

8. Davis, *Spearheads for Reform*, 12; Crocker, *Social Work and Social Order*, 2.

9. Davis, *Spearheads for Reform*, 33–34.

10. Davis, *Spearheads for Reform*, 35–36; quotation from published pamphlet "What Is the University Settlement Society?" (New York: University Settlement Society of New York, 1893), 1, https://archive.org/details/ldpd_9688487_000.

11. Davis, *Spearheads for Reform*, 35. Veiller's brother, Bayard, remembered his father as a domineering personality who insisted on his sons taking up careers in business—a factor that may have influenced Veiller's decision to pursue his own interests at City College of New York, a publicly funded institution. See Veiller, *Fun I've Had*, 1–30.

12. Waugh, "'Give This Man Work!,'" 232; Katz, *In the Shadow of the Poorhouse*, 147.

13. Veiller, "Recent Phase of Relief Work," 474.

14. Veiller, "Recent Phase of Relief Work," 474.

15. Veiller, "Recent Phase of Relief Work," 475.

16. Reynolds, "Report of Head Worker," 8.

17. For more on the conflicted "dual impulse" of settlement work, see Recchiuti, *Civic Engagement*, chapter 3.

18. Lowell, "Economic and Moral Effects," 89.

19. Lowell, "Five Months' Work for the Unemployed," 324.

20. Josephine Shaw Lowell, "East Side Relief Work," *New York Times*, December 14, 1893, 2.

21. For more on scientific charity, see Katz, *In the Shadow of the Poorhouse*, 58–84.

22. Hunter, "Social Settlements and Charity Organization," 81–82.

23. Taylor, "Chicago and the Social Settlement Movement," 76. These distinctions between settlements and organized charities did not always register prominently on the local level. In Ruth Crocker's study of social work in turn-of-the-twentieth-century Indianapolis, she characterizes the settlement as being more of an outgrowth of COS work than a departure from it, noting that each group's agenda contained a similar balance of "social control as well as social reform." See Crocker, *Social Work and Social Order*, 18, 46–47.

24. Veiller, "Recent Phase of Relief Work," 476.

25. Untitled document, box 12, Community Service Society (CSS) Collection,

Columbia RBML. Notably, Jacob Riis also experienced this ambivalence toward the impersonal, scientific approach of the COSCNY, and preferred the settlement as "the passenger bridge . . . upon which men go over, not down, to their duty from the mansion to the tenement." See Riis, "Blast of Cheer," 23. Lincoln Steffens recalled that Riis voiced criticisms similar to Veiller's in private, but then would "go right off to support it publicly with the passion of his rage at it." Steffens, "Jacob A. Riis," 420–21.

26. Julia Shaw Lowell to Richard Watson Gilder, February 9, 1898, box 11, Richard Watson Gilder papers, Manuscripts and Archives Division, New York Public Library.

27. Veiller, "Recent Phase of Relief Work," 477.

28. Lowell, "Methods of Relief for the Unemployed," 659. For a more thorough account of this shift in objectives, see Waugh, "'Give This Man Work!,'" 217–46.

29. Waugh, "'Give This Man Work!,'" 240–41.

30. For more on this transition from a personal perspective, see the autobiography of COSCNY official Edward T. Devine, *When Social Work Was Young.*

31. See O'Connor, *Poverty Knowledge,* 25–54.

32. Hunter, "Social Settlements and Charity Organization," 77.

33. Veiller, "Reminiscences," 3.

34. Lubove, *Progressives and the Slums,* 2. For more on this early wave of New York immigration, see Ernst, *Immigrant Life in New York City.*

35. Lubove, *Progressives and the Slums,* 2–3; Flagg, "New York Tenement-House Evil," 109.

36. Lin, "Changing Economy of the Lower East Side," 45.

37. Duffy, *Public Health in New York City, 1625–1866,* 302–3; Duffy, *Sanitarians,* 96. See also Chadwick, *Report on the Sanitary Condition.*

38. Griscom, *Annual Report of the Interments,* 156, 173.

39. By 1847 the New York Association for Improving the Condition of the Poor (NYAICP) associated the tenement house environment with "sickness and premature mortality"; because these outcomes often undermined working-class families' abilities to support themselves financially, the group also linked the tenement house environment to moral failings such as "wretchedness, pauperism, and crime." NYAICP, *Fourth Annual Report,* 13–14, 23. An NYAICP investigation of tenement house conditions in 1853 found the overcrowding situation to be, if anything, worse than what Griscom had described a decade earlier. Noting that the most overcrowded buildings were "invariably surrounded with disgusting filth, poisonous gases, and with various other local unhealthy influences," the committee concluded that "the number of persons on a given area of soil cannot be increased beyond a certain limit, without endangering health." NYAICP, *First Report,* 14–15, 16.

40. NYAICP, *First Report,* 24.

41. Griscom, *Annual Report of the Interments,* 176.

42. NYAICP, *Fifteenth Annual Report,* 52–53. While the NYAICP hoped to convince capitalists that working-class accommodations could be healthful as well as

profitable, the Working Men's Home degenerated into an unsightly, disorderly slum shortly after it passed into private hands. See de Forest and Veiller, *Tenement House Problem*, 1:86–87.

43. Griscom, *Annual Report of the Interments*, 188–207.

44. Declaring "pure air, light, and water [to be] indispensable to health and life," it proposed that if "tenements are so badly constructed as to preclude a proper supply of these . . . [that] the law should interpose for the protection of the sufferers, and either close up such dwellings, or cause them to be so remodeled as to be fit for human habitations." NYAICP, *Fourteenth Annual Report*, 36.

45. NYAICP, *First Report*, 4.

46. NYAICP, *First Report*, 4, 26.

47. Smith, "Riots and Their Prevention," 41–42.

48. Council of Hygiene, Citizens Association of New York, *Report*, xv, xliv–xlvi.

49. George Templeton Strong provides an especially vivid example. "What we need," he wrote in his diary in 1865, "is practical sanitary reformation of back streets, tenement houses, and pestiferous bone-boiling establishments. Thereby, and by nothing else, can the inevitable epidemic be mitigated. The city government will not do this . . . for it is rotten to the core. The 'Citizens' Association' will do what it can." Strong, *Diary of George Templeton Strong*, 4:44.

50. See Duffy, *Public Health in New York City, 1866–1966*, 6–15.

51. Plunz, *History of Housing*, 22. On the evolution of household plumbing arrangements, see Ogle, *All the Modern Conveniences*.

52. Day, *Urban Castles*, 27.

53. Plunz, *History of Housing*, 22–23.

54. Lubove, *Progressives and the Slums*, 22n33.

55. Burrows and Wallace, *Gotham*. Edward O'Donnell also provides a rich context for working-class agitation in *Henry George and the Crisis of Inequality*.

56. Smith, "Riots and Their Prevention," 42; Wingate, "Moral Side to the Tenement-House Problem," 160.

57. "Our Bad Tenement Houses," *New York Times*, March 1, 1879, 8.

58. Cadman, "Tenement House Reform," 588.

59. Daniel Czitrom offers a thoughtful and far-ranging survey of this genre in Yochelson and Czitrom, *Rediscovering Jacob Riis*, 45–58.

60. Smith, "Homes of the Poor," 510–12; Smith, "Mayor and the Tenements," 699.

61. Smith, "Homes of the Poor," 510.

62. Wingate, "Moral Side to the Tenement-House Problem,"162. This term seems to have come into use during the 1860s, when it circulated in official health reports before appearing in muckraking pieces. See Ezra Pulling, "Report of the Fourth Sanitary District," in Council of Hygiene, Citizens Association of New York, *Report*, lxviii, 64–65; Smith, "Report of the Sanitary Committee," 334; Gallatin, "Tenement House Reform," 309.

63. Wingate, "Moral Side to the Tenement-House Problem,"160.

64. "Some Supplementary Remarks," *Christian Union*, December 13, 1888, 681.

65. "Tenement House Reform: What the Government Should Do," *New-York Tribune*, March 10, 1884, 8. Adler would go on to lead a state-appointed Tenement House Commission later that year.

66. These amendments, passed in 1879 and 1887, slightly decreased the ratio of water closets to tenants from 1:20 to 1:15; they also outlined a more active role for the Board of Health in monitoring and enforcement, although the board did not have adequate numbers of inspectors for conducting these tasks. Lubove, *Progressives and the Slums*, 33.

67. Friess, *Felix Adler and Ethical Culture*, 94.

68. *Report of the Tenement House Committee*, 13.

69. "While technically supposed to be sewer-connected and flushed with water at intervals," Veiller recalled of these privies, "the flushing practically never happened. . . . [T]he stench arising from them into the windows of the bedrooms and the living rooms of the people living above them was horrible." Veiller, "Reminiscences," 4–5.

70. Day, *Urban Castles*, 27.

71. Gould, "Housing Problem in Great Cities," 378.

72. Tolman, "Tenement House Curse," 660–61.

73. Kessner, *Golden Door*, 136.

74. Wingate, "Moral Side to the Tenement-House Problem," 161.

75. Yochelson and Czitrom, *Rediscovering Jacob Riis*, 128–29.

76. Riis, *How the Other Half Lives*, 296.

77. *Report of the Tenement House Committee*, 6.

78. *Report of the Tenement House Committee*, 8, 11.

79. *Report of the Tenement House Committee*, 12.

80. de Forest and Veiller, *Tenement House Problem*, 1:106–7; "The New Tenement House Laws" (pamphlet), box 16, Richard Watson Gilder Papers.

81. de Forest and Veiller, *Tenement House Problem*, 1:106–7.

82. Marshall, "New York Tenements," 753–54.

83. Flagg, "New York Tenement-House Evil," 110.

84. Flagg, "New York Tenement-House Evil," 117.

85. Day, *Urban Castles*, 27.

86. Yochelson, in Yochelson and Czitrom, *Rediscovering Jacob Riis*, 190–204.

87. Lubove, *Progressives and the Slums*, 154, 127.

88. Veiller to Richard Watson Gilder, June 9, 1894, box 17, Richard Watson Gilder Papers. Veiller did not mention his failed bid to lead the 1894 investigation in conversations with Roy Lubove more than sixty years later, when he claimed to have "firmly rejected" Gilder's invitation to serve. Lubove, *Progressives and the Slums*, 127.

89. Upon taking office, Strong replaced all the Tammany-appointed city officials with patrician, public-minded administrators who, "unlike many of their predecessors

... left their private business and devoted their time to the institutions under their charge." Folks, "Reports from States," 73.

90. Lowell to Gilder, February 9, 1898, box 11, Richard Watson Gilder Papers.

91. Veiller, "Reminiscences," 6. Lowell to Gilder, February 6, 1898, box 11, Richard Watson Gilder Papers.

92. Veiller's abrupt termination occurred in conjunction with the return of Tammany to power in 1897. People of the State of New York ex rel. Lawrence Veiller v. Thomas J. Brady, 60–67. Veiller's dismissal was common knowledge among building advocates, who disparaged his subsequent housing-reform campaign as a quest for revenge. See "Building Code Argument," *New York Times*, September 24, 1899, 16.

93. Veiller, "Reminiscences," 5.

94. Lubove, *Progressives and the Slums*, 129.

95. Veiller, "Tenement House Reform in New York," 39; Tenement House Committee (THC) minutes, December 15, 1898, box 171, CSS Collection.

96. "Tenement House Reform," in COSCNY, *Eighteenth Annual Report*, 26.

97. Devine, *When Social Work Was Young*, 73.

98. "Tenement House Ordinances Proposed by the Tenement House Committee of the Charity Organization Society" (pamphlet), box 16, Richard Watson Gilder Papers.

99. Veiller, "Reminiscences," 9. The commission appointed by the municipal assembly to revise the building code consisted of employees from the city Building Department (including the commissioner); an iron contractor/engineer; builders; an architect; and "an Assistant to the Corporation Counsel." See "Report of the Tenement House Committee," in COSCNY, *Eighteenth Annual Report*, 42. Moreover, the resulting code revisions placed the Buildings Department commissioner in charge of interpreting and carrying out the regulations governing building construction—the same commissioner who was then in charge of revising the codes. See Day, *Urban Castles*, 64–65.

100. Veiller, "Reminiscences," 10–11. William J. Fryer, a builder who served on the Building Code Commission, appeared to verify Veiller's assessment. "I don't see why the public should listen to Veiller," he told the *New York Times*. "He has no property interests in the city, and he was quite recently discharged from the Department of Buildings. . . . The public will hardly believe that he and the little coterie for which he speaks have more at heart the best interests of this city than the men who have drawn the building code." "Building Code Attacked," *New York Times*, September 10, 1899, 15.

101. THC minutes, June 12, 1899, box 171, CSS Collection; see also Veiller, "New York's New Building Code," 388–91.

102. Veiller, "Tenement House Exhibit of 1899," 23.

103. Veiller, "Reminiscences," 11.

104. "Report of the Tenement House Committee," in COSCNY, *Eighteenth Annual Report*, 40.

105. Veiller, "Reminiscences," 13–14.

106. Veiller, "Reminiscences," 15. Notably, while the exhibition's disease maps purportedly reflect the number of tuberculosis cases reported to the Department of Health (NYCDOH) between 1894 and 1899, at least several of them contain fewer case dots than disease maps compiled by other tuberculosis studies for the same locations and time periods. In "The Lung Block: A New York City Slum and Its Forgotten Italian Immigrant Community," a 2019 exhibit hosted by the New York City Department of Records, co-curators Stefano Morello and Kerri Culhane uncovered considerable discrepancies between Veiller's tuberculosis map for Chinatown and the original map compiled by the NYCDOH. While Morello and Culhane attribute this example of Veiller's underreporting to extreme carelessness or an unscrupulous impulse to downplay Chinatown's tuberculosis problem in favor of the "Lung Block's," I am not convinced of these explanations. When comparing Veiller's disease map of the "Lung Block" with a tuberculosis map compiled by Hermann Biggs of the New York City Department of Health for the same area and time period, Veiller's map appears to underreport the cases here as well, a pattern that would appear to absolve him of intentionally manipulating the evidence to advance an agenda. While a much more extensive comparison is needed between these two sets of maps, the consistency of Veiller's underreporting in these two instances suggests that he was working from a smaller, possibly older data set; while his maps were completed in 1899, the total tuberculosis cases for 1895–1899 may not have been available for some time after that.

107. Veiller, "Tenement House Exhibition," 321–22; Veiller, "Tenement House Exhibit of 1899," 21.

108. Veiller, "Tenement House Reform in New York," 41. Both the exhibition's opening and succession of related events (evening lectures, design contests, and overall reviews) received steady coverage in citywide dailies like the *New York Post*, the *Sun*, the *Times*, the *World*, the *New-York Tribune*, the *Commercial Advertiser*, and the *Press*, in addition to reform publications like COSCNY's *Charities*, *Jewish Messenger*, and the *Evangelist*. Articles about the exhibition also appeared in the *Chicago Tribune* and *Boston Transcript*. THC scrapbook, box 176, CSS Collection.

109. Veiller, "Reminiscences," 17; Blake, *How New York Became American*, 209; Betts, "Tenement-House Exhibit," 589; Gould, "Housing Problem in Great Cities," 436.

110. "Tenement Ills," New York *Daily News*, February 21, 1900; "Diseases in Tenements," *New York Times*, February 21, 1900, both in THC scrapbook, box 176, CSS Collection. Knopf, "Tenement and Tuberculosis," 1151–54.

111. "Opened by the Governor," New York *Sun*, February 12, 1900, THC scrapbook, box 176, CSS Collection.

112. This contemporary observation supports Blake's assertion that Veiller and his fellow exhibition organizers expected visitors to "do the necessary work to move from one area of the exhibit to another," sifting through all of the proffered evidence

to arrive at the intended conclusions and "become inspired to act—or at least vote—in favor of further reforms." Blake, *How New York Became American*, 46.

113. "Tenement Exhibition," New York *Commercial Advertiser*, February 17, 1900, THC scrapbook, box 176, CSS Collection.

114. Veiller, "Reminiscences," 22. This map collection is housed at the New-York Historical Society.

115. Veiller, "Reminiscences," 11, 13. Historians have since upheld this bold assertion, agreeing that his display methods set the standard for similar efforts tackling a wide variety of social problems over the next several decades. See Yochelson in Yochelson and Czitrom, *Rediscovering Jacob Riis*, 224.

116. "Tenement House Committee," in COSCNY, *Eighteenth Annual Report*, 43–45.

117. Veiller, "Reminiscences," 21.

118. Veiller, "Reminiscences," 26; "Tammany Blocks Tenement Bill," *New York Herald*, March 31, 1900, THC scrapbook, box 176, CSS Collection.

119. By rewriting the bill to include Buffalo in the commission's investigations, Veiller circumvented the need to gain the consent of local New York City leaders. See Veiller, "Reminiscences," 24–26.

120. Veiller, *Housing Reform*, 160–61.

121. "Roosevelt Names a Tenement Board," *Evening Journal*, April 16, 1900; "Tenement Commission," New York *Evening Post*, April 16, 1900, both in THC scrapbook, box 176, CSS Collection.

122. "Need of Tenement House Reform Urged by the New Commissioners," New York *Evening Telegram*, April 20, 1900, THC scrapbook, box 176, CSS Collection.

123. Devine, *When Social Work Was Young*, 26; Pink, *New Day in Housing*, 93; "First Citizen of New York," New York *Sun*, May 7, 1931.

124. De Forest first declined the honor, suggesting that Elgin R. L. Gould take the position instead. When Gould refused to accept Veiller as his chief assistant on the project, de Forest eventually accepted the chairmanship in order to keep Veiller centrally involved, resulting in Gould's resignation. See Hijiya, "Four Ways of Looking at a Philanthropist," 415.

125. Veiller, "Reminiscences," 26–27.

126. de Forest and Veiller, *Tenement House Problem*, 1:5.

127. de Forest and Veiller, *Tenement House Problem*, 1:25.

128. Veiller, "Reminiscences," 27.

129. "Cherry Hill Tenements," New York *Evening Post*, May 2, 1900; "Ramble in Old New York," New York *Commercial Advertiser*, May 2, 1900; "Study Tenements at Close Range," *New York Herald*, May 3, 1900, all THC scrapbook, box 176, CSS Collection.

130. "Ramble in Old New York," New York *Commercial Advertiser*, May 2, 1900, THC scrapbook, box 176, CSS Collection.

131. "Many Evils Found in Tenement Houses," *New York World* (evening ed.),

May 3, 1900; "Tenement Laws are Violated," *New York Herald*, May 5, 1900, both in THC scrapbook, box 176, CSS Collection.

132. "Defy Tenement House Laws," *New York Journal*, May 5, 1900, THC scrapbook, box 176, CSS Collection.

133. Veiller, "Reminiscences," 29.

134. "Saw the Horrors of the Tenements," New York *World* (evening ed.), May 5, 1900; "Ramble in Old New York," New York *Commercial Advertiser*, May 2, 1900, both in THC scrapbook, box 176, CSS Collection.

135. "East Side Tenements Shock Commissioners," New York *Evening Telegram*, May 2, 1900; "Home Life of the East Side Poor," New York *World* (evening ed.), May 5, 1900; "Cherry Hill Tenements," New York *Evening Post*, May 2, 1900, all in THC scrapbook, box 176, CSS Collection.

136. "Cherry Hill Tenements," New York *Evening Post*, May 2, 1900; "Home Life of the East Side Poor," New York *World* (evening ed.), May 5, 1900, both in THC scrapbook, box 176, CSS Collection.

137. "Tour of Tenements," New York *Mail and Express*, May 2, 1900, THC scrapbook, box 176, CSS Collection.

138. "First Slum Trip of Tenement House Board," *Evening Journal*, May 2, 1900; "Tour of Tenements," New York *Mail and Express*, May 2, 1900; "Home Life of the East Side Poor," New York *World* (evening ed.), May 5, 1900; "Reformers Visit Slums and Are Hooted At," *New York Journal*, May 3, 1900, all in THC scrapbook, box 176, CSS Collection.

139. "Ramble in Old New York," New York *Commercial Advertiser*, May 2, 1900, THC scrapbook, box 176, CSS Collection.

140. "East Side Tenements Shock Commissioners," New York *Evening Telegram*, May 2, 1900; "Study Tenements at Close Range," *New York Herald*, May 3, 1900, both in THC scrapbook, box 176, CSS Collection.

141. Examples of coverage include "The Tuberculosis Danger: Disease Almost Wholly Confined to Tenement Districts," *New York Times*, November 17, 1900, 14; "Tenement House Commission Continues Its Hearings," *New York Times*, November 24, 1900, 6; "Conditions in Tenements," *New York Times*, November 17, 1900, 5; "Evil in the Tenements," *New York Times*, November 29, 1900, 3; "Evils of the Sweatshop," *New York Times*, December 1, 1900, 3; "Tenement Problems in the Big Cities," *New York Times*, December 9, 1900, 17; "Tenement House Abuses," *New York Times*, December 12, 1900, 5; "Absence of Fire Escapes," *New York Times*, December 14, 1900, 10; "Tenement House Conditions," *New York Observer*, December 27, 1900, 864. Coverage also extended to other cities: "The Tenement House Question," *Chicago Tribune*, October 17, 1900, 12, THC scrapbook, box 176, CSS Collection.

142. Biggs, "Tuberculosis and the Tenement House Problem," 1:447–48, 455.

143. Guerard, "Relation of Tuberculosis," 1:463–64.

144. de Forest and Veiller, *Tenement House Problem*, 1:10, 12, 35–36.

145. de Forest and Veiller, *Tenement House Problem*, 1:10.

146. The day after public health figures testified before the commission, the following stories ran on November 17, 1900: "Phthisis in Tenements," *World*; "Tuberculosis' Prey in City's Tenements," *New York Herald*; "Dying Like Flies in the Tenements," *New York Press*; "To Wipe Out Consumption," New York *Sun*; "The Tuberculosis Danger," *New York Times*; "Tuberculosis Prevalent," *Brooklyn Standard-Union*; "Disease Widespread," *New-York Tribune*; all in THC scrapbook, box 176, CSS Collection.

147. "Tenements and Tuberculosis" (editorial), *New-York Tribune*, November 19, 1900, THC scrapbook, box 176, CSS Collection.

148. Editorial, New York *Evening Post*, November 19, 1900, THC scrapbook, box 176, CSS Collection.

149. de Forest and Veiller, *Tenement House Problem*, 1:5.

150. de Forest and Veiller, *Tenement House Problem*, 1:11.

151. Veiller, "Reminiscences," 32.

152. Veiller, "Reminiscences," 33. Later, Veiller expressed it this way: "If you live in a boss-ridden state it is just as futile to ask the support of individual members of the legislature in that state as to ask the aid of the Mikado of Japan. Without the support of the boss all other support is of little value." Veiller, *Housing Reform*, 160.

153. Veiller, *Housing Reform*, 160.

154. Day, *Urban Castles*, 69; Lubove, *Progressives and the Slums*, 134–35. "Tenement Bills Signed," New York *Evening Post*, April 11, 1901; "Tenement Bill Hearing," *New York Times*, April 11, 1901; "Plan to Change Tenement Code," *New York Herald*, April 10, 1901, all in THC scrapbook, box 176, CSS Collection.

155. Edward T. Devine to Robert W. de Forest, November 7, 1901, box 4, CSS Collection.

156. After head worker James B. Reynolds pressed Veiller to finalize the dates for making the exhibition available to the University Settlement, Veiller offered a vague commitment to cooperate in the distant future, "provided the settlement society meets the expenses involved." This placed Reynolds in an awkward position, having used the prospect of hosting the exhibition to solicit favors and support from longtime volunteers and donors. Reynolds to Mariana Van Rensselaer, November 2, 1899, series 9, box 23, University Settlement Society of New York (hereafter USSNY), Wisconsin State Historical Society, Madison, WI; Reynolds to Veiller, November 2, 1899, and Veiller to Reynolds, January 8, 1900, both series 4, box 6, USSNY.

157. Upon learning that his published comments had offended many 1894 commission members, Veiller offered Richard Watson Gilder a curiously vague apology that, while assuming full responsibility, did not attempt to clarify or modify his position. Citing a "haste of preparation," he regretted that "some expressions were used which have evidently given cause for criticism." Veiller to Gilder, October 3, 1900, box 16, Richard Watson Gilder Papers. When Jacob Riis confronted him on the same

subject months earlier, Veiller took a stronger stance, dismissing the 1894 investigation's impact as "tremendously overestimated" and citing multiple examples of its "unscientific" approach that lacked "appreciation of the vital points." Perhaps in an attempt to make amends, Veiller then offered the patronizing comment, "Of course they did as well as they could with the imperfect knowledge they had when they started in." Veiller to Riis, May 22, 1900, Russell Sage Collection, City College of New York Archives.

158. Hijiya, "Four Ways of Looking at a Philanthropist," 415–16.

159. Veiller, "Reminiscences," 39. Historians have debated the significance of this "radical" charge against Veiller's appointment: Lubove, accepting Veiller's explanation uncritically, concluded that Veiller's independence and uncompromising nature jeopardized the conservative tone of Low's administration because it suggested "ideological unorthodoxy," although Veiller was in reality "no foe of the profit system." Lubove, *Progressives and the Slums*, 154. A decade later, Gerald Kurland dismissed Veiller's alleged radicalism as a factor in the decision altogether, asserting bluntly that de Forest was "simply the better man." See Kurland, *Seth Low*, 145–46. James Hijiya attributes de Forest's appointment to Veiller's brash and outspoken personality rather than his political leanings. Hijiya, "Four Ways of Looking at a Philanthropist," 415n56.

160. Veiller, "Reminiscences," 40–41.

161. Veiller, "Reminiscences," 39.

162. Pink, *New Day in Housing*, 96; Veiller, "Reminiscences," 38.

163. de Forest, "Tenement House Regulation," 85–86.

164. To Veiller, "the assumption that better housing was a basic, indeed, *the* basic need of the immigrant and working-class poor was so self-evident . . . that it apparently needed no further analysis." Lubove, *Progressive and the Slums*, 174–75.

165. Fairbanks, "From Better Dwellings to Better Neighborhoods," 30–35.

166. In the long run, Veiller's legacy also suffered on account of the limited effectiveness of his policies. The expense of building "new law" tenements resulted in higher rents, shutting out the poorer tenants whom Veiller and his fellow housing reformers were trying to help. According to Lubove, Veiller "never really examined or resolved this difficult question of how one applied the benefits of rising minimum standards in housing to those unable to afford them." Lubove, *Progressives and the Slums*, 181. Meanwhile, the "old law" tenements, which Veiller predicted would soon disappear on account of increased demand for "new law" housing, still persisted into the 1930s, with two million New Yorkers still living in conditions that COSCNY secretary Edward T. Devine deemed "unfit for human habitation." Devine, *When Social Work Was Young*, 77; Page, *Creative Destruction of Manhattan*, 96. By the late 1910s a new generation of housing reformers viewed restrictive legislation as an obstacle to obtaining wider support for the movement. "The best restrictive legislation is only negative," noted Edith Elmer Wood. "It will prevent the bad. It will not produce the good." See Wood, *Housing of the Unskilled Wage Earner*, 20.

167. Veiller, "Reminiscences," 26.

168. Veiller, "The Meaning of the Tenement House Exhibition," *Charities*, February 24, 1900, THC scrapbook, box 176, CSS Collection.

169. Biggs, "Tuberculosis and the Tenement House Problem," 1:449. "The Tuberculosis Danger," *New York Times*, November 17, 1900; "Phthisis in Tenements," *World*, November 17, 1900; "Disease Widespread," *New-York Tribune*, November 17, 1900, all THC scrapbook, box 176, CSS Collection.

170. Guerard, "Relation of Tuberculosis," 1:461; Veiller, "Meaning of the Tenement House Exhibition."

171. Veiller, "Tenement House Exhibit of 1899," 24.

172. de Forest and Veiller, *Tenement House Problem*, 1:12–13; Biggs, "Tuberculosis and the Tenement House Problem," 1:449.

CHAPTER 3: "THE PLAGUE IN ITS STRONGHOLD"

1. Klebs, review of *Handbook on the Prevention of Tuberculosis*, 353.

2. For a more detailed discussion of this etiological shift, see Ott, *Fevered Lives*; Rothman, *Living in the Shadow of Death*.

3. Otis, "Causes and Conditions of Pulmonary Tuberculosis," 534. The most significant of these setbacks involved tuberculin, a glycerin-extract substance derived from the tubercle bacillus that germ theory pioneer Robert Koch promoted as a cure for tuberculosis in 1890. Tuberculin turned out to be not only ineffective but harmful to many patients, damaging Koch's reputation in the scientific community for years afterward. See Teller, *Tuberculosis Movement*, 19.

4. Otis, "Causes and Conditions of Pulmonary Tuberculosis," 534.

5. Otis, "Causes and Conditions of Pulmonary Tuberculosis," 534.

6. Otis, "Significance of the Tuberculosis Crusade," 124–25.

7. "Review of the First Year," in Charity Organization Society of the City of New York (COSCNY), *Handbook for the Prevention of Tuberculosis*, 20–21.

8. Charles I. McBurney, "Report of the First District Committee," in COSCNY, *Twenty-First Annual Report*, 62.

9. "The Work of the City's Tenement House Department," *New York Times*, July 20, 1902, 24; Lawrence Veiller, "Reminiscences," Oral History Collection, Columbia Rare Book and Manuscript Library, 44–45. During their first year of setting up and managing the Tenement House Department, Veiller and de Forest defeated thirty-one bills in the state legislature intended to undermine various aspects of the Tenement House Act of 1901. See Tenement House Department of the City of New York (THD), *First Annual Report*, 1:259–82.

10. THD, *First Annual Report*, 1:86.

11. Quotation from Brandt, "Social Aspects of Tuberculosis Based on a Study of Statistics," 111, 112.

12. Devine, *When Social Work Was Young*, 91.

13. Although New York City in 1902 contained seven hundred thousand more people than in 1881 and had instituted a mandatory-reporting policy for contagious diseases, it still reported more than four hundred fewer tuberculosis deaths: a reduction of more than 45 percent. See Department of Health of the City of New York (NYCDOH), *Annual Report for 1902*, 31–32. This trend was part of a larger overall decline in infectious disease mortality, owing to improved sanitation and hygiene standards over the second half of the nineteenth century. See Bullough and Rosen, *Preventive Medicine in the United States*, 5; Bates, *Bargaining for Life*, 321–27.

14. Otis predicted in 1904 that if the downward trend continued, tuberculosis could be eradicated within another thirty to forty years. Otis, "Significance of the Tuberculosis Crusade," 120.

15. Biggs, "Tuberculosis and the Tenement House Problem," 1:455; Biggs, "Tuberculosis—Causation and Prevention," 166–67.

16. NYCDOH,. *Annual Report for 1902*, 10, 27–28; see also Knopf, *Tuberculosis as a Disease of the Masses*, 72, 200.

17. Biggs, "Tuberculosis—Causation and Prevention," 157.

18. COSCNY, *Twentieth Annual Report*, 30. The prototype for the Committee on the Prevention of Tuberculosis (CPT)—and the first voluntary antituberculosis organization in the country—was the Pennsylvania Society for the Prevention of Tuberculosis, founded by Flick in 1892. Bates, *Bargaining for Life*, 22–24; Walsh, "History of the Pennsylvania Society," 3–4.

19. Devine, *When Social Work Was Young*, 82–83; Veiller, "Reminiscences," 180.

20. COSCNY, *Twentieth Annual Report*, 31.

21. Knopf, "Tenement and Tuberculosis," 1153; NYCDOH. *Annual Report for 1902*, 10.

22. Biggs, "Tuberculosis—Causation and Prevention," 168.

23. COSCNY, *Twentieth Annual Report*, 4.

24. COSCNY, *Twentieth Annual Report*, 28–31.

25. COSCNY, *First Annual Report of the Committee on the Prevention of Tuberculosis*, 9–10, 137–42.

26. Prudden, "Tuberculosis and Its Prevention," 248–49, 253–55; Jacobi, "Tuberculosis and Children," 214–18; Biggs, "Tuberculosis—Causation and Prevention," 164–65.

27. Biggs, "Tuberculosis—Causation and Prevention," 162; Jacobi, "Tuberculosis and Children," 211; Prudden, "Tuberculosis and Its Prevention," 247–49; Knopf, "Duties of the Individual," 173–204.

28. Prudden, "Tuberculosis and Its Prevention," 253–55; Biggs, "Tuberculosis—Causation and Prevention," 167–69; Jacobi, "Tuberculosis and Children," 215; Knopf, "Duties of the Individual," 174–83.

29. Knopf, "Duties of the Individual," 164, 185, 192.

30. Biggs, "Tuberculosis—Causation and Prevention," 161, 163–64. An even more elaborate set of instructions for containing and destroying the bacillus exists

in a circular Biggs authored for the NYCDOH in the 1890s, which the CPT also distributed. See "Consumption Is a Preventable and Curable Disease," in COSCNY, *Handbook for the Prevention of Tuberculosis*, 267–68.

31. "Warfare against Consumption" (pamphlet), in COSCNY, *Handbook for the Prevention of Tuberculosis*, 261–64.

32. Prudden, "Tuberculosis and Its Prevention," 253–54.

33. Jacobi, "Tuberculosis and Children," 222.

34. Knopf, "Duties of the Individual," 200.

35. Affixing a monetary value of $1,500 to each human life, Biggs estimated that tuberculosis already cost New Yorkers $23 million every year, and $330 million for the country at large. Biggs, "Tuberculosis—Causation and Prevention," 166.

36. "Extent of the Anti-tuberculosis Crusade," 452. This concern fit into a larger pattern of anxiety and dissatisfaction among turn-of-the-century American scholars and professionals, many of whom compared their nation's infrastructure and institutions unfavorably with the centralized, "modern" examples of imperial Europe. See Rodgers, *Atlantic Crossings*, 12–17, 137–38, 224–26.

37. "Review of the First Year," in COSCNY, *Handbook for the Prevention of Tuberculosis*, 5; Biggs, "Tuberculosis—Causation and Prevention," 166; Loomis, "Climatic and Sanatorium Treatment of Consumption," 235; Prudden, "Tuberculosis and Its Prevention," 258.

38. Katz, "What Kind of a Problem Is Poverty?," 39. Personal inquiries and database searches at Columbia Rare Book and Manuscript Library, New York Public Library, New-York Historical Society, Municipal Archives, City College of New York Archives, and the Russell Sage Foundation yielded no personal correspondence, interview transcripts, or other unpublished material helpful for developing a fuller picture of Brandt. After her death in 1951, her longtime friend and companion, Helen Kelsey remembered her as "a sensitive spirit, a good friend, and in her quiet way a good companion." Clipping, Alumnae Biographical Files, Wellesley College Archives, Clapp Library, Wellesley College, Wellesley, MA.

39. "Brandt, John Baughman," 142; Manuscript Census Returns, Eighth Census of the United States, 1860, Fairfield County, Greenfield Township, Ohio, National Archives and Records Administration (NARA) microfilm publication M653, Roll 960, p. 101, accessed through Ancestry.com..

40. Research undertaken by Allen Davis reveals that of 120 settlement workers whose fathers' occupations could be determined, thirty-three were ministers, twenty-one were teachers, fifteen were lawyers, fourteen were business owners, and seven were doctors. Davis, *Spearheads for Reform*, 271n27.

41. In the decades following the Civil War, the number of American colleges and universities admitting both men and women increased from one-third to two-thirds; by the turn of the century, the number of women enrolled in college approached eighty-five thousand, which accounted for 36 percent of American undergraduates

and 13 percent of graduate students. Rothman, *Woman's Proper Place*, 106; Muncy, *Creating a Female Dominion*, 4.

42. Sheila Rothman refers to this trend as "educated motherhood," which departed from the Cult of True Womanhood in that women's insights into child development were encouraged to take precedence over their virtuous and maternal instincts. Rothman, *Woman's Proper Place*, 5.

43. Coman, "Preparation for Citizenship," 342.

44. These colleges' different tones and objectives also manifested in the paths their students took following graduation. In *Collegiate Women*, Roberta Frankfort points out that in a given year, 13–25 percent of Bryn Mawr's graduates carved out careers in social work, whereas only 2–4 percent of Wellesley's graduates selected such a life course (57–61). Meanwhile, John Rousmaniere defined "cultural hybrid" in this context as "modified true womanhood . . . educated, certainly, but they would be educated *women*, superior to their less-disciplined sisters because they were hybrids of intellect and virtue." See Rousmaniere, "Cultural Hybrid in the Slums," 54. For more on the development of women's colleges in the United States, see Horowitz, *Alma Mater*.

45. Hart and Fallows, "Women's Colleges and Their Student Life," 170.

46. The list of courses Brandt took in Wellesley is available in her biographical file, located at Wellesley College Archives; Palmieri, *In Adamless Eden*, 168.

47. For a deeper discussion, see Palmieri, *In Adamless Eden*, particularly chapter 5.

48. Coman, "Preparation for Citizenship," 344–46. On Coman's intellectual influences, see Vaughn, "Katharine Coman."

49. In one contemporary statistical report on the career paths of female college graduates, more than half of survey participants had gone into teaching. Van Kleeck, "Census of College Women," 560. On the general dissatisfaction and restlessness among women college graduates, see Claghorn, "Problem of Occupation," 217–25, and Solomon, *In the Company of Educated Women*, chapter 8. "Alumnae Notes," (1896), 354; "Alumnae Notes," (1898), 308; *American College and Public School Directory*, 151.

50. Brandt taught at Bradford until June 1900. *Handbook of the American Academy*, 39. According to a 1918 survey of women college graduates, 8.5 percent had earned a master's degree. Van Kleeck, "Census of College Women," 570.

51. Palmieri, *In Adamless Eden*, 170. Balch would go on to cofound the Women's Trade Union League, serve on several labor-related state commissions, and be the second woman to receive the Nobel Peace Prize. See Randall, *Improper Bostonian*, 170; and Johnston, "Disappearance of Emily G. Balch," 175, 184.

52. Faver, "Creative Apostle of Reconciliation," 338.

53. In *In Adamless Eden*, Palmieri describes the Wellesley community during Balch's time as "a hothouse for reformers" (52). A reference to Brandt's graduate settlement activity appears in "Alumnae Notes," *Wellesley Magazine*, May 20, 1899, 448. Wellesley was also home to the College Settlement Association (CSA), which Kath-

arine Coman cofounded in 1890 with Wellesley colleagues Vida Scudder and Katherine Lee Bates. See Coman, "Influence of the College Settlement," 53–58. By the turn of the century, the CSA had established chapters at twelve colleges and opened settlements in Boston, Philadelphia, and New York. Brandt would remain active in the CSA throughout her career; her early postgraduate involvement is documented in College Settlements Association, *Seventeenth Annual Report*, 7.

54. Brandt's passport application, roll 557 (18 Jun 1900–22 Jun 1900), NARA, Washington, DC. Brandt included her European itinerary in a 1905 survey she completed for Wellesley's Alumni Association. "Alumnae Record," Lilian Brandt file, Alumnae Biographical Files, Wellesley College Archives.

55. Brandt, "Negroes of St. Louis," 205.

56. Brandt, "Negroes of St. Louis," 232, 268.

57. Library of Congress, *Select List of References*, 49.

58. Brandt, "Negroes of St. Louis," 205–6.

59. Brandt, "Negroes of St. Louis," 226. See Claghorn, "Use and Misuse of Statistics," 164–65.

60. Brandt, "Negroes of St. Louis," 227.

61. Brandt, "Negroes of St. Louis," 227.

62. A representative sample from this period includes McKie, "Brief History of Insanity and Tuberculosis," 537–38; Mays, "Increase of Insanity and Consumption," 538–40; Coleman, "Tuberculosis among the Dark-Skinned Races," 118–30. For more on how turn-of-the-century physicians medicalized the "Negro Problem" in their writings on tuberculosis, see Hunter, *To 'Joy My Freedom*, 187–98; Roberts, *Infectious Fear*, chapter 2.

63. Brandt, "Negroes of St. Louis," 264.

64. Brandt, "Negroes of St. Louis," 267.

65. Greeley, *Beyond Benevolence*, 302–3.

66. Quoted in Devine, *When Social Work Was Young*, 125.

67. "The Wise Dispensing of Charity Taught as a Profession," New York *Sun*, December, 4 1904, 9.

68. Kellor's involvement is discussed in Fitzpatrick, *Endless Crusade*, 80, 132–33; quotation from Brandt, "Characteristics of Social Work," 105.

69. Greeley, *Beyond Benevolence*, 308. In *Woman's Proper Place*, Rothman observes that while "women quickly dominated the field of social work . . . the same process that operated in the nineteenth century to make women the typists and men the managers, to make women the salesclerks and men the supervisors, reappeared here as well" (154). This was true for New York, where as late as 1907, COSCNY staff listings reveal men heading most of the bureaus and women filling the assistant, stenographer, nurse, and case-visitor positions. Women who held leadership positions tended to work at the district level, such as supervising case workers. Brandt, who headed the Bureau of Statistics by that time, presents a rare exception. Brandt, *Twenty-Fifth Annual Report*, 233–45. This gender imbalance had modified somewhat by 1915, when a

study of four thousand social service employees in New York revealed that 70 percent were women and that women occupied supervisory positions by a ratio of roughly three to one; however, men still outnumbered women in executive positions by a ratio of approximately six to four. In other large cities (Chicago, Boston, Baltimore, Philadelphia, and Minneapolis), women were more involved at every level of social work. Chambers, "Women in the Creation of the Profession," 7–8, 27n14.

70. Brandt, "Social Aspects of Tuberculosis Based on a Study of Statistics," 31. This anecdote appears several times in popular Western literary journals over a fifty-year span, each time accompanied by commentary promoting it as a succinct example of the strengths and weaknesses of Eastern and Western mindsets. "British and Continental Characteristics," 48–49; Greg, "Life at High Pressure," 626; Merriam, "Census in Foreign Countries," 885–86.

71. Brandt, "Social Aspects of Tuberculosis Based on a Study of Statistics," 36–38, 74.

72. Brandt, "Social Aspects of Tuberculosis Based on a Study of Statistics," 33, 36–41, 48–49, 66–67. Brandt's findings concerning occupations paralleled those advanced in 1901 by noted statistician Frederick L. Hoffman of the Prudential Insurance Company, based on three years' worth of data. See Hoffman, "Industrial Insurance and the Prevention of Tuberculosis."

73. Brandt, "Social Aspects of Tuberculosis Based on a Study of Statistics," 35.

74. Beyond the limited "registration area"—a conglomeration of cities and states that kept the most accurate records, according to US Census officials—reporting methods remained quite primitive at the turn of the century. According to Brandt, "Social Aspects of Tuberculosis Based on a Study of Statistics," 33, the registration area in 1900 included only ten northern states and a handful of large cities, accounting for 38 percent of the total national population. While other cities and states outside the registration area also generated vital statistics during this period, no systematic collection method existed until well into the twentieth century. Ott, *Fevered Lives*, 3. Including tuberculosis mortality figures from both registration and nonregistration areas rendered regional comparisons difficult—a fact that Brandt acknowledged ("Social Aspects of Tuberculosis Based on a Study of Statistics," 33, 80). On the murky nature of late nineteenth-century and early twentieth-century mortality statistics, see Smith, *Retreat of Tuberculosis*; Wilson, "Historical Decline of Tuberculosis," 366–96; Condran and Crimmins, "Description and Evaluation of Mortality Data," 1–23.

75. Brandt, "Social Aspects of Tuberculosis Based on a Study of Statistics," 71.

76. Brandt, "Social Aspects of Tuberculosis Based on a Study of Statistics," 86.

77. Brandt, "Social Aspects of Tuberculosis Based on a Study of Statistics," 33–34.

78. Brandt, "Social Aspects of Tuberculosis Based on a Study of Statistics," 61, 86–87, 102. In actuality, these immigrant groups owed much of their low tuberculosis mortality to their relatively short residency in the United States; within several years,

New York physicians and nurses would observe rising numbers of tuberculosis cases developing among these groups. See Wald, *House on Henry Street*, 53–54; Sachs, "Tuberculosis in the Jewish District of Chicago," 393; Fishberg, "Health Problems of the Jewish Poor," 86; Stella, "Tuberculosis and the Italians," 486–89.

79. Brandt, "Social Aspects of Tuberculosis Based on a Study of Statistics," 49–50, 53–54. For instance, while maintaining that fully understanding the difference in tuberculosis death rates among large American cities required a much closer investigation into "the climatic and sanitary conditions of each city, the composition of its population as to race, sex, and age, the industrial situation, and the method of registering deaths," Brandt nevertheless felt comfortable speculating that "the large negro element in New Orleans and the Chinese population of San Francisco would go far toward accounting for their position at the head of the list" (56).

80. Brandt, "Social Aspects of Tuberculosis Based on a Study of Statistics," 89–91.

81. A number of exceptionally fine studies explore how such "discourses of civilization" laid the groundwork for late nineteenth-century imperialist policies, including Bederman, *Manliness and Civilization*; Lears, *No Place of Grace*; and Jacobson, *Barbarian Virtues*.

82. Brandt, "Social Aspects of Tuberculosis Based on a Study of Statistics," 88–91.

83. Brandt, "Social Aspects of Tuberculosis Based on a Study of Statistics," 85–92; quotation on 112.

84. Notably, in other Progressive Era cities, women commenting publicly on urban reform issues from more established positions of expertise and leadership—often from within a women's organization—promoted solutions that diverged substantially from those of male-dominated organizations. One prominent example of this involves public debates over developing Chicago's lakefront, which exposed differing visions and priorities between the (male) City Club and Woman's City Club, led by Sophonsiba Breckinridge. Flanagan, "City Profitable, the City Livable," 178–79.

85. "Red Light Warnings against Consumption," New York *Herald*, July 19, 1903, 12; "Politics in Charities," *New-York Daily Tribune*, November 20, 1903, 6; "Gleanings," New York *Tribune*, October 31 1904, 7; Brandt, "Social Aspects of Tuberculosis" (1903), 65–76.

86. Historians from the 1990s onward have discussed these interpretive patterns in their own works. In *Bargaining for Life*, Barbara Bates notes that "observers have often seen what they wanted to see" in tuberculosis rates, citing questionable inconsistencies in antituberculosis crusader Lawrence Flick's work as a prime example. She suggests that Flick, rather than being deliberately deceptive, "was so convinced that his views were right—intellectually, socially, and morally—that he adjusted the figures to match his beliefs" (313–18).

87. Poole's long and prolific literary career included twenty-four novels, three plays, more than two hundred newspaper and magazine articles, and America's first

Pulitzer Prize for fiction; yet his work had receded into near-obscurity by his death in 1950. Few of his personal papers survive; one early biographer speculated that Poole's private nature, his tendency to be "a listener instead of a talker," and his lack of eccentricities resulted in few of his friends or associates retaining distinct memories of him later on. See Keefer, "Literary Career," 486–531. Beyond his most famous work, *The Harbor* (1915), scholarly interest in Poole's life and literary legacy has languished since the 1960s. See Penn, "Ernest Poole," 1. While historians tend to rely heavily on Poole's autobiography, *The Bridge*, Keefer's research uncovered multiple inaccuracies and inconsistencies in Poole's version of events. For a partial list of examples, see Keefer, "Literary Career," 3, 8n7, 54n33, 56n37, 73n15, 135–36, 339n55, 468n15. Likewise, *The Bridge*'s strong focus on national and international events—supplemented with lighthearted anecdotes and excerpts from Poole's previously published works—do little to further illuminate the personality of its author. For a more detailed critique of *The Bridge*, see Keefer, "Literary Career," 456–59.

88. Poole, *Bridge*, 34–36.

89. Poole, *Bridge*, 9, 15–30; Keefer, "Literary Career," 6n4.

90. Keefer, "Literary Career," 2–6; Keefer, *Ernest Poole*, 19.

91. Poole, *Bridge*, 7; Keefer, "Literary Career," 8–13.

92. Keefer, "Literary Career," 13.

93. Poole, *Bridge*, 26–27.

94. Poole, *Bridge*, 38–41.

95. Poole, *Bridge*, 11.

96. Poole, *Bridge*, 63, 56. Not everyone agreed with this dim assessment of Poole's gifts: one of his professors, John Huston Finley, recommended Poole as "one of our best Princeton men" to New York's University Settlement Society in 1902, although he did not venture beyond "agreeable and helpful" when listing Poole's attributes. Finley to Robert Hunter, n.d., 1902, University Settlement Society of New York (hereafter cited as USSNY), series 5, box 17, Wisconsin State Historical Society, Madison, WI. Poole graduated cum laude, having earned fourteen of his eighteen A's during his last two years, a fact bearing out his account of having been an intellectual late bloomer. Keefer, "Literary Career," 39n26; "Honors, 1901–02," 297.

97. Poole, *Bridge*, 48.

98. Brooks, *Autobiography*, 160. These critiques of elite education likewise resonated among Poole's elders; see Adams, *Education of Henry Adams*, 54–55, 317.

99. Poole, *Bridge*, 65.

100. Poole, *Bridge*, 66.

101. Poole, *Bridge*, 66.

102. For an overview of late-1800s popular representations of tenement life, see Czitrom in Yochelson and Czitrom, *Rediscovering Jacob Riis*, 44–81.

103. Poole shared his European itinerary with Robert Hunter in a letter dated July 20, 1902. USSNY, series 5, box 17.

104. Poole, *Bridge*, 71. In a letter to the CPT, Hunter confirmed that Poole was

"independent in means" and worked for the settlement "voluntarily and at his own expense." Hunter to de Forest, April 22, 1903, USSNY, series 5, box 17.

105. Davis, *Spearheads for Reform*, 129; Barbuto, *American Settlement Houses*, 101; Carson, *Settlement Folk*, 97–98.

106. At the time Poole began writing in New York, at least six University Settlement workers were writing about social problems for local and national publications, not including Hunter himself. Hunter, Report to the Council of the University Settlement Society, May 19, 1903, USSNY, series 1, box 3.

107. Poole, *Bridge*, 73. Later in life, Poole claimed that he took up settlement work as a means of pursuing his literary ambitions rather than advocating for social reforms; this statement contradicts a letter he wrote to Hunter months before his settlement residence began. In it, he discusses devoting a significant part of his European vacation to meeting with labor politicians and reformers, as well as touring settlements and model tenements in London and Berlin. Poole to Hunter, July 20, 1902, USSNY, series 5, box 17.

108. Poole, *Bridge*, 67, 72.

109. Poole, *Bridge*, 72–73.

110. Poole, *Bridge*, 74.

111. Poole, *Bridge*, 68. The child labor investigation originated with the Association of Neighborhood Workers, a multisettlement coalition that included prominent reformers Florence Kelley, Lillian Wald, Felix Adler, and others. Barbuto, *American Settlement Houses*, 150–51.

112. Poole, *Bridge*, 68; "Waifs of the Street," 40.

113. Poole, "Waifs of the Street," 40–43. Similar examples include "Newsboy Wanderers Are Tramps in the Making," New York *Evening Post*, January 26, 1903; "Child Labor Reform in New York," 55–56. Later on, Poole admitted bribing many of his subjects for the details he wanted, and "in true reformer fashion . . . center[ing] on the worst ones, the toughest and the wildest." Poole, *Bridge*, 68.

114. Poole, "Waifs of the Street," 45. David Nasaw argues that reformers' portrayals of victimized, corrupted "newsies" overlooked the benefits of labor from the children's perspective, most notably the opportunity to develop initiative and to earn and manage their own money independently. Although the dangers were real enough, reformers were "too worried by the potential dangers of city life to notice how well the children handled their environment." Nasaw, *Children of the City*, chapters 4 and 5, 144.

115. Poole, *Bridge*, 68–69. The New York City child labor investigation, led by Hunter, also paved the way for permanent state as well as national child labor committees. Barbuto, *American Settlement Houses*, 150–51.

116. Hunter to de Forest, April 22, 1903, USSNY, series 5, box 17.

117. Poole, *Bridge*, 78.

118. Poole, *Plague in Its Stronghold*, 3.

119. Poole, *Plague in Its Stronghold*, 7.

120. Poole, *Plague in Its Stronghold*, 3.

121. Poole, *Plague in Its Stronghold*, 7–8.

122. Poole, *Plague in Its Stronghold*, 8, 10.

123. Poole, *Plague in Its Stronghold*, 7, 9, 10, 15–19.

124. Poole, *Plague in Its Stronghold*, 11–12.

125. Poole, *Bridge*, 13, 27.

126. Poole, *Bridge*, 20, 27–28.

127. Poole, *Bridge*, 8, 9, 11, 13, 16.

128. This parallel was especially evident in Riis's more recently published *Battle with the Slum*, which referenced Veiller's housing reform campaign, as well as the CPT's work. In it, he framed urban problems in stark terms of survival: "We win, or we perish. There is no middle way" (7).

129. Poole, *Plague in Its Stronghold*, 20.

130. Poole, *Plague in Its Stronghold*, 22.

131. Poole, *Plague in Its Stronghold*, 21, 22, 24.

132. Koch, "Aetiology of Tuberculosis," 311. This is an English translation of the original, which originally appeared in 1882.

133. "Plans for a Hospital for Consumptive Poor," *New York Times*, July 11, 1903. The city's first sanitarium, founded in nearby Otisville, eventually opened its doors in 1906; the National Association for the Study and Prevention of Tuberculosis, founded in 1905, drew heavily upon the CPT's organizational structure and research. "Report of the Committee on the Prevention of Tuberculosis," in COSCNY, *Twenty-Third Annual Report*, 108.

134. This window of cooperation between the two fields would not last. From the 1910s onward, as both sets of fields continued to specialize, medicine and public health found it politically expedient to steer away from championing broader social missions. Starr, *Social Transformation of American Medicine*, 190–91.

135. COSCNY, *Handbook for the Prevention of Tuberculosis*, 5.

136. Knopf, "Duties of the Individual," 198–200; Jacobi, "Tuberculosis and Children," 221–24; Brandt, "Social Aspects of Tuberculosis Based on a Study of Statistics," 113.

137. Brandt, "Social Aspects of Tuberculosis Based on a Study of Statistics," 111, 113. Quotation attributed to former French president Jean Casimir-Perier in "Whole World Wars with Tuberculosis," 176.

138. Notably, Katherine Ott identifies the same process at work among late twentieth-century health professionals when identifying at-risk populations: "Ideological frameworks are imported into medicine, and the resulting interpretations become naturalized, accepted as scientific truths; the complexity of the ways in which people become sick is lost." As in Brandt's time, this tendency to rely on popular assumptions is exacerbated by ongoing issues concerning case-reporting reliability and periodic reclassifications of the disease. Ott, *Fevered Lives*, 161, 164–65; Comstock, "Frost Revisited," 366.

139. "Statistics Her Work," *New-York Daily Tribune*, January 8, 1905, 4. Greeley, *Beyond Benevolence*, 306–7. For more on the public minefield that early female social workers navigated between the images of warm, womanly inefficiency and cold, unwomanly efficiency, see Tice, *Tales of Wayward Girls and Immoral Women*, 48–49.

140. Brandt, "Report of the Committee on Social Research," 86.

141. Poole, "Lung Block," 199.

142. Poole, *Plague in Its Stronghold*, 23.

143. Poole, *Bridge*, 79, 81.

144. Poole, *Bridge*, 79. It is not clear whether Poole personally funded these interventions. While gathering information for *Plague in Its Stronghold* Poole often accompanied Herman ("Harry") Lorber—a young Jewish immigrant physician—on his rounds to tubercular patients. In a letter to philanthropist Jacob H. Schiff several months later, Lorber mentioned that the University Settlement had provided him with $1,000 for sending working-class consumptives to the country. Lorber to Schiff, September 12, 1903, USSNY, series 9, box 23.

145. Poole, *Bridge*, 83.

146. Poole, "April, 1903," 394; Poole, "April, 1904," 395; Poole, "Song That Failed," 418. From there, he moved on to covering radical organizing activities, a violent packinghouse strike in Chicago in 1904, and the aftermath of the failed 1905 revolution in Russia. Poole and Hard, "Stockyard Strike," 884–89. By 1908, he had become an avowed socialist: Poole, "Harnessing Socialism," 427–32.

147. Poole, *Bridge*, 89.

148. Poole, "Lung Block," 199; Poole, *Plague in Its Stronghold*, 14–15.

149. Poole, *Plague in Its Stronghold*, 6; Poole, *Bridge*, 78.

150. Poole, *Plague in Its Stronghold*, 6.

151. Brandt, "Wanted: A Breathing Space," 200.

152. NYCDOH, *Annual Report* (1896), 246. Knopf concurred in 1899, stating, "When a thorough sanitary overhauling does not suffice to stamp out these centres of infection, the destruction of such dwellings seems the only remedy." Knopf, *Pulmonary Tuberculosis*, 57.

153. COSCNY, *Twenty-First Annual Report*, 62.

154. Poole, *Bridge*, 82.

CHAPTER 4: "LUNG BLOCK OR PARK-PLAYGROUND—WHICH?"

Portions of this chapter originally appeared in "'Letting in the Light': Jacob Riis's Crusade for Breathing Spaces on the Lower East Side," *Journal of Urban History* 46, no. 4 (2020): 775–93.

1. For a more detailed look at New York's economic expansion during this period and its impact on both demographics and built environment, see Scobey, *Empire City*, 55–88, and Hobsbawm, *Age of Capital*, 27–71.

2. The phase "city wilderness" originates with Robert Woods's 1898 South End settlement study of Boston working-class neighborhoods. This juxtaposition of city wildernesses with imperialism and the closing of the Western frontier draws on the work of Matthew Frye Jacobson, who reimagines the relationship between late nineteenth-century American immigration and imperialism as "two sides of the same coin." Jacobson, *Barbarian Virtues*, 4. New York arguably provides a microcosm for Jacobson's arguments, both with regard to its own preoccupations with expansion (incorporation of Brooklyn in 1898) and its struggles to resolve its image of white "old-stock" Americans as the basis for a reliable, well-informed citizenry with its growing dependence on imported labor from southern and eastern Europe. For more on these themes in a national context, see Jacobson, 179–219.

3. Whether mid- and late nineteenth-century generations of park activism were connected, and the nature of that connection, have occupied historians for decades. In the 1970s Thomas Bender argued that the small parks and playgrounds movement abandoned Olmsted's "social vision and moral commitment in favor of administrative energy and bureaucratic adjustment"; by contrast, Paul Boyer stressed moral environmentalism and social control as key guiding influences that linked both generations of park advocates. Bender, *Toward an Urban Vision*, 192–93; Boyer, *Urban Masses and Moral Order*, 239–40, 356n26. Subsequent historical works have followed this pattern: see Ethan Carr, *Wilderness by Design*, as well as Hague and Siegel, "Municipal Parks in New York City." Viewing this debate through the lens of Jacob Riis's small-parks activism, as this chapter does, demonstrates how Riis himself embodies a philosophical and methodological bridge connecting two seemingly disparate park movements into successive waves of the same movement.

4. Fellow muckraking journalist Lincoln Steffens described Riis as a man of childlike faith who was guided chiefly by his emotions: "Far deeper than any intellectual faculty," he told *McClure's* readers in 1903, "lay [Riis's] sympathy." He added that Riis possessed "an undisciplined mind that grasps facts as he himself sees them, an imagination to reconstruct, emotion to suffer, and a kind, fighting spirit, to weep, whoop, laugh, and demand." Steffens, "Jacob A. Riis," 422. Similarly affectionate yet condescending portrayals later appeared in the work of scholars such as Roy Lubove, who remarked that Riis was "an incorrigible romantic" whose "perception was that of the poet not the scholar." Lubove, *Progressives and the Slums*, 63–64.

5. Lubove, *Progressives and the Slums*, 64.

6. When historians discuss Riis's parks activism, they either refer to it briefly or limit their discussions to his campaign against Mulberry Bend, although this was one of many small-parks projects he championed in New York. Ware, *Jacob Riis*, 160–64; Lubove, *Progressives and the Slums*, 75–80; Lane, *Jacob Riis and the American City*, 113–15; Yochelson and Czitrom, *Rediscovering Jacob Riis*, 193–201. By the late 1890s major newspapers referred to Riis as "leader of the small-parks movement"; see "Move for Slum Parks," *Chicago Times-Herald*, November 12, 1899, box 10, Jacob A. Riis Papers, Library of Congress (hereafter LC). Likewise, the brand-new Playground and

Recreation Association identified Riis as "father of the small parks movement" when appointing him an honorary vice president in 1906. Ware, *Jacob Riis*, 165n22.

7. Riis devoted progressively more space in his reform writings to parks and playgrounds: from several pages in *How the Other Half Lives* (1890) and *Children of the Poor* (1892), to nearly fifty in his *Ten Years' War* (1900) and *Battle with the Slum* (1902). His growing interest in parks also manifested in newspaper coverage and lectures during the same period; see Box 10, Riis Papers, LC.

8. Riis, *Battle with the Slum*, 274. Today, historians regard Mulberry Bend as "one of the first slum clearance projects on a modern scale in New York City"; see Plunz, *History of Housing*, 52; Page, *Creative Destruction of Manhattan*, 75.

9. In *The Creative Destruction of Manhattan*, Max Page frames New York City housing reform as a struggle between competing ideologies. Taking his timeline into account, the Lung Block campaign marks the point where the nineteenth-century creative reform impulse (resources, services) tipped toward twentieth-century destructive impulses (slum clearance).

10. Riis, *Making of an American*, 12–13.

11. Riis, *Old Town*, 7–12, 24–25.

12. Riis, *Making of an American*, 22; Riis, *Old Town*, 50; Ware, *Jacob Riis*, 5.

13. Riis, *Making of an American*, 30–100.

14. Assigning Riis's Danish upbringing a high importance in shaping his personality and views on America is a trend persisting among historians through most of the twentieth century. Louise Ware attributes Riis's tenacity to "the fighting temper of hero Danes"; Roy Lubove and James B. Lane credit Danish culture with Riis's love of nature, belief in hard work, and the character-building virtues of family and religion. Ware, *Jacob Riis*, 1; Lubove, *Progressives and the Slums*, 56, 60; Lane, *Jacob Riis and the American City*, 13–14. Likewise, David Ward attributes Riis's guiding vision to "an ideal rooted in his sentimental recollections of his own Danish childhood rather than a coherent description of the realities of the American city." Ward, *Poverty, Ethnicity, and the American City*, 73. By contrast, twenty-first-century scholars devote little if any discussion to Riis's Danish origins, a departure reflecting their break from the traditional social reform angle through comparative literary analysis, urban planning, and photography, respectively. See Gandal, *Virtues of the Vicious*; Hague and Siegel, "Municipal Parks in New York City"; and Yochelson and Czitrom, *Rediscovering Jacob Riis*. Consistent with those of earlier scholars, my assessment is based on the considerable emphasis that Riis himself gave his Danish upbringing throughout his writings, particularly *The Making of an American* and *The Old Town*.

15. Riis, *Old Town*, 60.

16. Riis, *Old Town*, 143–68.

17. Yochelson and Czitrom, *Rediscovering Jacob Riis*, 119.

18. In Ware's 1938 biography, Riis's son, Roger, confirmed that Riis's reform impulse stemmed from experiential rather than intellectual influences. "The mainspring of his hostility to the slum was a simple one," he explained. "On Denmark's North

Sea coast, the universe is only two parts: the high-arched blue sky, and the green and blue world. Going directly from that to a city's tenements, back alleys, and windowless rooms, father reacted indignantly and wholly." Ware, *Jacob Riis*, xii.

19. Riis, *Making of an American*, 197–99.

20. "Jail Sermons in Stones," New York *World*, July 15, 1883; "Some Oddities in Low Life," New York *Mail and Express*, May 18, 1883; "He Never Returned," New York *Sunday Mercury*, June 14, 1885; "Keeping an Empty Chair," *New-York Tribune*, March 21, 1886; "The Little Tin Box," *Evening Sun*, April 21, 1887, all in box 12, Riis Papers, LC.

21. Riis, *Making of an American*, 204, 223.

22. "Removing the Dead," *New York Morning Journal*, April 4, 1883; "The City's Virus Farm," *New York Morning Journal*, April 26, 1883; "Epidemic Dangers," *New York Morning Journal*, April 14, 1883; "Secrets of the River," New York *World*, May 25, 1883; "Life in the Pest House," New York *Mail and Express*, May 26, 1883; "Pestilence Nurseries," New York *World*, June 11, 1883; "What It Costs to Keep Rats," New York *Mail and Express*, June 25, 1884; "A Hidden Danger," New York *Sunday Mercury*, November 1, 1885; "An Odorous Subject," New York *Sunday Mercury*, June 17, 1888, all in box 12, Riis Papers, LC.

23. Riis, *Making of an American*, 228–30; "Dr. Cyrus Edson on Food Adulteration," *Herald of Health*, June 1887, 143–45.

24. Riis, *Battle with the Slum*, 62.

25. "The Tenement House Question," *New-York Tribune*, February 4, 1884, 3; "Room for a Great Agitation," *New-York Tribune*, February 18, 1884, 3; "Tenement-House Reform," *New-York Tribune*, March 3, 1884, 2; "Red Tape Extravagance," New York *Sunday Mercury*, April 6, 1884; "Violating City Laws," New York *Mail and Express*, August 17, 1884; "The Miseries of Poverty," *New York Times*, December 15, 1884, 8; "Evils in Tenement Houses," *New-York Tribune*, February 18, 1885, 2, all in box 12, Riis Papers, LC.

26. Riis, "Flashes from the Slums," *Sun*, February 12, 1888; "Visible Darkness," *New York Morning Journal*, February 12, 1888; "Tenement Life as Seen by a Police Reporter," *Brooklyn Daily Eagle*, April 13, 1888; "The Other Half," New Bedford *Mercury*, May 30, 1888; "A Successful Lecturer," *Jamaica (L.I.) Times*, March 28, 1889; "Reporter Riis in Stamford," *Stamford Community News*, March 30, 1889; "The Other Half," *Jamestown Journal*, June 14, 1889, all in box 12, Riis Papers, LC.

27. Riis, "Homeless Waifs of the City," 204–5; "The Tenement-House Question," *Churchman*, May 1889; review of *How the Other Half Lives*, by Jacob Riis, *Scribner's Magazine*, December 1889, 643–63.

28. Riis, *How the Other Half Lives*, 10–13, 62, 152, 299–301 (appendix).

29. Riis, *How the Other Half Lives*, 265. Kate Sampsell-Willmann has observed that other "social" photographers operating during this time period did not fully share Riis's emphasis on the role of environment. Where Riis's photographs asserted direct connections between individuals and their physical surroundings, Lewis

Hine's stayed firmly trained on the individuals; this had the effect of elevating them "from object in the photographer's narrative to subject in his or her own story, thus denying the determinism of ones' surroundings." Sampsell-Willmann, *Lewis Hine as Social Critic*, 32.

30. Riis, *How the Other Half Lives*, 181–82.

31. "The Seamy Side," *New-York Tribune*, November 25, 1890; "Literary Brevities," *Chicago Times*, December 20, 1890. Reviews appeared in the *Sun*, November 18, 1890; *New York Herald*, November 23, 1890, 10; *Chicago Tribune*, January 24, 1891; *Washington Star*, January 5, 1891; *San Francisco Chronicle*, December 9, 1890; *Indianapolis News*, December 24, 1890; *Christian Union*, November 27, 1890, 706–7; *Churchman*, December 13, 1890, 767; *Evangelist*, January 15, 1891; and *Epoch*, January 16, 1891, 383, all in box 10, Riis Papers, LC.

32. Reviews, *Critic*, December 27, 1890, 332, *Sun*, November 18, 1890, and *New York Press*, November 23, 1890, 13, all in box 10, Riis Papers, LC. Over many shorter publications and public lectures, Riis perfected the balance between hard facts and entertainment, leavening his statistics, gritty descriptions, and moralizing with colorful flourishes and even jokes. Over the past twenty years, scholars have examined this touristic, slum-as-spectacle aspect of Riis's reform writings more closely, particularly Gandal in *Virtues of the Vicious*. For more on slumming in a general context, see Heap, *Slumming*.

33. After being appointed New York City police commissioner several years later, Roosevelt often accompanied Riis on his rounds through East Side tenement districts, absorbing firsthand impressions of working-class conditions. Riis, *Making of an American*, 242; Riis, *Theodore Roosevelt*, 131.

34. This antipathy is exemplified in William Dean Howells's determination to only "speak tenderly of the poor"; he conceded that "it is useless to pretend that they are other than offensive in aspect, and I have to take my sympathy in both hands when I try to bestow it upon them." Howells, *Impressions and Experiences*, 277. Historians have discussed this angle of Riis's work more critically in recent years. "Riis conceived of [the poor] . . . as victims deserving pity and charity, as historical objects rather than the subjects of their own lives," Daniel Czitrom observes; "for all his talk of arousing the public conscience, his public tuned out to be quite narrow, excluding the very people he wrote about." Yochelson and Czitrom, *Rediscovering Jacob Riis*, 119.

35. Riis, *How the Other Half Lives*, 273.

36. One early and dramatic example of Riis's reliance on ethnic stereotypes is "The Ambulance Service," an article featuring brief, largely unflattering portraits of how German, Irish, Italian, Jewish, and Chinese immigrants behaved in the police station. New York *World*, August 1883, box 12, Riis Papers, LC.

37. Riis, *How the Other Half Lives*, 26–27, 49. Sensitive contemporaries noted Riis's "warped sense of justice" on this topic: "The 'Heathen Chinee,' and the Russian Jew fleeing from persecution in his own land," one remarked dryly, "finds no mercy in Mr. Riis's creed." Review of *How the Other Half Lives*, *Critic*, December 27, 1890,

332. For a concise twenty-first-century analysis of Riis's use of ethnic stereotypes, see Yochelson and Czitrom, *Rediscovering Jacob Riis*, 109–15.

38. Although Riis himself was foreign-born and left for America with few marketable skills, he adopted an unforgiving stance toward fellow immigrants who had not "risen" since arriving. In future years, Riis continued to blame long-term poverty on idleness or ineptitude, offering himself as proof that any man in America could "get shaken into the corner where he belonged if he took a hand in the game." Riis, *Making of an American*, 21.

39. Until the early 1800s, New York's park development was meager and haphazard, accomplished through "accidents of history, rather than any explicit plan." Weber, "Social Function of New York Municipal Parks," 6–7.

40. Downing, "New York Park," 159. For more on European trends in municipal ownership and their impact on American cities, see Rodgers, *Atlantic Crossings*.

41. As the Romantic movement inspired American poet-philosophers such as Ralph Waldo Emerson and Henry David Thoreau to extol the transcendent qualities of natural settings, New York's emergence as a global industrial and commercial center evoked an imperative to match European cities in cultural refinement and resources as well as in economic productivity. Hague and Siegel, "Municipal Parks in New York City," 159; Kasson, *Amusing the Million*, 11.

42. Downing, "Talk about Public Parks and Gardens," 154; Downing, "Public Cemeteries and Public Gardens," 1–12. Later, when designing Yosemite Park, Frederick Law Olmsted charged government with the responsibility of ensuring public access to beautiful natural scenery for Americans' "pursuit of happiness." See Olmsted and Kimball, *Forty Years of Landscape Architecture*, 45–46.

43. Rybczynski, *Clearing in the Distance*, 177. A concise discussion of Olmsted's guiding influences and motives can be found in Boyer, *Urban Masses and Moral Order*, 236–39.

44. Downing, "New York Park," 163. In his transatlantic study of the Progressive Era, Daniel Rodgers maintains that Central Park, once completed, in turn provided a fresh source of inspiration for European cities. Rodgers, *Atlantic Crossings*, 131–32.

45. Olmsted, *Public Parks*, 34. Such remarks generally support Thomas Bender's assessment of Olmsted's approach as "combin[ing] a sincere feeling for the less fortunate with a somewhat manipulative concern for raising them up to middle-class standards." Bender, *Toward an Urban Vision*, 179.

46. By the 1860s Baltimore, Philadelphia, and Brooklyn had embarked upon the design phases of major parks; by the 1870s Buffalo and Chicago had also followed suit. Carr, *Wilderness by Design*, 24–25; Rauch, *Report on Public Parks*; Boyer, *Urban Masses and Moral Order*, 236.

47. Howells, *Impressions and Experiences*, 227.

48. The park's construction involved the obliteration of houses, churches, schools, and other traces of several stable African American and Irish communities. See Rosenzweig and Blackmar, *Park and the People*, 63–77 (quotation on 233).

49. Strong, *Diary of George Templeton Strong*, 3:567; Browne, *Great Metropolis*, 124. See also Rosenzweig and Blackmar, *Park and the People*, 212–25.

50. Even as Olmsted touted the park's health and civilizing benefits for working-class visitors in 1870, he acknowledged that "for practical every-day purposes . . . the park might as well be a hundred miles away." Olmsted, *Public Parks*, 31–32. Olmsted had intended for park supervision to be more instructive than coercive, believing that the greatest danger to the grounds lay in visitors' ignorance rather than deliberate malice. See Thacher, "Olmsted's Police," 577–620.

51. This observation applied especially to Lower East Side residents. New York governor and onetime presidential candidate Alfred E. Smith, who grew up a short distance from the "Lung Block" neighborhood, relied upon the docks and the nearby East River for his playground; he remembered roller skating in City Hall Park as "something of a luxury," and a trip to Central Park as "something that came to you on your birthday if you were lucky." Smith, *Up to Now*, 18.

52. Americans' promotion of the "strenuous life" through outdoor-living publications, physical education classes, team sports, and community organizations such as the Boy Scouts supported larger discourses aimed at preserving white Anglo-Saxon Protestant hegemony in the face of immigration from within and imperialism from abroad. See Jacobson, *Barbarian Virtues*; Green, *Fit for America*; Roosevelt, "Value of an Athletic Training," 1236.

53. Gould, "Park Areas and Open Spaces," 53.

54. Gould, "Park Areas and Open Spaces," 50–51.

55. Edward Clarke, testimony in "Report of Joint Special Committee," 105, 6–7; Gould, "Park Areas and Open Spaces," 52.

56. A detailed discussion of Hall's recapitulation theory in the context of immigration and urbanization appears in Bederman, *Manliness and Civilization*, chapter 3.

57. Vrooman, "Playgrounds for Children," 286; Gould, "Only Cure for Slums," 499.

58. Wald, *House on Henry Street*, 72.

59. Addams, *Twenty Years at Hull House*, 17.

60. Vrooman, "Playgrounds for Children," 284; Vrooman, "Municipal Playgrounds," 501–2; Tsanoff, "Children's Playgrounds," 294–99. In *Children of the City*, David Nasaw substantiates these concerns with vivid eyewitness accounts from street children themselves, which attest to the corruption and persecution of law enforcement.

61. Juvenile Court of the City and County of Denver, *Problem of the Children*, 22; Gould, "Only Cure for Slums," 499.

62. For a concise history of New York's gridiron pattern of land development, see Plunz, *History of Housing*, 11–13.

63. Weber, "Social Function of New York Municipal Parks," 94–96.

64. Weber, "Social Function of New York Municipal Parks," 97; Vrooman, "Play-

grounds for Children," 286. Gould also decried the "keep-off-the-grass air" of large parks; see "Park Areas and Open Spaces," 61.

65. Although most New York City housing codes and proposed reforms included the prospect of demolition in some form, eminent domain remained "mainly a stock rhetorical device rather than a tool of public policy" until the 1890s. See Page, *Creative Destruction of Manhattan*, 75.

66. Felix Adler, "Tenement House Reform," *New-York Daily Tribune*, March 10, 1884; Gould, "Only Cure for Slums," 495.

67. In 1865, for example, the Citizens Association noted the Bend's sanitary ills and appalling disease prevalence in its investigation of the Sixth Ward. Council of Hygiene, Citizens Association of New York, *Report*, 73–84.

68. Riis, *Making of an American*, 173.

69. Quotation in "The Miseries of Poverty," *New York Times*, December 15, 1884, 8. That year, under Adler's supervision, state Tenement House Commission investigators found 659 deaths recorded in Mulberry Bend over the previous three years, 65 percent of them children under five. Calling the houses "nests of moral and physical disease," the commission added that the area hosted "some of the lowest stale beer shops and places of ill-fame." New York State Senate, *Documents of the Senate of the State of New York*, 14, 232–35.

70. Riis, *How the Other Half Lives*, 55, 57, 60.

71. Riis, *How the Other Half Lives*, 183.

72. Riis, "Clearing of Mulberry Bend," 172–73.

73. Riis, *Battle with the Slum*, 39.

74. Riis, *Battle with the Slum*, 274.

75. Boyer, *Urban Masses and Moral Order*, 236–37.

76. Designing the park, determining costs, and condemning each of the forty-one lots took city officials ten years—much of which Riis attributed to "endless delays and red tape." Riis, "Clearing of Mulberry Bend," 175.

77. "Awful Mulberry Bend," *Sun*, September 29, 1895, 3. Riis later remarked that "My scrap-book from 1883–1896 is one running comment on the Bend and upon the official indolence that delayed its demolition nearly a decade." Riis, *Making of an American*, 275.

78. Riis, "Clearing of Mulberry Bend," 177. Such statements echoed Adler's arguments: "It is next to useless to try to disinfect 'The Bend.' The whole of it should be torn down." Adler, "The Miseries of Poverty," *New York Times*, December 15, 1884, 8.

79. *Report of the Tenement House Committee*, 36.

80. Riis, *Battle with the Slum*, 264, 275.

81. After Riis goaded the city to vacate and destroy the houses, the empty lot became a neglected dumping ground. Ultimately, it took a deadly accident involving two children on the razed Bend site for construction of the park to finally begin in earnest. Riis, *Ten Years' War*, 178–79.

82. Riis, "Clearing of Mulberry Bend," 177.

83. Lee, "Preventive Work," 181.

84. Riis, "Clearing of Mulberry Bend," 176; "Good-By to Mulberry Bend," *Sun*, May 25, 1895.

85. Riis, *Ten Years' War*, 185.

86. Riis, "Clearing of Mulberry Bend," 177. Emphasis added.

87. City of New York, *Report of Committee on Small Parks*, 1. Former New York mayor and early small-parks champion Abram S. Hewitt, who led the committee, advised Riis that "you will have to do most of the work." Hewitt to Riis, June 3, 1897, box 4, Riis Papers, LC.

88. City of New York, *Report of Committee on Small Parks*, 2.

89. City of New York, *Report of Committee on Small Parks*, 20–22; "Parks and Playgrounds," *Commercial Advertiser*, July 3, 1897; "Land for First Playground," *Sun*, July 2, 1897; "Sites for More Playgrounds," *Sun*, July 9, 1897; Riis, *Ten Years' War*, 189.

90. Stover, "Playground Progress in Seward Park," 386–93; Stover, "Seward Park Playground at Last a Reality," 127–33.

91. "Want Daylight in Slums," *Chicago Tribune*, November 12, 1899; "Move for Slum Parks," *Chicago Times-Herald*, November 12, 1899; box 10, Riis Papers, LC.

92. Riis, *Ten Years' War*, 202.

93. Veiller, "The Meaning of the Tenement House Exhibition," *Charities*, February 24, 1900, found in THC scrapbook, box 176, Community Service Society Collection, Columbia Rare Book and Manuscript Library (hereafter Columbia RBML).

94. Veiller, "Parks and Playgrounds," in de Forest and Veiller, *Tenement House Problem*, 2:5–6, 7, 12.

95. Veiller to Riis, May 22, 1900, Russell Sage Collection, City College of New York Archives.

96. In the 1900 Tenement House Commission report, Veiller touched only lightly on the achievements of the previous 1894 commission in which Riis participated—most notably legislation granting the city's Health Department the power to condemn private property, which Riis felt to be "the biggest part of the progress." Riis to Richard Watson Gilder, December 19, 1903, box 13, Richard Watson Gilder Papers, Manuscript and Archives Division, New York Public Library (hereafter NYPL).

97. "Corlears Hook Park," New York *Daily News*, March 3, 1895; Citizens Union, "Small Parks and Recreation Piers for the People" (pamphlet), Russell Sage Collection.

98. Howe, "Parks for Street Dwellers," 637.

99. "New Places for Tots to Play," *New York Herald*, June 18, 1897; Parks and Playgrounds Association, *Statement Relating to Recreation*, 25; "Fruits of Reform Rule," *New-York Daily Tribune*, October 10, 1903, 4.

100. Howe, "Parks for Street Dwellers," 627.

101. "Good-By, 'Bone Alley,'" *New York World*, March 28, 1897; "Bone Alley Club Revenges Itself," *New York Herald*, August 8, 1897, 13.

102. "Famous Raggery to Go," *New York Press*, March 29, 1896, 2.

103. "Famous Raggery to Go," 2; "The Passing of Bone Alley," *Evening Post*, April 11, 1896; "Bone Alley Is Doomed," *Sun*, April 12, 1896, 8; "Good-By, 'Bone Alley,'" New York *World*, March 28, 1897.

104. By 1905, park systems in thirty-five cities would join New York in including municipally owned playgrounds. Carr, *Wilderness by Design*, 36.

105. Riis, speech notes, box 6, Jacob A. Riis Papers, Manuscript and Archives Division, NYPL.

106. Brandt, "Wanted," 201.

107. Brandt, "Wanted," 200–201.

108. Brandt, "Wanted," 202–3.

109. Brandt, "Wanted," 201, 203, 204–5.

110. According to Nasaw, Brandt's observation overlooked the fact that city children's highly developed sense of "turf" prevented them from using playgrounds in nearby neighborhoods, or that parents were loath to let their children travel too far out of range. Despite police harassment and many other dangers of playing in the street, "children . . . felt safer on their home blocks than anywhere else." Notably, when interviewed in the 1910s, some children expressed their disdain for the supervised-play model: "I can't go to the playground now," one of them said; "they get on me nerves with so many men and women around telling you what to do." Nasaw, *Children of the City*, 36–38.

111. Brandt, "Wanted," 201–2. Emphasis added.

112. The Board of Estimate was then still a relatively new institution, having developed out of the charter revisions that occurred with the city's consolidation of Brooklyn and Staten Island in 1898. Sayre and Kaufman, *Governing New York City*, 626–56.

113. Brandt, "Wanted," 204.

114. "'Lung Block' for East Side Park," New York *World* (evening ed.), September 30, 1903, 2; "Would Raze Lung Block for Park," *New-York Tribune*, October 1, 1903, 4; "Would Raze Lung Block," *New York Times*, October 1, 1903; "Would Raze the 'Lung' Block," *Sun*, October 1, 1903, 3.

115. "'Lung Block' for East Side Park," New York *World* (evening ed.), September 30, 1903. Quotation in Robert W. de Forest to Board of Estimate and Apportionment, September 29, 1903, reprinted in Board of Estimate and Apportionment of the City of New York, *Minutes*, March 3, 1905, 520. The East Side Civic Club was founded in 1901 by settlement and social workers seeking to organize Lower East Side residents to take action on political, social, and economic issues of local importance. Box 18, Lillian F. Wald Papers, Columbia RBML.

116. Board of Estimate and Apportionment of the City of New York, *Minutes*, 520.

117. Board of Estimate and Apportionment of the City of New York, *Minutes*, 520–21.

118. Board of Estimate and Apportionment of the City of New York, *Minutes*, 520.

119. Board of Estimate and Apportionment of the City of New York, *Minutes*, 520.

120. "A City Wilderness Park," *Evening Post*, September 5, 1903, 3; "New East Side Park," *New York Herald*, September 6, 1903, 6; "More Breathing Space," *New-York Daily Tribune*, September 6, 1903, 5; "For a New Playground," *New York Times*, September 6, 1903, 21.

121. "A City Wilderness Park," *Evening Post*, September 5, 1903, 3; "New East Side Park," *New York Herald*, September 6, 1903, 6; "For a New Playground," *New York Times*, September 6, 1903, 21; "100,000 Cry for East Side Park," New York *World* (evening ed.), September 11, 1903, 3.

122. "100,000 Cry for East Side Park," 3; "The Cherry Hill Park" (editorial), New York *World* (evening ed.), September 12, 1903, 8.

123. "Dread Consumption Has Hold on New York," Brooklyn *Daily Eagle*, September 13, 1903, 1; "City Block a Plague Hotbed," *New York Herald*, September 13, 1903, 5; "Call to Combat the Mighty Plague of Consumption," *New York Press*, September 13, 1903, 3; "Lesson of the Lung Block," *Sun*, September 13, 1903, 3; "Some Plague Spots in New York," *New-York Tribune*, September 13, 1903, 1.

124. "Park to Rise in City Plague Spot," New York *World* (evening ed.), October 1, 1903, 11; "Would Raze 'Lung Block,'" *New York Times*, October 1, 1903; "Would Raze Lung Block for Park," *New-York Daily Tribune*, October 1, 1903, 4; "Would Raze the 'Lung' Block," *Sun*, October 3, 1903, 8. "Lung Block or Park-Playground—Which?" 335–7.

125. "Horrors of 'Lung Block,' Where Consumption Holds Sway, Described by an Investigator," New York *Evening Telegram*, October 17, 1903, 9; "Away with Manhattan's 'Lung Block,'" *New York Herald*, October 25, 1903, 4.

126. "Horrors of 'Lung Block,'" 9; "Away with Manhattan's 'Lung Block,'" 4.

127. "Away with Manhattan's 'Lung Block,'" 4.

128. "Horrors of 'Lung Block,'" 9.

129. "100,000 Cry for East Side Park," New York *World* (evening ed.), September 11, 1903, 3.

130. "Away with Manhattan's 'Lung Block,'" 4.

131. "Would Raze The 'Lung Block,'" *Sun*, October 1, 1903, 7. At some point during September 1903, park supporters shifted their proposed site one block east from their original site of Hamilton, Catherine, Monroe, and Market Streets. While de Forest attributed this change to a desire for more acreage, the impact of Poole's article may have encouraged de Forest and his colleagues to ask for the larger, more expensive parcel of Cherry, Catherine, Hamilton, and Market streets. See de Forest to Board of Estimate and Apportionment, 519.

132. "Lung Block or Park-Playground—Which?," 335.

133. "Away with Manhattan's 'Lung Block,'" *New York Herald*, October 25, 1903, 4; "100,000 Cry for East Side Park," New York *World* (evening ed.), September 11, 1903, 3.

134. "Park to Rise in City Plague Spot," New York *World* (evening ed.), October 1, 1903, 11.

135. "All Agree the Lung Block Shall Go," New York *World* (evening ed.), November 11, 1903, 10.

136. "All Agree the Lung Block Shall Go," 10.

137. Based on the map that appeared in Brandt's "Breathing Space" article in *Charities*, it is possible that Marks referred to Seward and Corlears Hook Parks. Both were located in the same ward as the "Lung Block" neighborhood, although Brandt's map states they were a mile and three-quarters of a mile away, respectively. Alternatively, Marks may have been referring to City Hall and Mulberry Bend parks; although these were situated much more closely at one-quarter and half of a mile, respectively, reaching them required crossing busy thoroughfares. See Brandt, "Wanted," 200–201.

138. "All Agree the 'Lung Block' Shall Go," New York *World* (evening ed.), November 11, 1903, 10; Brandt, "Wanted," 200–201.

139. "All Agree the 'Lung Block' Shall Go," New York *World* (evening ed.), November 11, 1903, 10. Brandt also alluded vaguely to a "Political Power" who had initially declined to support the project with the incredulous "You're innocent, don't you see that you'll be scattering the votes?" She reported that he eventually came around after park supporters appealed to his self-interest, reassuring him that "the scattering could not take place before the fall elections, and that if the playground became a fact more babies would survive who could be trained up into good Tammany voters." Brandt, "Wanted," 204.

140. "All Agree the 'Lung Block' Shall Go," New York *World* (evening ed.), November 11, 1903, 10.

141. Riis to Nathan Strauss, November 14, 1897, reel 3, Riis Papers, LC.

142. Steffens, "Jacob A. Riis," 420.

143. Johnson, "Marks, Isaac, 1875–," 463–64; Murlin, *New York Red Book*, 81.

CHAPTER 5: "MY POOR PEOPLE NEED HOMES, NOT PARKS"

1. Most "official" sources from the Lung Block campaign can be traced back directly to the Charity Organization Society of the City of New York (COSCNY), particularly its Committee on the Prevention of Tuberculosis. Additional references appear in works by individuals and groups that worked with the COSCNY for specific causes, such as Ernest Poole and James Graham Phelps Stokes of the University Settlement, or in city newspapers from the period. Some individuals acted in the campaign as private citizens and public officials, such as Lawrence Veiller and Robert de Forest, COSCNY members who also led the city's Tenement House Department.

2. Miller, *Emigrants and Exiles*, 291–92. Approximate arrival dates for Peter and Ellen Curry (1848 and 1846, respectively) appear in the New York State Census for 1855, New York City, Ward 21, Election District 2, microfilm, various county clerk offices, New York, accessed via Ancestry.com. Of the 5.5 million immigrants who arrived in America between 1820 and 1860, 3.7 million—roughly two-thirds—disembarked in New York City. Of these, two million arrived during the 1850s alone. Albion, *Rise of New York Port*, 337, 418. By 1855, Irish immigrants constituted 53.9 percent of New York's foreign-born population, 87 percent of its manual laborers, and 74 percent of its domestic servants. Ernst, *Immigrant Life in New York City*, 54, 192–93, 214–18.

3. Diner, "'Most Irish City in the Union,'" 93–94. Hester Street residence appears in an obituary for Anna Curry, New York *Sun*, August 7, 1851. In the Twenty-First Ward, where the Currys lived, 41 percent of residents in 1855 were foreign-born. Of these, 72 percent were Irish; Ernst, *Immigrant Life in New York City*, 193–94.

4. Entries for Peter Curry and Cornelius Horgan in *Rode's New York City Directory*, 133, 336. On the rarity of Irish immigrant butchers in mid-nineteenth-century New York, see Anbinder, *City of Dreams*, 160; and Anbinder, *Five Points*, 112–13.

5. William Perris, *Maps of the City of New York*, vol. 5 (New York: Perris & Browne, 1859), plate 70, Lionel Pincus and Princess Firyal Map Division, New York Public Library. Separate domiciles first appear for Peter Curry and Cornelius Horgan in *Trow's New York City Directory, 1857–58*, 198, 398.

6. Council of Hygiene, Citizens Association of New York, *Report*, 269, 273–75, 276–78. Peter Curry's slaughterhouse attracted at least one complaint to health officials: "Meeting of the Board of Health Commissioners," New York *Morning Courier and New-York Enquirer*, June 4, 1859.

7. During the cholera epidemic of 1832, for instance, New York doctors blamed the high death toll among Irish immigrants to their "being exceedingly dirty in their habits, much addicted to intemperance and crowded together into the worst portions of the city." New York City Board of Health, *Reports of Hospital Physicians*, 14–15, 93. Similar observations exist in subsequent sanitary reports: Griscom, *Sanitary Condition*, 16; New York Association for Improving the Condition of the Poor (NYAICP), *Seventeenth Annual Report*, 50–51.

8. A list of tenants in the home occupied by the Curry family appears in the New York State Census for 1855, New York City, Ward 21, Election District 2; and Bureau of the United States Census (1860), New York City, Ward 21, District 5; both accessed through Ancestry.com. The conditions in Curry's neighborhood likely paralleled those of famed labor leader Samuel Gompers, who also grew up in a New York tenement near a slaughterhouse: "All day long we could see the animals being driven into the slaughter-pens and hear the turmoil and he cries of the animals. The neighborhood was filled with the penetrating, sickening odor." His family procured water from a common pump in the yard, where the toilets were also located. Gompers, *Seventy Years of Life and Labor*, vol. 1, 493–94.

9. The Currys placed the following death notices in New York newspapers over fifteen years: Anna, eleven months (*Sun*, August 7, 1851); Timothy, three years, seven months (*New-York Daily Tribune*, July 25, 1862, 5); Catharine, six months (*Sun*, February 8, 1866). A census entry from 1855 includes six-month-old Ellen, who presumably died before 1860. New York State Census, 1855, New York City, Ward 21, Election District 2.

10. Shannon, *American Irish*, 37. One Irish American in 1860 estimated the average immigrant's lifespan after landing in America to be about six years; another observed that "a man who labours steadily for 10 to 12 years in America is of very little use afterward, he becomes old before his time and generally dies unheeded." Miller, *Emigrants and Exiles*, 319.

11. "Real Estate," *New-York Daily Tribune*, August 20, 1869, 6; US Census Bureau, Ninth Census of the United States (1870), New York Ward 18 District 2 (2nd Enum), 26, NARA microfilm publication M593, accessed via Ancestry.com. Widows, who presided over 20 percent of Irish immigrant households in some American cities, often turned to housekeeping or running boardinghouses as a means of support. Diner, *Erin's Daughters in America*, 52, 61, 96.

12. Margaret Curry's obituary appeared in the New York *World*, February 24, 1871, 8. By 1900 James and his younger brother, Peter, remained the only two of eight original Curry children to survive to adulthood. US Census Bureau, Twelfth Census of the United States (1900), Manhattan, Roll 1112, Supervisor's District 1, Election District 701, accessed via Ancestry.com.

13. Many prominent Irish American leaders assumed breadwinning responsibilities at a young age. "Big" Tom Foley, left fatherless at thirteen, quit school and found work as a blacksmith, then broke into Tammany politics as a saloon owner; he in turn opened doors for Al Smith, whose father's death forced him to begin working one month before he was slated to complete the eighth grade. Golway, *Machine Made*, xviii–xix; Smith, *Up to Now*, 6–7.

14. As late as 1870, nearly 40 percent of the Irish-born immigrants in the United States still toiled as manual laborers or domestic servants; the same figure holds true in 1900 for New York. See Miller, *Emigrants and Exiles*, 319; McCaffrey, "Forging Forward and Looking Back," 229. For more on different categories of Irish American labor, see Stott, *Workers in the Metropolis*, 54–60.

15. Reppetto, *American Police*, 47.

16. Shannon, *American Irish*, 49–50. An estimated 90 percent of Irish Catholics had joined the Democratic fold by 1844; see Clark's *Hibernia America*, 52. Tammany Hall then maintained its grip on city government by naturalizing immigrants at an incredible rate—9,207 per year between 1856 and 1867. These immigrants, mostly Irish, then supported Tammany with votes. Erie, *Rainbow's End*, 26–27, 51.

17. For working-class immigrant families, public jobs often brought higher pay and prestige than similar work in the private sector. For example, policemen earned higher wages than skilled mechanics, and their long hours were offset by lax super-

vision and abundant graft; Reppetto, *American Police*, 43. Recalling the 1880s, Al Smith recalled, "Few bank clerks . . . received as much salary as a policeman or fireman." Such practical considerations played a role in his choosing a career in politics: "I had a choice of hard labor at a small wage of ten dollars a week . . . or easier work at a greater wage." Smith, *Up to Now*, 26, 56.

18. Ernst, *Immigrant Life in New York City*, 163–65, 216–17; Valentine, *Manual of the Corporation of the City of New York for 1855*, 55–57, 120–47; Valentine, *Manual of the Corporation of the City of New York for 1860*, 90–91, 276–79. To arrive at the percentage of Irish Americans in New York City law enforcement for 1860, I compared the number of police officers in the 1860 census with Irish surnames or birthplaces against the total number of police officers in the city, yielding a proportion of roughly 36 percent.

19. Erie, *Rainbow's End*, 2, 5.

20. Miller, *Emigrants and Exiles*, 319. By 1900, New Yorkers hailing from Irish backgrounds filled approximately 10 percent of the city's high-white-collar occupations, and at least 20 percent of clerical, skilled, and semiskilled occupations, respectively; the largest proportion of Irish Americans, at 39 percent, remained laborers. Irish American advancement was greatest in the West and Midwest, least in New England, and considerable in New York and Pennsylvania, where 35 percent of all Irish Americans lived in 1900. Miller, *Emigrants and Exiles*, 495–96; Hammack, *Power and Society*, 69, 84–85.

21. In 1852, the NYAICP observed that increased immigration worked against "the native laboring and mechanic classes in this city, both by crowding them out of employment, and diminishing the rewards of industry." NYAICP, *Ninth Annual Report*, 22. For a more expansive discussion of the factors restricting Irish immigrant upward mobility in the 1850s, see Miller, *Emigrants and Exiles*, 320–22.

22. For vivid examples of election-day violence, see Anbinder, *Five Points*, 150–57; Anbinder, *City of Dreams*, 190–95; and Reppetto, *American Police*, 50.

23. One common objection to Catholics rested upon the nativist belief that Catholics did not vote as individuals, but according to their church leaders' commands. "Religion and Party," *New York Evening Express*, September 10, 1855, 1.

24. *Evangelist*, January 4, 1849; quoted in Rosenberg, *Cholera Years*, 141.

25. Crosby, "Letter to the People of New York," 427.

26. Brownson, "Native Americanism," 82.

27. Strong, *Diary of George Templeton Strong*, 1:244–45, 348; Roosevelt in Kohn, *Most Glorious Ride*, 214.

28. Miller, *Emigrants and Exiles*, 322–24; Dolan, *Irish Americans*, 96–97; Dolan, *American Catholic Parish*, 1:20–21; Dolan, *American Catholic Experience*, 202–3. See also Curtis, *Apes and Angels*, 3, 5.

29. Dolan, *Immigrant Church*, 53–54. According to Miller, the church's primary function was "to insulate [the Irish] from native animosity and from despair engendered by their own deplorable condition," and "bolster the emigrants' shattered pride

in their Irishness." At the same time, the church provided a parallel, but separate track to respectability, fending off anti-American criticisms with its promotion of patriotism, temperance, industry, thrift, sobriety, and self-control. Miller, *Emigrants and Exiles*, 333.

30. Casino, "From Sanctuary to Involvement," 1:15; Bayley, *Brief Sketch*, 160; McDannell, "Going to the Ladies' Fair," 243–44.

31. Hammack, "Nonprofit Organizations," 218.

32. Dolan, *Immigrant Church*, 22. By 1900, two-thirds of America's Catholic bishops were of Irish birth or descent, including those in New York, Baltimore, Boston, Philadelphia, Detroit, Saint Paul, and San Francisco. Kenny, *American Irish*, 164.

33. Kenny, *American Irish*, 65–66. In 1850s New York, a Catholic pastor's salary was $600, the same figure promoted in city newspapers as the base-level income for supporting a family of four. Stansell, *City of Women*, 111, 262n25.

34. In the Irish community, individual and family reputations were indelibly linked: "A man was judged not only on his own merits but also on the merits of his entire family." Shannon, *American Irish*, 37.

35. Dolan, *Irish Americans*, 125.

36. "St. Stephen's Church," *World*, February 23, 1888, 6; Shea, *Catholic Churches of New York City*, 664–65.

37. Colleen McDannell argues that this means of escape is precisely what motivated working-class Irish Americans to fund elaborate churches: "Paid choirs, orchestras, processions both inside and outside the church, and the ever-increasing number of statues and stained-glass windows made the church . . . a journey into another world." McDannell, "Going to the Ladies' Fair," 245.

38. Since McGlynn's death in 1900, historians have focused on the controversy that his radical views generated among late nineteenth-century American Catholics regarding wealth distribution, education, and stronger state control of the economy. This radical emphasis overshadows McGlynn's considerable accomplishments as a "priest-reformer" in promoting the social gospel from a Catholic perspective in earlier decades. See Shanaberger, "Edward McGlynn," 23–47.

39. Malone, *Dr. Edward McGlynn*, 1.

40. Malone, *Dr. Edward McGlynn*, 111.

41. Shelley, "Ubiquitously Useful," 470, 475; University of the State of New York, *92nd Annual Report of the Regents*, 181.

42. Brann, *History of the American College*, 530, 553.

43. Kenny, *American Irish*, 165–71; Miller, *Emigrants and Exiles*, 528–32.

44. Shannon, *American Irish*, 114–30; Kenny, *American Irish*, 165–71; Dolan, *American Catholic Experience*, 270–93; Carey, *Catholics in America*, 55–66; Roohan, *American Catholics and the Social Question*, chapters 8–10.

45. McLeod, *Piety and Poverty*, 120–25; a longer account appears in Roohan, *American Catholics and the Social Question*, 332–83.

46. Shea, *Catholic Churches*, 400. In 1880, residents of the "Lung Block" area

consisted generally of Irish American laborers and their children. Younger children attended school, while older children and young adults worked as store clerks or domestic servants. The block also contained a sizable German population. US Census Bureau, Tenth Census of the United States (1880), Manhattan, Enumeration District 82, accessed via Ancestry.com.

47. Al Smith's daughter, Emily Smith Warner, recalled the neighborhood surrounding Saint James church and rectory as stable and heavily Catholic in the 1900s. "There was no wealth," she wrote, "but neither was there any grinding poverty." Referring to the slums made infamous by Jacob Riis and others, she protested that "nothing of this nature existed in our neighborhood, and we children were never permitted to wander to other vicinities where we might come upon them." These vicinities existed nearby, however; as Warner grew more aware of her surroundings, she "looked askance" at the tenements located across a busy side street and felt "trepidation as I passed certain doubtful addresses." Warner, *Happy Warrior*, 14–15, 20.

48. Graham, *Al Smith, American*, 12; Smith, *Up to Now*, 40–41; Hapgood and Moskowitz, *Up from the City Streets*, 9, 33; Diner, *Erin's Daughters in America*, 114; Shea, *Catholic Churches*, 399–400.

49. Shea, *Catholic Churches*, 400–401; Smith, *Up to Now*, 40–41. For more on fundraising activities in New York parishes, see McDannell, "Going to the Ladies' Fair," 234–51.

50. Slayton, *Empire Statesman*, 26.

51. Meehan, "Right Rev. John J. Kean," 195.

52. "Practical Christianity," Duluth *News-Tribune*, August 27, 1905.

53. "Dope Plague Scourges while Priest Combats," New York *World* (evening ed.), August 27, 1906, 10.

54. Margaret Dwyer, "St. James School," in *Golden Jubilee of St. James School, 1854–1904* (souvenir pamphlet), 14, box 21, Parish History Collection, Archives of the Archdiocese of the City of New York, Saint Joseph's Seminary, Dunwoodie (hereafter AACNY); "City Shift Dooms St. James," New York *Evening Telegram*, January 30, 1921, 7.

55. "Pledge Signed Not to Drink," Duluth *Evening Herald*, December 3, 1903, 2; "Live Well on $12 a Week," *Columbia* (Hudson, NY) *Republican*, December 1, 1907.

56. "Cherry Hill Priest Opens War on Liquor," *World*, July 22, 1905, 2.

57. "Captain O'Reilly Makes His Debut as Lecturer," Brooklyn *Standard-Union*, June 10, 1902, 3; "Recreation Piers Demoralizing, Priest Says," *Chicago Tribune*, June 6, 1904, 4; "Rowdyism on the Recreation Piers," *New York Herald*, June 8, 1904, 7.

58. "Practical Christianity," Duluth *News-Tribune*, August 27, 1905. Curry considered his own authority to outweigh that of parents; at one point, he advised parish children to skip school in favor of attending a special mass, even if it meant disobeying their parents' wishes. "Priest Advises Playing 'Hooky,'" *New York Times*, December 4, 1904, 2.

59. "Priest Calls Captain Liar," *Evening Telegram*, April 7, 1902, 12.

60. Curry to Archbishop Michael A. Corrigan, September 15, 1901, folder 13, box 21, Parish History Collection, AACNY.

61. "Complains of Chatham Square," *Sun*, July 7, 1901, 7.

62. New York City police officers tended to view prostitution as a necessary evil. "I can't govern them," remarked police commissioner Charles Murphy in 1901; "I don't see who could . . . we've kept 'em under the surface, out of the public eye, and I think that's all the public wants us to do." "Commissioner Murphy Talks," *New York Times*, August 18, 1901, 3. This lax approach enabled police officers to charge brothels "protection fees" for continuing to operate illegally. Gilfoyle, *City of Eros*, chapter 12. Curry's remarks appeared in the following newspapers on April 7, 1902: "Priest Attacks the Police," *Sun*, 2; "Priest Calls Captain Liar," *Evening Telegram*, 12; "Priest Denounces Police from Altar," *New York Herald*, 10; "Priest Flays Police Gang," *New York Press*, 2; and "Priest Accuses New York Police," *Chicago Tribune*.

63. "Priest Attacks the Police," *Sun*, April 7, 1902, 2.

64. "Policy Raid by Jerome," New York *Tribune*, April 9, 1902, 1; "'Shake Up' Bears Fruit," New York *Tribune*, June 11, 1902, 6; "Captain O'Reilly Makes His Debut as a Lecturer," Brooklyn *Standard-Union*, June 10, 1902, 3.

65. "To Help on Cherry Hill," *Evening Post*, December 17, 1904, 6.

66. "Priest Accuses New York Police," *Chicago Tribune*, April 7, 1902; "Priest Flays Police Gang," *New York Press*, April 7, 1902, 2.

67. This pattern becomes clearer in subsequent years: When speaking out against unsupervised socializing on nearby piers, Curry clarified that he was not interested "in any but the one [pier] here in my parish." "Rowdyism on the Recreation Piers," *New York Herald*, June 8, 1904, 7. Curry issued similar disclaimers when cracking down on local saloons selling beer to children: "Fewer Tots Buy Liquor," *New-York Tribune*, August 8, 1905, 5.

68. As Curry explained the brothel closure to a reporter, "I had a political friend who enforced it on [Police] Commissioner Murphy." "Calls Priest's Charges Part of Political Plot," *World*, April 7, 1902, 6. Divver and Foley each served as the area's district leader during the early 1900s, with Foley defeating Divver in the 1902 municipal election. When Divver died several months later, his funeral filled Saint James with dozens of former and current Tammany-affiliated city officials. "Thousands at Divver's Bier," *Sun*, February 1, 1903, 6.

69. For example, in 1902, Curry complained to the mayor about mission workers taking advantage of the Jewish and Catholic children at the nearby Mariner's Temple, which was being used as a public school annex. "Church Used as School," *Sun*, November 28, 1902.

70. James B. Curry to Charlotte A. Waterbury, January 28, 1903, box 9, Jacob A. Riis Neighborhood Settlement Records, Manuscripts and Archives Division, New York Public Library.

71. "Changes in City Hall," *New York Times*, August 13, 1902, 3; "Secret Stairway in New York City Hall," *Los Angeles Herald*, July 31, 1903, 4.

72. *City Record* (New York), November 28, 1903, 9823; weather details from *Sun*, November 14, 1903, 3; "A Tammany Landslide," *New-York Tribune*, November 4, 1903, 1; "Sketches of the Successful Men," *Evening Telegram*, November 3, 1903, 3.

73. "Fight Is on Today to Abolish Lung Block," *World*, November 13, 1903, 6; "Would Save the 'Lung Block,'" *New York Times*, November 14, 1903.

74. "Fight Is on Today to Abolish Lung Block," 6.

75. "Example of Neighborhood Inertia," 566.

76. To arrive at a rough estimate of how many people living on the "Lung Block" belonged to Curry's parish in 1903, I counted residents from the 1900 census who were born in Ireland or Italy. In families with one Irish- or Italian-born spouse, I counted the children if their mother was Irish or Italian. This yielded a rough estimate of 1,800 out of 2,800 residents, or 64 percent. It is impossible to know how many of these residents were active members of Saint James Catholic Church; nevertheless, the 1,800 estimate is likely conservative, given that Ernest Poole estimated the block's total population to be nearly 4,000 three years later. Bureau of the US Census (1900), Manhattan, Enumeration District 62, 1–56; Poole, "Lung Block," 193.

77. "Would Save 'Lung Block,'" *New York Times*, November 14, 1903; "Example of Neighborhood Inertia," 567.

78. *City Record*, November 28, 1903, 9823–24.

79. *City Record*, November 28, 1903, 9823–24.

80. *City Record*, November 28, 1903, 9823–24. Emphasis added.

81. *City Record*, November 28, 1903, 9823–24.

82. *City Record*, November 28, 1903, 9823–24.

83. *City Record*, November 28, 1903, 9824.

84. "In War on Park Defends the 'Gap,'" *New York Herald*, November 14, 1903, 6.

85. "Millions to Widen Street," *New York Press*, November 14, 1903, 3; "Would Save the 'Lung Block,'" *New York Times*, November 14, 1903; "Poor Want Homes, Not Parks," *Sun*, November 14, 1903, 11.

86. "Attacked by a Priest," *New-York Tribune*, November 14, 1903, 4.

87. "Example of Neighborhood Inertia," 566–67.

88. The editorial then issued the tongue-in-cheek observation that "a habitual purchaser of reporters would laugh at the very idea of giving for them 'any price from a glass of beer to a dollar.' The regular rate is six reporters, three copy readers, and a city editor for a glass of beer, and for a dollar two managing editors, one editor-in-chief, a writer of paragraphs, the foreman of the composing room, and the head bookkeeper are always expected." "Topics of the Times," *New York Times*, November 16, 1903, 6.

89. "Example of Neighborhood Inertia," 567.

90. "Tenement House Babies," *World*, November 16, 1903.

91. "Topics of the Times," *New York Times*, November 18, 1903, 8.

92. "Example of Neighborhood Inertia," 567.

93. "Topics of the Times," *New York Times*, November 18, 1903, 8.

94. *New-York Daily Tribune*, December 8, 1903, 20; "Lung Block' Park Is De-

layed," *Evening Telegram*, December 4, 1903, 14; "No Park in 'Lung Block,'" *World*, December 4, 1903, 13; "To Continue Gas Fight," *New-York Daily Tribune*, December 5, 1903.

95. "Paragraphs in Philanthropy," 600–601.

96. These officials included Isaac Marks, who represented the block in city government as district alderman, and John F. Ahearn, the block's Tammany district leader. Ahearn, also the incoming Manhattan Borough president, had already made his disapproval of the project known to fellow Board of Estimate members. "'Lung Block' Park Is Delayed," *Evening Telegram*, December 4, 1903, 14; "No Park in 'Lung Block,'" *World*, December 4, 1903, 13; "To Continue Gas Fight," *New-York Daily Tribune*, December 5, 1903; "News of the Districts," *Tammany Times*, November 7, 1903, 10.

97. "Paragraphs in Philanthropy," 600.

98. "Paragraphs in Philanthropy," 600.

99. Poole to S. J. Mar, December 5, 1903, University Settlement Society of New York (USSNY), series 5, box 17, Wisconsin State Historical Society, Madison, WI. The *New York American* had already featured a similar pro-park piece submitted by fellow University Settlement resident James Graham Phelps Stokes several weeks earlier. "Asks 'American' to Help to Make 'Lung Block' a Park," *New York American*, November 14, 1903. Shortly before Poole's unsigned editorial appeared, Mar promised Stokes "to see that your movement gets full sway" in its coverage. Mar to Stokes, December 3, 1903, box 16, James G. Phelps Stokes Papers, Columbia Rare Book and Manuscript Library.

100. Curry to Archbishop Michael A. Corrigan, September 15, 1901, folder 13, box 21, Parish History Collection, AACNY.

101. Curry was not alone among New York's Catholic clergy in harboring these concerns. Archbishop Corrigan, known for his unyieldingly conservative interpretations of the church's role in modern American life, nevertheless supported tenement house reform publicly while Lawrence Veiller and others fought for stricter housing regulations in Albany. "Archbishop Corrigan Protests against Tenement System," *New York Journal*, March 27, 1901.

102. "Says 'Lung Block' Should be Cured," *New-York Tribune*, November 19, 1903.

103. "The Lung Block," *Sun*, November 16, 1903, 4.

104. The Fusion Party consisted of Republicans, anti-Tammany Democrats, German American political organizations, and the nonpartisan Citizens' Union. By 1903, Democrats felt that Low had gone too far in enforcing the city's blue laws and forfeited his claims to nonpartisanship by supporting Republicans for state and national elections. Meanwhile, Republicans felt Low had not gone far enough in enforcing the city's blue laws and resented his rewarding Democrats with more than a third of key government positions, despite Republicans having supplied 80 percent of the Fusion vote. Kurland, *Seth Low*, 147, 170–71. For a detailed analysis of the Low administration's strengths and weaknesses, see Swett, "Test of a Reformer."

105. In recent years, historians such as Kenneth Finegold, *Experts and Politicians*, have argued that Fusion's 1903 defeat reflected New Yorkers' return to preexisting voting patterns, rather than an explicit rejection of reform. Running in the incumbent position, however, necessarily placed Seth Low's reform-friendly administration and policies on the defensive—a situation that contemporary writers and previous historians have characterized as reform on trial. Swett, "Test of a Reformer," 21.

106. Low, *Seth Low*, 90.

107. Low's historians have characterized his 1901 mayoral victory as somewhat accidental, "less an endorsement of his brand of reform than a public reaction against the excesses of Tammany." Holli, "Social and Structural Reform," 227; Swett, "Test of a Reformer," 10–14, 16–18.

108. James E. Reynolds, a University Settlement worker who became Low's private secretary at City Hall, declined one supporter's request for patronage by explaining that it would be impossible, "*if Low desired to do so*, to reward one-fourth of those who rendered good service during the campaign." Swett, "Test of a Reformer," 21, emphasis added. This rigid denial of patronage not only failed to adequately reward his supporters but left the city government riddled with Tammany-appointed holdovers from previous administrations. Kurland, *Seth Low*, 147, 170–71.

109. "Personalities of Prominent People," *Successful American*, May 1903, 270.

110. "Leaders in the Fight for the City," *Independent*, October 29, 1903, 2565.

111. Lowry, "Reform Results in New York," 3907.

112. "President on Jerome's Charge," *World*, September 16, 1903, 1.

113. Steffens, "Good Government in Danger," 126–27. Low's 1903 mayoral opponent, George B. McClellan, shared similar impressions later: "Seth Low was entirely devoid of any sense of humor. Had he been a man of extraordinary ability, he might have overcome this terrible handicap, but unfortunately for him he was a dull, obstinate man with an excellent opinion of himself. He never could see a joke, especially at his own expense." McClellan, *Gentleman and the Tiger*, 171.

114. Villard, "Low Administration," 6. Forty percent of Low's appointments hailed from the native-born Protestant upper classes, and the proportion of them with job-oriented skills was lower in Low's administration than in those of his predecessor, Robert Van Wyck, or of any of his successors, reform or machine. Kurland, *Seth Low*, 146; Finegold, *Experts and Politicians*, 42.

115. When running for mayor in 1901, Low promised to interpret the law "in a liberal spirit and in a just one. All will have to obey the laws, but none will be oppressed by them." "Mark Twain and Seth Low Speak," *New York Times*, October 31, 1901. When Low later hired a new police commissioner who enforced the state excise law aggressively, Germans protested; "Low a Menace to the City," *Tammany Times*, May 16, 1903, 1. For a more extensive and nuanced discussion of the Low administration's vacillating position on the excise question, see Kurland, *Seth Low*, 149–57.

116. For a Tammany-centered critique of civil service, see Riordon, *Plunkitt of Tammany Hall*, 19–29.

117. "Low Administration Attacked," *New-York Tribune*, May 26, 1902, 4.

118. "Is Low the Only Candidate? Asks Spokesman for Reform," *New York Herald*, April 14, 1903, 5. The *Herald* described the author as "a man who took a conspicuous part in the reform movement of 1901 and whose views represented those of other influential reformers who participated in drafting the letter."

119. Wardman, "Men and Issues," 553

120. Steffens, "Good Government in Danger," 92.

121. Mulrine, *Price of Honor*, 44.

122. McClellan, *Gentleman and the Tiger*, 174.

123. "New City Administration," *Review of Reviews*, February 1902, 139; Kurland, *Seth Low*, 165–68.

124. "Leaders in the Fight for the City," *Independent*, October 29, 1903, 2565.

125. Throughout October of 1903, the *New-York Tribune* compared the legacies of Tammany unfavorably with reform administrations across a host of topics; see "Fruits of Reform Rule," *New-York Tribune*, October 7, 8, 9, 15, and 17, p. 3; October 13 and 20, p. 4. The *New York Press* ran a similar series titled "A Century of Tammany Graft," October 12–17, 19–24, 26–30.

126. "Sources of Tammany's Power," 420. These arbitrary, socially constructed distinctions have led twenty-first-century historians to view Irish American assimilation as more complicated than simply "becoming white"; it also involved the right to cultural pluralism, to forge American identities on their own terms. Golway, *Machine Made*, xx–xxi.

127. "A Century of Graft," *New York Press*, October 30, 1903, 6.

128. Steffens, "Good Government in Danger," 85.

129. Riis, "Has Reform Made Good?," 23.

130. "The Fusion Ticket," *New-York Tribune*, September 10, 1903, 8.

131. "Against a Fusion Ticket," *New York Times*, July 5, 1903.

132. "Plain People Will Defeat Low," *Brooklyn Daily Eagle*, October 28, 1903, 18.

133. "Against a Fusion Ticket," *New York Times*, July 5, 1903. This letter appeared in response to an editorial from June 14, which asked, "How could the leaders of any of the organizations that supported Mr. Low two years ago frame an excuse for not supporting the Reform candidate for mayor this year that would not instantly raise a public question as to their sanity or their morality?" *New York Times*, June 14, 1903, 6.

134. New York *Evening Journal*, November 2, 1903; quoted in Kurland, *Seth Low*, 192.

135. "McClellan Talks Excise and Low," *New York Herald*, October 21, 1903, 4.

136. "Several Reasons Why Seth Low Was Defeated," *Tammany Times*, November 7, 1903, 8.

137. "Democrats Sweep the City," *Evening Telegram*, November 3, 1903, 1.

138. "Tammany Buries Fusion under Avalanche of Votes," *New York Herald*, November 4, 1903, 3.

139. "Street Crowds Wild at Result," New York *Evening Telegram*, November 3, 1903, 1.

140. Low, *Seth Low*, 70–71.

141. "Fusion Banner Burned in Bowery," *New York Herald*, November 4, 1903, 4.

142. "Along the White Way it was a Night of Revelry," *New York Herald*, November 4, 1903, 3.

143. "McClellan and Tammany Win with a Plurality of 63,462 and New York Makes Merry," New York *Morning Telegraph*, November 4, 1903, 1.

144. Jacob A. Riis to Elgin Gould, November 7, 1903, Jacob A. Riis Collection, Duane Norman Diedrich Collection, William L. Clements Library, University of Michigan, Ann Arbor.

145. Theodore Roosevelt to Nicholas Murray Butler, November 4, 1903, in Morison, *Letters of Theodore Roosevelt*, 3:839.

146. The number of registered Fourth Assembly District voters in the first and second election districts with "Lung Block" addresses amounted to 54 percent, constituting a representative sample. "Transcript of the Enrollment Books for the Enrollment of 1905," *City Record*, December 30, 1905, supplement.

147. "Election Notice," *New-York Daily Tribune*, October 9, 1903, 13.

148. "Official Canvass of the County of New York," *City Record*, December 31, 1903, 9304, supplement; "Election Notice," *New-York Daily Tribune*, October 9, 1903, 13

149. "Transcript of the Enrollment Books for the Enrollment of 1905," *City Record*, December 30, 1905, supplement.

150. "Crain to His Critics," *Evening Post*, June 1904.

151. Riordon, *Plunkitt of Tammany Hall*, 168.

152. Riordon, *Plunkitt of Tammany Hall*, 168–69.

153. Stead, "Mr. Croker and Greater New York," 346.

154. Steffens, "Good Government in Danger," 89.

155. Addams, "Why the Ward Boss Rules," 880.

156. Riis, *Battle with the Slum*, 429–30.

157. Addams, "Why the Ward Boss Rules," 882.

158. Riis, *Battle with the Slum*, 429–30, 439.

159. "Priest on Pier Lovemaking," *New-York Tribune*, June 6, 1904, 8; "Against Selling Beer to Minors," *New-York Tribune*, July 23, 1905, 5; "Priest Tours Saloons in Children's Cause," *New York Times*, July 23, 1905; "Selling Rum to Minors: One Priest's Uphill Fight to Prevent It in His Parish," *Evening Post*, July 25, 1905, 1; "Children in Saloons," *New-York Tribune*, July 27, 1905, 6. Quotation from "Fewer Tots Buy Liquor," *New-York Tribune*, August 8, 1905, 5.

160. Curry's activism made headlines in other large cities: "Anti-growler Crusade," *Illustrated Buffalo Express*, August 27, 1905, 30; "Checking a Bad Trade," *Los Angeles Herald*, November 12, 1905, 4; "Practical Christianity," Duluth *News-Tribune*, August 27, 1905; "Cocaine Prohibited," Honolulu *Pacific Commercial Advertiser*, October 13,

1907, 6. In New York, his efforts also gained traction among Protestant-based groups like the Women's Christian Temperance Union, and eventually resulted in his being made a deputy sheriff. "Priest and Deputy Sheriff," *Sacred Heart Review*, October 12, 1912, 4; "Women Fight for Children," *New-York Tribune*, August 1, 1905, 5.

161. "Checks Cocaine Sale: New Law Operative," *New-York Tribune*, September 1, 1907, 10.

162. Curry, *What Settlement Clubs Stand For*, 7.

CONCLUSION: REDEMPTION(?) OF THE LUNG BLOCK

1. "Bad Tenement House Conditions Found," *New York Press*, November 21, 1906, 6; "Tenement Houses Foul," *New-York Daily Tribune*, November 16, 1906, 3.

2. Tenement House Department of the City of New York (THD), *Fourth Annual Report*, 191–92. These renovations were carried out under Edmond J. Butler, a New York City philanthropist, Democrat, and loyal Catholic who served as secretary of the city's Vincent De Paul Society. McClellan appointed Butler in 1905 to succeed Thomas Crain, a Tammany-backed attorney whose eighteen-month tenure had crippled the department's efficiency and given it a reputation for laxness and corruption. After former THD deputy commissioner Lawrence Veiller took McClellan on a tour of the most egregious Tenement House Law violations, McClellan replaced Crain with Butler, whom Veiller described as "an honest intelligent man of high ideals." Crain's swift dismissal reflects McClellan's growing rejection of Tammany influence late in his second term. Mulrine, *Price of Honor*, 112–13; Lawrence Veiller, "Reminiscences of Lawrence Veiller," 66–67, Oral History Collection, Columbia Rare Book and Manuscript Library (hereafter Columbia RBML); McClellan, *Gentleman and the Tiger*, 27n41, 234–39.

3. Dinwiddie, "Redemption of 'Lung Block,'" 581.

4. Finley, "Congestion of Manhattan," 15.

5. Arguing that "excessive incidence of tuberculosis on certain houses is no proof of house infection," public health official Charles V. Chapin identified "exposure to living cases . . . [as] a much more likely source of the disease than exposure to bacilli on the walls." Chapin, *Sources and Modes of Infection*, 178–79; also see Hillier, "Nature of the Infectivity of Phthisis," 596.

6. "To Show Congested New York to New Yorkers," *New York Press*, March 1, 1908, 1.

7. For example, in 1905, the CPT sent the city's Board of Estimate a copy of Robert de Forest's original letter from September 1903, reminding them that "so long as buildings known to be infected with tuberculosis are permitted to be occupied, just so long will the effort and the money spent by this city and by private citizens fail to accomplish commensurate results." Paul Kennaday (CPT secretary) to Mayor George B. McClellan, February 3, 1905, in Board of Estimate and Apportionment of the City of New York, *Minutes*, 518–19.

8. Special Committee of the Metropolitan Parks Association, "Report as to Playground Localities" (1905), box 28, Lillian D. Wald Papers, Columbia RBML. A basic description of the group's goals appears in Charity Organization Society of the City of New York (COSCNY), *Twenty-Third Annual Report*, 114–15.

9. "J .G. P. Stokes, Socialist," *Washington Post*, July 13, 1906, 4.

10. "Public School Teaching False, says Mr. Stokes," New York *Evening Telegram*, March 10, 1904, 6; "A Talk to Civitas," *New-York Tribune*, March 10, 1904, 7; "Should Use Its Eminent Domain," *New-York Tribune*, March 7, 1904, 4.

11. "The Lung Block and Bad Government," New York *World* (evening ed.), February 12, 1906, 10.

12. Pink, *Old Tenements and the New Law*, 10–11.

13. Jacob Riis "To Our Supporters" (pamphlet), 1908, Jacob A. Riis Neighborhood Settlement Records, Manuscripts and Archives Division, New York Public Library (hereafter NYPL).

14. James Curry, "What Settlement Clubs Stand For," 6–7, 9–10, box 9, Jacob A. Riis Neighborhood Settlement Records.

15. Riis, *Making of an American*, 272.

16. Riis, "What Settlements Stand For," 72.

17. Riis, *Making of an American*, 272–77.

18. Miller, *Emigrants and Exiles*, 332.

19. Mitchell, *Bottom of the Harbor*, 67.

20. "Knickerbocker Village," *Time*, October 15, 1934.; "Jones Here Urges 500-Acre Housing," *New York Times*, October 3, 1934, 23; Federal Writers Project, *WPA Guide to New York City*, 115.

21. "Mgr. J. B. Curry, Noted Pastor, Dead," *New York Times*, June 26, 1932, 30.

22. Veiller, "Reminiscences," 39. A contemporary newspaper article quoted Veiller as follows: "That the Federal Government should invade, not merely the fields of trade, but even of the municipalities throughout the country, and go into a given community and with Federal funds, taken from the citizens of other parts of the country through the taxing power, proceed to develop housing enterprises to serve as the homes of individual families, marks a most astounding departure from accepted principles of government." "A New City Landlord," *New York Times*, June 28, 1934, 22.

23. Poole, *Bridge*, 83.

24. Likewise, Lillian Wald made no public statements; yet she kept abreast of the project, accumulating a large clippings file on its progress. Box 43, Lillian D. Wald Papers, Manuscripts and Archives Division, NYPL.

25. The East Side Is Awakening to the Glory of Its Olden Days," *New York Times*, May 3, 1931, 23.

26. "$50,000,000 to Build Homes on East Side," *New York Times*, December 13, 1931, 1.

27. Page, *Creative Destruction of Manhattan*, 100–104; Fogelson, *Downtown*, 339.

28. French, "Housing in Lower Manhattan" (address to the Department of Eco-

nomics and Social Institutions, Princeton University, 24 April 1934), typescript, p. 8, quoted in Page, *Creative Destruction of Manhattan*, 101.

29. Box 3, folder 1, Fred F. French Companies Records, Manuscripts and Archives Division, NYPL.

30. Box 3, folder 1, Fred F. French Companies Records.

31. Box 3, folder 1, Fred F. French Companies Records.

32. Williams, "White Collar Neighbors," 78.

33. "Modern Housing Development Proposed in New York City through Loan of Reconstruction Finance Corporation to Fred. F. French Operators, Inc.," *Commercial and Financial Chronicle*, April 8, 1933, 2357–58.

34. Box 9, folder 1, Fred F. French Companies Records.

35. Williams, "White Collar Neighbors," 70–71.

36. Rosner, "RFC Subsidizes Fred F. French," 439.

37. "Slum Work Begun by Smith's Sledge," *New York Times*, October 11, 1933, 25; "Few in Slums Are Able to Try New Homes," *New York Times*, December 22, 1933, 23; "Jones Here Urges 500-Acre Housing," *New York Times*, October 3, 1934, 23.

38. War on Slums Proceeds Steadily," *New York Times*, June 17, 1934, 22; "Jones Here Urges 500-Acre Housing," 23; "Tenements," *Time*, April 2, 1934. "Knickerbocker Village," observes Max Page in *The Creative Destruction of Manhattan*, "revealed how the conflict between reformers and property owners could be mended with the introduction of the federal government into the housing business. Suddenly, slum clearance meant new profits." From then on, slum clearance "would no longer require the enthusiasm of a single, vociferous champion, but would become institutionalized in law in government programs and in state and federal budgets, driven forward not by revealing photographs but by planning logic" (87, 101).

39. "Jones Here Urges 500-Acre Housing," *New York Times*, October 3, 1934, 23; "Proceedings at Formal Opening of Knickerbocker Village, October 2, 1934," box 2, folder 9, Fred F. French Companies Records.

40. According to the statistical breakdown, 45 percent of displaced families had lived in the same "Lung Block" apartment for at least ten years prior to moving. Fred L. Lavanburg Foundation, *What Happened to 386 Families*, 2–3.

41. Williams, "White Collar Neighbors," 76–78.

BIBLIOGRAPHY

ARCHIVES

Alumnae Biographical Files. Wellesley College Archives, Clapp Library, Wellesley College, Wellesley, MA

Columbia Rare Book and Manuscript Library, New York
> Community Service Society (CSS) Collection
> Oral History Collection
> Stokes, James G. Phelps. Papers
> Wald, Lillian F. Papers

National Archives and Records Administration (NARA), Washington, DC

New-York Historical Society

New York City Municipal Archives

New York Public Library
> Fred F. French Companies Records. Manuscripts and Archives Division
> Gilder, Richard Watson. Papers. Manuscript and Archives Division
> Jacob A. Riis Neighborhood Settlement Records. Manuscripts and Archives Division
> Lionel Pincus and Princess Firyal Map Division
> Riis, Jacob A. Papers. Manuscript and Archives Division
> Wald, Lillian D. Papers. Manuscripts and Archives Division

Parish History Collection, Archives of the Archdiocese of the City of New York (AACNY)

Riis, Jacob A. Collection. Duane Norman Diedrich Collection, William L. Clements Library, University of Michigan, Ann Arbor

Riis, Jacob A. Papers. Library of Congress, Washington, DC

Russell Sage Collection, City College of New York Archives

University Settlement Society of New York (USSNY). Wisconsin State Historical Society, Madison, WI

BIBLIOGRAPHY

NEWSPAPERS

Boston Transcript
Brooklyn Daily Eagle
Chicago Daily Tribune
Chicago Times
Chicago Times-Herald
Chicago Tribune
Columbia Republican (Hudson, NY)
Commercial Advertiser (New York)
Commercial and Financial Chronicle
Daily News (Batavia, NY)
Daily News (New York)
Evening Express (New York)
Evening Herald (Duluth)
Evening Journal (New York)
Evening Post (New York)
Evening Sun (New York)
Evening Telegram (New York)
Herald Tribune (New York)
Illustrated Buffalo Express
Independent
Indianapolis News
Jamaica (L.I.) Times
Jamestown (NY) Journal
Los Angeles Herald
Mail and Express (New York)
Mercury (New Bedford, MA)
Morning Courier and New-York Enquirer (New York)
Morning Telegraph (New York)
New York American
New York Herald
New York Journal
New York Morning Journal
New York Observer
New York Post
New York Press
New York Times
News-Tribune (Duluth)
New-York Daily Tribune
New-York Tribune

Pacific Commercial Advertiser (Honolulu)

San Francisco Chronicle

Stamford Community News

Standard-Union (Brooklyn)

Sun (New York)

Sunday Mercury (New York)

Tammany Times

Washington Post

Washington Star

World (New York)

ANNUAL REPORTS

Brandt, Lilian. *Charity Organization Society of the City of New York, 1882–1907, Twenty-Fifth Annual Report.* New York: Charity Organization Society, 1907.

Charity Organization Society of the City of New York (COSCNY). *Eighteenth Annual Report.* New York: Charity Organization Society, 1900.

Charity Organization Society of the City of New York (COSCNY). *First Annual Report of the Committee on the Prevention of Tuberculosis.* New York: Charity Organization Society, 1903.

Charity Organization Society of the City of New York (COSCNY). *A Handbook for the Prevention of Tuberculosis.* New York: Charity Organization Society, 1903.

Charity Organization Society of the City of New York (COSCNY). *Twentieth Annual Report.* New York: Charity Organization Society, 1902.

Charity Organization Society of the City of New York (COSCNY). *Twenty-First Annual Report.* New York: Charity Organization Society, 1903.

Charity Organization Society of the City of New York (COSCNY). *Twenty-Third Annual Report.* New York: Charity Organization Society, 1905.

College Settlements Association. *Seventeenth Annual Report.* New York: A. G. Sherwood, 1906.

Department of Health of the City of New York. *Annual Report for 1902.* New York: Martin B. Brown, 1904.

Department of Health of the City of New York. *Annual Report of the Board of Health of the Health Department of the City of New York for the Year Ending December 31, 1893.* New York: Martin B. Brown, 1897.

Department of Health of the City of New York. *Annual Report of the Board of Health of the Health Department of the City of New York for the Year Ending December 31, 1896.* New York: Martin B. Brown, 1897.

Griscom, John H. *Annual Report of the Interments in the City and County of New-York, for the Year 1842, with Remarks thereon, and a Brief View of the Sanitary Condition of the City.* New York: James Van Norden, 1843.

New York Association for the Improvement of the Condition of the Poor (NYAICP). *Fifteenth Annual Report*. New York: John F. Trow, 1858.

New York Association for the Improvement of the Condition of the Poor (NYAICP). *First Report of a Committee on the Sanitary Condition of the Laboring Classes in New York*. New York: John F. Trow, 1853.

New York Association for the Improvement of the Condition of the Poor (NYAICP). *Fourteenth Annual Report*. New York: John F. Trow, 1857.

New York Association for the Improvement of the Condition of the Poor (NYAICP). *Fourth Annual Report*. New York: John F. Trow, 1847.

New York Association for the Improvement of the Condition of the Poor (NYAICP). *Ninth Annual Report*. New York: John F. Trow, 1852.

New York Association for the Improvement of the Condition of the Poor (NYAICP). *Seventeenth Annual Report*. New York: John F. Trow, 1860.

New York Board of Education. *46th Annual Report*. New York: De Leeuw & Oppenheimer, 1887.

New York Board of Education. *49th Annual Report*. New York: De Leeuw & Oppenheimer, 1891.

New York City Board of Health. *Reports of Hospital Physicians*. New York: 1832.

New York State Senate. *Documents of the Senate of the State of New York, One Hundred and Eighth Session*. Albany: Weed, Parsons, 1885.

Smith, Stephen. "Report of the Sanitary Committee." In *Second Annual Report of the Board of Health of the Health Department, City of New York*, 333–47. New York: David H. Gildersleeve, 1872.

Tenement House Department of the City of New York (THD). *First Annual Report*. New York: Martin B. Brown, 1903.

Tenement House Department of the City of New York (THD). *Fourth Annual Report*. New York: Martin B. Brown, 1908.

University of the State of New York. *92nd Annual Report of the Regents*. Albany: Van Benthuysen & Sons, 1879.

University of the State of New York. *101st Annual Report of the Regents*. Albany: Troy, 1888.

University of the State of New York. *104th Annual Report of the Regents*. Albany: James. B. Lyon, 1892.

PRIMARY AND SECONDARY SOURCES

Abel, Emily K. "Medicine and Morality: The Health Care Program of the New York Charity Organization Society." *Social Service Review* 71, no. 4 (1997): 634–51.

Abel, Emily K. *Tuberculosis and the Politics of Exclusion: A History of Public Health and Migration to Los Angeles*. New Brunswick, NJ: Rutgers University Press, 2007.

Abrams, Jeanne E. "'Spitting Is Dangerous, Indecent, and Against the Law!': Legislating Health Behavior during the American Tuberculosis Crusade." *Journal of the History of Medicine and Allied Sciences* 68, no. 3 (2013): 416–50.

Adams, Henry. *The Education of Henry Adams.* Boston: Houghton Mifflin, 1918.

Addams, Jane. *Twenty Years at Hull House.* New York: Macmillan, 1910.

Addams, Jane. "Why the Ward Boss Rules." *Outlook* 58 (1898): 880.

Albion, Robert. *The Rise of New York Port, 1815–1860.* New York: Charles Scribner's Sons, 1939.

"Alumnae Notes." *Wellesley Magazine* 4, no. 6 (March 14, 1896), 349–56.

"Alumnae Notes." *Wellesley Magazine* 6, no. 6 (March 19, 1898), 307–13.

"Alumnae Notes." *Wellesley Magazine* 7, no. 8 (May 20, 1899), 446–48.

American College and Public School Directory. Saint Louis: C. H. Evans, 1897.

Anbinder, Tyler. *City of Dreams: The 400-Year Epic History of Immigrant New York.* Boston: Mariner Books, 2016.

Anbinder, Tyler. *Five Points: The 19th-Century New York City Neighborhood That Invented Tap Dance, Stole Elections, and Became the World's Most Notorious Slum.* New York: Plume, 2001.

"Bacteriology in Medical Colleges." *Bacteriological World and Modern Medicine* 1, no. 6 (April 1892): 210–11.

Barbuto, Domenica M. *American Settlement Houses and Progressive Social Reform: An Encyclopedia of the American Settlement Movement.* Phoenix, AZ: Oryx, 1999.

Bates, Barbara. *Bargaining for Life: A Social History of Tuberculosis, 1876–1938.* Philadelphia: University of Pennsylvania Press, 1992.

Bayley, J. R. *A Brief Sketch of the Early History of the Catholic Church on the Island of New York.* New York: Catholic Publication Society, 1870.

Bederman, Gail. *Manliness and Civilization: A Cultural History of Gender and Race in the United States, 1880–1917.* Chicago: University of Chicago Press, 1995.

Bender, Thomas. *Toward an Urban Vision: Ideas and Institutions in Nineteenth-Century America.* Baltimore, MD: Johns Hopkins University Press, 1975.

Betts, Lillian W. "The Tenement-House Exhibit." *Outlook* 64 (1900): 589–92.

Biggs, Hermann. "History of the Recent Outbreak of Epidemic Cholera in New York." *American Journal of the Medical Sciences* 105 (1893): 63–72.

Biggs, Hermann. "The Municipal Sanatorium at Otisville." *Monthly Bulletin of the Department of Health of the City of New York* 2 (1912): 265–83.

Biggs, Hermann. "Preventive Medicine in the City of New York." *British Medical Journal* 2 (1897): 629–38.

Biggs, Hermann. "The Registration of Tuberculosis." *Philadelphia Medical Journal* 6 (1900): 1023–29.

Biggs, Hermann. "To Rob Consumption of Its Terrors." *Forum* 16 (1894): 758–67.

Biggs, Hermann. "Tuberculosis and the Tenement House Problem." In *The Tenement House Problem,* ed. Robert W. de Forest and Lawrence Veiller, vol. 1, 447–55. New York: Lea & Febiger, 1901.

BIBLIOGRAPHY

Biggs, Hermann. "Tuberculosis—Causation and Prevention." In Charity Organization Society of the City of New York, *Handbook for the Prevention of Tuberculosis*, 153–69.

Biggs, Hermann, and John Henry Huddleston. "The Sanitary Supervision of Tuberculosis as Practised by the New York City Board of Health." *American Journal of Medical Science* 109, no. 1 (1895): 109.

Blake, Angela M. *How New York Became American, 1890–1924*. Baltimore, MD: Johns Hopkins University Press, 2006.

Blancher, David Anthony. "Workshops of the Bacterial Revolution: A History of the Laboratories of the New York City Department of Health, 1892–1912." PhD diss., City University of New York, 1979.

Board of Estimate and Apportionment of the City of New York. *Minutes of the Board of Estimate and Apportionment* 1 (1905): 520.

Bocock, Kemper. "Tenement Houses and their Tenants." *Social Economist* 6 (1894): 111.

Bonner, Thomas Neville. *American Doctors and German Universities: A Chapter in International Intellectual Relations, 1870–1914*. Lincoln: University of Nebraska Press, 1963.

Bonner, Thomas Neville. *Becoming a Physician: Medical Education in Britain, France, Germany, and the United States, 1750–1945*. New York: Oxford University Press, 1995.

Boyer, Paul. *Urban Masses and Moral Order in America, 1820–1920*. Cambridge, MA: Harvard University Press, 1978.

"Brandt, John Baughman." In *Encyclopedia of American Biography of the Nineteenth Century*, ed. Thomas W. Herringshaw, 142. Chicago: American Publishers' Association, 1905.

Brandt, Lilian. "Characteristics of Social Work in the United States." *Chautauquan* 60 (1910): 102–12.

Brandt, Lilian. "The Negroes of St. Louis." *Publications of the American Statistical Association* 8 (1903): 203–68.

Brandt, Lilian. "Social Aspects of Tuberculosis." *Annals of the American Academy of Political and Social Science* 21, no. 3 (1903): 65–76.

Brandt, Lilian. "The Social Aspects of Tuberculosis Based on a Study of Statistics." In Charity Organization Society of the City of New York, *Handbook for the Prevention of Tuberculosis*, 29–115.

Brandt, Lilian. "Wanted: A Breathing Space." *Charities* 11 (1903): 200–205.

Brandt, Lilian. "Report of the Committee on Social Research." In Charity Organization Society of the City of New York, *Annual Report* 23 (1904–05): 86.

Brann, Henry A. *History of the American College of the Roman Catholic Church of the United States, Rome, Italy*. New York: Benziger Brothers, 1910.

"British and Continental Characteristics." *North British Review* 21, no. 41 (May 1854): 45–68.

BIBLIOGRAPHY

Brooks, Van Wyck. *Autobiography*. New York: E. P. Dutton, 1965.

Browne, Junius Henri. *The Great Metropolis: A Mirror of New York*. Hartford: American Publishing, 1869.

Brownson, Orestes. "Native Americanism." *Brownson's Quarterly Review* 2 (1845): 76–98.

Bullough, Bonnie, and George Rosen. *Preventive Medicine in the United States, 1900–1990: Trends and Interpretations*. Canton, MA: Science History Publications, 1992.

Burrows, Edwin G., and Mike Wallace. *Gotham: A History of New York City to 1898*. New York: Oxford University Press, 1999.

Cadman, S. Parkes. "Tenement House Reform in New York City." *Chautauquan* 25 (1897): 587–92.

Camp, Stephanie M. H. *Closer to Freedom: Enslaved Women and Everyday Resistance in the Plantation South*. Chapel Hill: University of North Carolina Press, 2004.

Carey, Patrick W. *Catholics in America: A History*. Westport, CT; Praeger, 2004.

Carr, Ethan. *Wilderness by Design: Landscape Architecture and the National Park Service*. Lincoln: University of Nebraska Press, 1998.

Carson, Mina. *Settlement Folk: Social Thought and the American Settlement Movement, 1885–1930*. Chicago: University of Chicago Press, 1990.

Casino, Joseph. "From Sanctuary to Involvement: A History of the Catholic Parish in the Northeast." In *The American Catholic Parish: A History from 1850 to the Present*, edited by Jay Dolan, vol. 1, 7–116. New York: Paulist, 1987.

"The Causation of Pulmonary Consumption." *Science* 7, no. 155 (1886): 86–88.

Chadwick, Edwin. *Report on the Sanitary Condition of the Labouring Population of Great Britain*. London: W. Clowes and Sons, 1843.

Chambers, Clarke A. "Women in the Creation of the Profession of Social Work." *Social Service Review* 60, no. 1 (1986): 1–33.

Chapin, Charles V. "The End of the Filth Theory of Disease." *Popular Science Monthly* 60, no. 3 (1902): 234–39.

Chapin, C[harles]. V. "The Fetich of Disinfection." *Journal of the American Medical Association* 47, no. 8 (1906): 574–77.

Chapin, Charles V. *The Sources and Modes of Infection*. New York: John Wiley & Sons, 1910.

Chapin, Charles. "Tribute to Dr. Biggs from Some of His Colleagues." *Health News* 18, no. 7 (1923): 178–79.

Chapin, Charles V. *What Changes Has the Acceptance of the Germ Theory Made in Measures for the Prevention of Consumption?* Providence, RI: Providence, 1888.

"Child Labor Reform in New York." *Charities* 10, no. 2 (1903): 52–56.

City of New York. *Report of Committee on Small Parks*. New York: Martin B. Brown, 1897.

Claghorn, Kate Holladay. "The Problem of Occupation for College Women." *Education Review* 15 (1898): 217–25.

BIBLIOGRAPHY

Claghorn, Kate Holladay. "The Use and Misuse of Statistics in Social Work." *Publications of the American Statistical Association* 11, no. 82 (1908): 150–67.

Clark, Dennis. *Hibernia America: The Irish and Regional Cultures.* Westport, CT: Greenwood, 1986.Coleman, Thomas. "Tuberculosis among the Dark-Skinned Races." In *Tuberculosis: A Treatise by American Authors*, edited by Eugene Klebs, 118–30. New York: Appleton, 1909.

Coman, Katharine E. "Influence of the College Settlement." *Wellesley Magazine* 6 (1897): 53–58.

Coman, Katharine E. "Preparation for Citizenship at Wellesley College." *Education* 10 (1890): 341–47.

Comstock, George W. "Frost Revisited: The Modern Epidemiology of Tuberculosis." *American Journal of Epidemiology* 101, no. 5 (1975): 363–82.

Condran, Gretchen A., and Eileen Crimmins. "A Description and Evaluation of Mortality Data in the Federal Census, 1850–1900." *Historical Methods* 12, no. 1 (1979): 1–23.

Cornet, Georg. "Uber das Verhalten der Tuberkelbazillen Im Tierischen Organismus unter dem Einfluss entwicklungshemmen der Stoffe." *Zeitschrift fur Hygiene und Infektions krankheiten* 5 (1888): 98–133.

Cornet, Georg. *Ueber Tuberculose.* Leipzig: Veit, 1890.

Council of Hygiene, Citizens Association of New York. *Report.* New York: 1865.

Craddock, Susan. *City of Plagues: Disease, Poverty, and Deviance in San Francisco.* Minneapolis: University of Minnesota Press, 2000.

Crocker, Ruth Hutchinson. *Social Work and Social Order: The Settlement Movement in Two Industrial Cities, 1889–1930.* Urbana: University of Illinois Press, 1992.

Crosby, Howard. "A Letter to the People of New York." *Forum* 2 (1886): 420–28.

Curry, James B. *What Settlement Clubs Stand For.* New York: Italian-American Press, 1909.

Curtis, L. Perry. *Apes and Angels: The Irishman in Victorian Caricature.* Washington, DC: Smithsonian Institution Press, 1977.

Davis, Allen. *Spearheads for Reform: The Social Settlements and the Progressive Movement 1890–1914.* New Brunswick, NJ: Rutgers University Press, 1967.

Davis, N. S. "Report of the Committee on Practical Medicine and Epidemics." *Journal of the American Medical Association* 1 (1883): 409–16.

Dawley, Alan. *Changing the World: American Progressives in War and Revolution.* Princeton, NJ: Princeton University Press, 2005.

Day, Jared N. *Urban Castles: Tenement Housing and Landlord Activism in New York City, 1890–1943.* New York: Columbia University Press, 1999.

de Forest, Robert W. "Tenement House Regulation: The Reasons for It—Its Proper Limitations." *Annals of the American Academy of Political and Social Science* 20, no. 1 (1902): 83–95.

de Forest, Robert Weeks, and Lawrence Veiller, eds. *The Tenement House Problem: In-*

cluding the Report of the New York State Tenement House Commission of 1900. New York: Macmillan, 1903.

Department of Health of the City of New York. *The Action of the Health Department in Relation to Pulmonary Tuberculosis.* Albany: Wynkoop Hallenbeck Crawford, 1897.

Devine, Edward T. *When Social Work Was Young.* New York: Macmillan, 1939.

Diner, Hasia R. *Erin's Daughters in America: Irish Immigrant Women in the Nineteenth Century.* Baltimore, MD: Johns Hopkins University Press, 1983.

Diner, Hasia R. "'The Most Irish City in the Union': The Great Migration, 1844–1877." In *The New York Irish,* edited by Ronald H. Bayor and Timothy J. Meagher, 87–106. Baltimore, MD: Johns Hopkins University Press, 1996.

Dinwiddie, Emily. "The Redemption of 'Lung Block.'" *Charities* 20 (1908): 579–81.

Dolan, Jay P. *The American Catholic Experience: A History from Colonial Times to the Present.* Garden City, NY: Doubleday, 1985.

Dolan, Jay P. *The American Catholic Parish: A History from 1850 to the Present.* New York: Paulist, 1987.

Dolan, Jay P. *The Immigrant Church: New York's Irish and German Catholics, 1815–1865.* South Bend, IN: University of Notre Dame Press, 1975.

Dolan, Jay P. *The Irish Americans: A History.* New York: Bloomsbury, 2008.

Downing, Andrew. "The New York Park." In *First Annual Report on the Improvement of the Central Park,* by New York Board of Commissioners of Central Park, 159–64. New York: Charles W. Baker, 1857.

Downing, Andrew. "Public Cemeteries and Public Gardens." *Horticulturalist* 4, no. 1 (1849): 1–12.

Downing, Andrew. "A Talk about Public Parks and Gardens." *Horticulturalist* 3, no. 4 (1848): 154–56.Draper, William H. "On the Relations of Scientific and Practical Medicine." *Transactions of the Association of American Physicians* 3 (1888): 1–8.

Duffy, John. *A History of Public Health in New York City, 1625–1866.* New York: Russell Sage Foundation, 1966.

Duffy, John. *A History of Public Health in New York City, 1866–1966.* New York: Russell Sage Foundation, 1968.

Duffy, John. *The Sanitarians: A History of American Public Health.* Urbana: University of Illinois Press, 1990.

Dunglison, Robley. *A Dictionary of Medical Science.* Philadelphia: Henry C. Lea, 1874.

Erie, Steven P. *Rainbow's End: Irish-Americans and the Dilemmas of Urban Machine Politics, 1840–1985.* Berkeley: University of California Press, 1988.

"An Example of Neighborhood Inertia." *Charities* 11, no. 24 (1903): 566–67.

"The Extent of the Anti-tuberculosis Crusade." *Charities* 8, no. 20 (1902): 452–55.

Ernst, Robert. *Immigrant Life in New York City, 1825–1863.* New York: King's Crown, 1949.

BIBLIOGRAPHY

Fairbanks, Robert B. "From Better Dwellings to Better Neighborhoods: The Rise and Fall of the First National Housing Movement." In *From Tenements to the Taylor Homes: In Search of an Urban Housing Policy in Twentieth-Century America*, edited by John F. Bauman, Roger Biles, and Kristin M. Szylvian, 21–29. University Park: Pennsylvania State University Press, 2010.

Faver, Catherine A. "Creative Apostle of Reconciliation: The Spirituality and Social Philosophy of Emily Greene Balch." *Women's Studies* 18, no. 4 (1991): 335–51.

Federal Writers Project. *The WPA Guide to New York City*. New York: Random House, 1939.

Fee, Elizabeth, and Evelynn M. Hammonds. "Science, Politics, and the Art of Persuasion: Promoting the New Scientific Medicine in New York City." *Hives of Sickness: Public Health and Epidemics in New York City*, edited by David Rosner, 155–198. New Brunswick, NJ: Rutgers University Press, 1995.

Finegold, Kenneth. *Experts and Politicians: Reform Challenges to Machine Politics in New York, Cleveland, and Chicago*. Princeton, NJ: Princeton University Press, 1995.

Finley, Harold M. "The Congestion of Manhattan." *Federation* 5, no. 3 (1908): 10–18.

Fishberg, Maurice. "Health Problems of the Jewish Poor." *Menorah* 35 (1903): 79–93.

Fitzpatrick, Ellen. *Endless Crusade: Women Social Scientists and Progressive Reform*. New York: Oxford University Press, 1990.

Flagg, Ernest. "The New York Tenement-House Evil and Its Cure." *Scribner's Magazine* 16, no. 1 (July 1894): 108–17.

Flanagan, Maureen A. "The City Profitable, the City Livable: Environmental Policy, Gender, and Power in Chicago in the 1910s." *Journal of Urban History* 22, no. 2 (1996): 163–90.

Flexner, Simon. *William Henry Welch and the Heroic Age of American Medicine*. New York: Viking, 1941.

Flick, Lawrence. "The Contagiousness of Phthisis (Tubercular Pulmonitis)." *Transactions of the Medical Society of the State of Pennsylvania* 20 (1888): 164–86.

Flick, Lawrence. *The Control of Tuberculosis*. Philadelphia: Clarence M. Busch, 1897.

Flick, Lawrence. "Discussion on the Advisability of the Registration of Tuberculosis." *Transactions of the College of Physicians in Philadelphia* 16 (1894): 1–27.

Flick, Lawrence. "House Infection of Tuberculosis." *Medical News* 84 (1904): 345–50.

Flint, Austin. *A Treatise on the Principles and Practice of Medicine*. Philadelphia: H. C. Lea, 1881.

Flügge, Carl. "Die Verbreitung der Phthise durch staubtörmiges Sputum und durch beim Husten verspritzte Tröpfchen," *Zeitschrift fur Hygiene und Infektionskrankheiten* 30 (1899): 107–24.

Fogelson, Robert M. *Downtown: Its Rise and Fall, 1880–1950*. New Haven, CT: Yale University Press, 2001.

Folks, Homer. "Reports from States: New York." In *Proceedings of the National Con-*

ference of Charities and Correction, Twenty-Third Annual Session, 71–78. Boston: George H. Ellis, 1896.

Formad, H. F. "The Bacillus Tuberculosis and the Aetiology of Tuberculosis: Is Consumption Contagious?" *Journal of the American Medical Association* 2, no. 6 (1884): 141–51.

Formad, H. F. "The Bacillus Tuberculosis and the Aetiology of Tuberculosis: Is Consumption Contagious? Second Communication." *Journal of the American Medical Association* 2, no. 17 (1884): 449–63. https://jamanetwork.com/journals/jama/article-abstract/422370

Fox, Daniel M. "Social Policy and City Politics: Tuberculosis Reporting in New York, 1889–1900." *Bulletin of the History of Medicine* 49, no. 2 (1975): 169–95.

Frankfort, Roberta. *Collegiate Women: Domesticity and Career in Turn-of-the-Century America.* New York: New York University Press, 1977.

Fred L. Lavanburg Foundation. *What Happened to 386 Families Who Were Compelled to Vacate Their Slum Dwellings to Make Way for a Large Housing Project.* New York: Fred L. Lavanburg Foundation, 1933.

Friess, Horace L. *Felix Adler and Ethical Culture: Memories and Studies.* New York: Columbia University Press, 1981.

Fronc, Jennifer. *New York Undercover: Private Surveillance in the Progressive Era.* Chicago: University of Chicago Press, 2009.

Gaertner, Frederick. "The Microscope from a Medical, Medico-Legal, and Legal Point of View." *Arena* 4 (1891): 615–16.

Gallatin, James. "Tenement House Reform in the City of New York." In American Public Health Association, *Public Health Papers and Reports,* vol. 6, 309–17 (Boston: Franklin, 1881).Gallup, George. *The Gallup Poll,* vol. 1, 1935–48. New York: Random House, 1972.

Gandal, Keith. *Virtues of the Vicious: Jacob Riis, Stephen Crane, and the Spectacle of the Slum.* New York: Oxford University Press, 1997.

Gilfoyle, Timothy J. *City of Eros: New York City, Prostitution, and the Commercialization of Sex, 1790–1920.* New York: W. W. Norton, 1992.

Golway, Terry. *Machine Made: Tammany Hall and the Creation of Modern American Politics.* New York: Liveright, 2014.

Gompers, Samuel. *Seventy Years of Life and Labor: An Autobiography,* vol. 1. New York: E. P. Dutton, 1925.

Gorham, Frederic P. "The History of Bacteriology and Its Contribution to Public Health Work." In *A Half Century of Public Health: Jubilee Historical Volume of the American Public Health Association,* edited by Mazÿck P. Ravenel, 66–93. New York: American Public Health Association, 1921.

Gould, Elgin. "The Housing Problem in Great Cities." *Quarterly Journal of Economics* 14, no. 3 (1900): 378–93.

Gould, Elgin. "The Only Cure for Slums." *Forum* 19 (1895): 495–500.

BIBLIOGRAPHY

Gould, E[lgin] R. L. "Park Areas and Open Spaces in Cities." *Publications of the American Statistical Association* 1, no. 2/3 (1888): 49–61.

Graham, Frank. *Al Smith, American: An Informal Biography.* New York: G. P. Putnam's Sons, 1945.

Greg, W. R. "Life at High Pressure." *Contemporary Review,* vol. 25, March 1875, 623–35.

Greeley, Dawn M. *Beyond Benevolence: The New York Charity Organization Society and the Transformation of American Social Welfare, 1882–1935.* Bloomington: Indiana University Press, 2022.

Green, Harvey. *Fit for America; Health, Fitness, Sport, and American Society.* Baltimore, MD: Johns Hopkins University Press, 1986.

Griscom, John H. *The Sanitary Condition of the Laboring Population of New York.* New York: Harper & Brothers, 1845.

Guerard, Arthur R. "Relation of Tuberculosis to the Tenement House Problem." In *The Tenement House Problem,* edited by Robert W. de Forest and Lawrence Veiller, vol. 1, 461–70. New York: Macmillan, 1903.

Guerard, Arthur R. "Report on the Distribution of Tuberculosis in New York City." In *The Action of the Health Department in Relation to Pulmonary Tuberculosis,* Board of Health of the City of New York, 34–46. Albany: Wynkoop Hallenbeck Crawford, 1897.

Hague, Mary, and Nancy Siegel. "Municipal Parks in New York City: Olmsted, Riis, and the Transformation of the Urban Landscape, 1858–1897." In *Transformations of Urban and Suburban Landscapes: Perspectives from Philosophy, Geography, and Architecture,* edited by Gary Backhaus and John Murungi. New York: Lexington Books, 2002, 153–91.

Hammack, David C. "Nonprofit Organizations, Philanthropy, and Civil Society." In *A Companion to the Gilded Age and Progressive Era,* edited by Christopher McKnight Nichols and Nancy C. Unger, 215–28. Malden, MA: John Wiley and Sons, 2017.

Hammack, David C. *Power and Society: Greater New York at the Turn of the Century.* New York: Russell Sage Foundation, 1982.

Hammonds, Evelynn Maxine. *Childhood's Deadly Scourge: The Campaign to Control Diphtheria in New York City, 1880–1930.* Baltimore, MD: Johns Hopkins University Press, 1999.

Handbook of the American Academy of Political and Social Science. Philadelphia: American Academy of Political and Social Science, 1901.

Hapgood, Norman, and Henry Moskowitz. *Up from the City Streets: A Life of Alfred E. Smith.* New York: Grosset and Dunlap, 1927.

Harley, J. B. "Deconstructing the Map." *Cartographica* 26, no. 2 (1989): 1–20.

Hart, Lavina, and Alice Katherine Fallows. "Women's Colleges and Their Student Life." *Bay View Magazine* 15 (1907): 165–78.

Harvey, David. *Justice, Nature, and the Geography of Difference*. Oxford: Blackwell, 1996.

"The Health Board and Compulsory Reports," *Medical Record* 51, no. 3 (1897): 126–27.

Heap, Chad. *Slumming: Sexual and Racial Encounters in American Nightlife, 1885–1940*. Chicago: University of Chicago Press, 2009.

Hijiya, James A. "Four Ways of Looking at a Philanthropist: A Study of Robert Weeks de Forest." *Proceedings of the American Philosophical Society* 124, no. 6 (1980): 404–18.

Hillier, Alfred. "The Nature of the Infectivity of Phthisis: A Study of the Views of Koch, Flügge, and Others." *British Medical Journal* 1, no. 2202 (1903): 593–96.

Hobsbawm, Eric J. *The Age of Capital, 1848–1875*. New York: Scribner, 1975.

Hoffman, Frederick L. "Industrial Insurance and the Prevention of Tuberculosis." *Medical Examiner* 11 (1901): 692–720.

Hofstadter, Richard. *The Age of Reform: From Bryan to F.D.R.* New York: Vintage Books, 1955.

Holli, Melvin G. "Social and Structural Reform." In *Bosses and Reformers: Urban Politics in America, 1880–1920*, edited by Blaine A. Brownell and Warren E. Stickle, 220–43. Boston: Houghton Mifflin, 1973.

Holt, L. Emmett. "Tribute to Dr. Biggs from Some of His Colleagues." *Health News* 18 (1923): 170.

"Honors, 1901–02." In *Princeton University Catalogue*, 297–304. Princeton, NJ: Princeton University Press, 1903.

Horowitz, Helen Lefkowitz. *Alma Mater: Design and Experience in the Women's Colleges from Their Nineteenth-Century Beginnings to the 1930s*. New York: Knopf, 1984.

Howe, Samuel. "Parks for Street Dwellers." *Harper's Weekly*, April 18, 1903, 637.

Howells, W. D. *Impressions and Experiences*. New York: Harper and Brothers, 1896.

Hunter, Robert. "The Relation between Social Settlements and Charity Organization." *Journal of Political Economy* 11, no. 1 (1902): 75–88.

Hunter, Tera W. *To 'Joy My Freedom: Southern Black Women's Lives and Labors after the Civil War*. Cambridge, MA: Harvard University Press, 1997.

Hutchinson, Woods. *Preventable Diseases*. Boston: Houghton Mifflin, 1909.

Jacobi, Abraham. "Inaugural Address." *Transactions of the New York Academy of Medicine* 6 (1885): 163–64.

Jacobi, Abraham. "Tuberculosis and Children." In Charity Organization Society of the City of New York, *Handbook for the Prevention of Tuberculosis*, 207–24.

Jacobson, Matthew Frye. *Barbarian Virtues: The United States Encounters Foreign Peoples at Home and Abroad, 1876–1917*. New York: Hill and Wang, 2000.

Johnson, Willis Fletcher. "Marks, Isaac, 1875–." In *New York University: Its History, Influence, Equipment, and Characteristics*, edited by Joshua L. Chamberlain, vol. 2, 463–64. Boston: R. Herndon, 1903.

Johnston, Andrew M. "The Disappearance of Emily G. Balch, Social Scientist." *Journal of the Gilded Age and Progressive Era* 13, no. 2 (2014): 166–99.

Jordan, E. O., G. C. Whipple, and C.-E. A. Winslow. *A Pioneer of Public Health: William Thompson Sedgwick.* New Haven, CT: Yale University Press, 1924.

Juvenile Court of the City and County of Denver. *The Problem of the Children and How Colorado Cares for Them.* Denver, CO: Merchants, 1904.

Kasson, John F. *Amusing the Million: Coney Island at the Turn of the Century.* New York: Hill and Wang, 1978.

Katz, Michael B. *In the Shadow of the Poorhouse: A Social History of Welfare in America.* New York: Basic Books, 1986.

Katz, Michael B. "What Kind of a Problem Is Poverty? The Archaeology of an Idea." In *Territories of Poverty: Rethinking North and South,* edited by Ananya Roy and Emma Shaw Crane, 39–78. Athens: University of Georgia Press, 2015.

Kaufman, Martin. *American Medical Education: The Formative Years, 1765–1910.* Westport, CT: Greenwood, 1976.

Keefer, Truman Frederick. *Ernest Poole.* New York: Twayne, 1966.

Keefer, Truman Frederick. "The Literary Career and Literary Productions of Ernest Poole, American Novelist." PhD diss., Duke University, 1961.

Kenny, Kevin. *The American Irish: A History.* Harlow, Essex, UK: Longman, 2000.

Kessner, Thomas. *The Golden Door: Italian and Jewish Immigrant Mobility in New York City, 1880–1915.* New York: Oxford, 1977.

Klebs, Arnold. Review of *A Handbook on the Prevention of Tuberculosis,* by Charity Organization Society of the City of New York. *Charities* 12 (1904): 353.

Knopf, S. A. "The Duties of the Individual and the Government in the Combat of Tuberculosis." In Charity Organization Society of the City of New York, *Handbook for the Prevention of Tuberculosis,* 173–204.

Knopf, S. A. "A Plea for Justice to the Consumptive." *Medical Record* 65 (1904): 1–7.

Knopf, S. A. *Pulmonary Tuberculosis: Its Modern Prophylaxis and the Treatment in Special Institutions and at Home.* Philadelphia: P. Blakiston's Son, 1899.

Knopf, S. A. "The Tenement and Tuberculosis." *Journal of the American Medical Association* 34, no. 19 (1900): 1151–54.

Knopf, S. A. *Tuberculosis as a Disease of the Masses and How to Combat It.* New York: M. Firestack, 1901.

Koch, Robert. "The Aetiology of Tuberculosis." *American Review of Tuberculosis* 25, no. 3 (1932): 285–323.

Kohn, Edward P., ed. *A Most Glorious Ride: The Diaries of Theodore Roosevelt, 1877–1886.* Albany: State University of New York Press, 2014.

Kraut, Alan M. *Silent Travelers: Germs, Genes, and the "Immigrant Menace".* Baltimore, MD: Johns Hopkins University Press, 1994.

Kurland, Gerald. *Seth Low: The Reformer in an Urban and Industrial Age.* New York: Twayne, 1971.

BIBLIOGRAPHY

Lane, James B. *Jacob Riis and the American City*. Port Washington, NY: Kennikat, 1974.

Lears, T. J. Jackson. *No Place of Grace: Antimodernism and the Transformation of American Culture, 1880–1920*. Chicago: University of Chicago Press, 1981.

Leavitt, Judith Walzer. *Typhoid Mary: Captive to the Public's Health*. Boston: Beacon, 1996.

Lee, Joseph. "Preventive Work." *Charities* 6 (1901): 176–85.

LeFebvre, Henri. *The Production of Space*. Translated by Donald Nicholson-Smith. Oxford: Blackwell, 1991.

Library of Congress. *Select List of References on the Negro Question*. Washington, DC: Government Printing Office, 1906.

"A Life of Service." *Health News*, 18, no. 7 (July 1923): 161–63.

Lin, Jan Chien. "The Changing Economy of the Lower East Side." In *From Urban Village to East Village: The Battle for New York's Lower East Side*, edited by Janet L. Abu-Lughod, 43–62. Cambridge: Blackwell, 1994.

Loomis, Henry P. "The Climatic and Sanatorium Treatment of Consumption." In Charity Organization Society of the City of New York, *Handbook for the Prevention of Tuberculosis*, 227–39.

Low, Benjamin R. C. *Seth Low*. New York: AMS, 1971.

Lowell, Josephine Shaw. "The Economic and Moral Effects of Public Outdoor Relief." *Proceedings of the Seventh Annual National Conference of Charities and Correction*, 81–91. Boston: George H. Ellis, 1890.

Lowell, Josephine Shaw. "Five Months' Work for the Unemployed in New York City." *Charities Review* 3 (1894): 323–42.

Lowell, Josephine Shaw. "Methods of Relief for the Unemployed." *Forum* 16 (1894): 655–62.

Lowry, Edward. "Reform Results in New York." *World's Work* 6, no. 5 (1903): 3904–8.

Lubove, Roy. *The Progressives and the Slums: Tenement House Reform in New York City, 1890–1917*. Pittsburgh: University of Pittsburgh Press, 1962.

Ludmerer, Kenneth M. *Learning to Heal: The Development of American Medical Education*. New York: Basic Books, 1985.

"Lung Block or Park-Playground—Which?" *Charities* 11, no. 15 (1903): 335–37.

Malone, Sylvester L., ed. *Dr. Edward McGlynn*. New York: Dr. McGlynn Monument Association, 1918.

Markel, Howard. "The Extraordinary Dr. Biggs." *Journal of the American Medical Association* 305, no. 23 (2011): 2473–74.

Markel, Howard. *Quarantine! East European Jewish Immigrants and the New York City Epidemics of 1892*. Baltimore, MD: Johns Hopkins University Press, 1997.

Marshall, Edward. "New York Tenements." *North American Review* 157, no. 445 (1893): 753–56.

Mays, Thomas J. "Increase of Insanity and Consumption among the Negro Population of the South since the War." *Boston Medical and Surgical Journal* 136, no. 22 (June 3, 1897): 537–40.

McCabe, James D. *Lights and Shadows of New York Life; or, The Sights and Sensations of the Great City*. Philadelphia: National, 1872.

McCaffrey, Lawrence. "Forging Forward and Looking Back." In *The New York Irish*, edited by Ronald H. Bayor and Timothy J. Meagher, 213–33. Baltimore, MD: Johns Hopkins University Press, 1996.

McClellan, George B. Jr. *The Gentleman and the Tiger: The Autobiography of George B. McClellan, Jr.*, edited by Harold C. Syrett. Philadelphia: J. B. Lippincott, 1956.

McDannell, Colleen. "Going to the Ladies' Fair: Irish Catholics in New York City, 1870–1900." In *The New York Irish*, edited by Ronald H. Bayor and Timothy J. Meagher. Baltimore, MD: Johns Hopkins University Press, 1996.

McGerr, Michael. *A Fierce Discontent: The Rise and Fall of the Progressive Movement in America, 1870–1920*. Oxford: Oxford University Press, 2005.

McKie, T. J. "A Brief History of Insanity and Tuberculosis in the Southern Negro." *Journal of the American Medical Association* 28, no. 12 (March 20, 1897): 537–38.

McLeod, Hugh. *Piety and Poverty: Working-Class Religion in Berlin, London, and New York, 1870–1914*. New York: Holmes & Meyer, 1996.

Meehan, Thomas F. "Right Rev. John J. Kean." In *Historical Records and Studies* 10, edited by Rev. Joseph F. Delany, Stephen Farrelly, and Thomas F. Meehan, 194–95. New York: United States Catholic Historical Society, 1917.

Merriam, W. R. "The Census in Foreign Countries." *Century Illustrated Magazine* 66 (October 1903): 879–86.

Miller, Kerby A. *Emigrants and Exiles: Ireland and the Irish Exodus to North America*. New York: Oxford University Press, 1985.

Mitchell, Joseph. *The Bottom of the Harbor*. New York: Knopf Doubleday, 2008.

Morgenthau, Henry. "A National Constructive Programme for City Planning." *First National Conference on City Planning*, 59–60. Washington, DC: Government Printing Office, 1909.

Morison, Elting, ed. *The Letters of Theodore Roosevelt*. Cambridge, MA: Harvard University Press, 1951.

Mulrine, M. Barbara. *The Price of Honor: The Life and Times of George Brinton McClellan Jr.* Madison, NJ: Fairleigh Dickinson University Press, 2011.

Muncy, Robyn. *Creating a Female Dominion in American Reform, 1890–1935*. New York: Oxford University Press, 1991.

Murlin, Edgar L. *New York Red Book*. Albany: J. B. Lyon, 1912.

Nasaw, David. *Children of the City: At Work and at Play*. Garden City, NY: Doubleday, 1985.

Nicoli, Matthias. "Foreword." *Health News* 18, no. 7 (1923): 159–61.

O'Connor, Alice. *Poverty Knowledge: Social Science, Social Policy, and the Poor in Twentieth-Century U.S. History*. Princeton, NJ: Princeton University Press, 2001.

O'Donnell, Edward T. *Henry George and the Crisis of Inequality: Progress and Poverty in the Gilded Age.* New York: Columbia University Press, 2015.

Ogle, Maureen. *All the Modern Conveniences: American Household Plumbing, 1840–1890.* Baltimore, MD: John Hopkins University Press, 1996.

Olmsted, Frederick L. *Public Parks and the Enlargement of Towns.* Cambridge, MA: Riverside, 1870.

Olmsted, Frederick L., and Theodora Kimball, eds. *Forty Years of Landscape Architecture: Central Park.* Cambridge: MIT Press, 1973.

Oshinsky, David. *Bellevue: Three Centuries of Medicine and Mayhem at America's Most Storied Hospital.* New York: Doubleday, 2016.

Otis, Edward O. "The Causes and Conditions of Pulmonary Tuberculosis, and How to Avoid Them." *American Journal of the Medical Sciences* 116, no. 5 (1898): 534–39.

Otis, Edward O. "The Significance of the Tuberculosis Crusade and Its Future." *Journal of the American Social Science Association* 42 (1904): 120–32.

Ott, Katherine. *Fevered Lives: Tuberculosis in American Culture since 1870.* Cambridge, MA: Harvard University Press, 1996.

Page, Max. *The Creative Destruction of Manhattan, 1900–1940.* Chicago: University of Chicago Press, 1999.

Palmieri, Patricia Ann. *In Adamless Eden: The Community of Women Faculty at Wellesley.* New Haven, CT: Yale University Press, 1995.

"Paragraphs in Philanthropy." *Charities* 11, no. 26 (1903): 595–602.

Park, William H. "Tribute to Dr. Biggs from Some of His Colleagues." *Health News* 18 (1923): 164–65.

Parks and Playgrounds Association. *Statement Relating to Recreation in Greater New York.* New York: Parks and Playgrounds Association, 1910.

Penn, Susan A. "Ernest Poole: Novelist as Social Interpreter, 1902–1950." PhD diss., University of Wisconsin, 1968.

People of the State of New York ex rel. Lawrence Veiller v. Thomas J. Brady. In *Reports of Cases Heard and Determined in the Appellate Division of the Supreme Court of the State of New York,* vol. 43, 60–67. Albany, NY: Banks, 1899.

Pink, Louis H. *The New Day in Housing.* New York: John Day, 1928.

Pink, Louis H. *Old Tenements and the New Law.* New York: University Settlement Society, 1907.

Plunz, Richard. *A History of Housing in New York City.* New York: Columbia University Press, 1990.

Poole, Ernest. "April, 1903: The Prayer of the Tenement." *Charities* 12, no. 15 (1904): 394.

Poole, Ernest. "April, 1904: The Prayer Unanswered." *Charities* 12, no. 15 (1904): 395.

Poole, Ernest. *The Bridge: My Own Story.* New York: Macmillan, 1940.

Poole, Ernest. "Harnessing Socialism." *American Magazine* 66 (1908): 427–32.

Poole, Ernest. "The Lung Block: Some Pictures of Consumption in Its Stronghold." *Charities* 11 (1903): 193–99.

Poole, Ernest. *The Plague in Its Stronghold: Tuberculosis in the New York Tenement.* New York: Charity Organization Society, 1903.

Poole, Ernest. "The Song That Failed." *Charities* 12, no. 16 (1904): 418.

Poole, Ernest. "Waifs of the Street." *McClure's*, May 1903, 40–48.

Poole, Ernest, and William Hard. "The Stockyard Strike: Competitive Wages and the Right to Live." *Outlook* 77 (1904): 884–89.

Prudden, T. Mitchell. *Dust and Its Dangers.* New York: G. P. Putnam, 1899.

Prudden, T. Mitchell. *The Story of the Bacteria and Their Relations to Health and Disease.* New York: G. P. Putnam, 1889.

Prudden, T. Mitchell. "Tuberculosis and Its Prevention." In Charity Organization Society of the City of New York, *Handbook for the Prevention of Tuberculosis,* 243–59.

Randall, Mercedes M. *Improper Bostonian: Emily Greene Balch, Nobel Peace Laureate, 1946.* New York: Twayne, 1964.

Rauch, John H. *Report on Public Parks: Their Effects upon the Moral Physical and Sanitary Condition of the Inhabitants of Large Cities.* Chicago: S. C. Griggs, 1869.

Recchiuti, John Louis. *Civic Engagement: Social Science and Progressive-Era Reform in New York City.* Philadelphia: University of Pennsylvania Press, 2007.

"Report of Joint Special Committee Appointed to Confer with Park Commissioners, in Relation to Public Parks." In *Documents of the City of Boston for the Year 1876,* 1–14. Boston: Rockwell and Churchill, 1877.

Report of the Special Committee of the Assembly, Appointed to Investigate the Public Offices and Departments of the City of New York. Albany, NY: James B. Lyon, 1900.

"Report of the Committee on Hygiene." *Medical Record* 51, no. 13 (1897): 462.

Report of the Tenement House Committee as Authorized by Chapter 479 of the Laws of 1894. Albany, NY, 1895.

Reppetto, Thomas A. *American Police: The Blue Parade, 1845–1945.* New York: Enigma Books, 2011.

Reynolds, James B. "Report of Head Worker." In *University Settlement Society: Report of the Year's Work, December, 1894,* by University Settlement Society of New York, 7–10. New York, 1894.

Riis, Jacob. *The Battle with the Slum.* New York: Macmillan, 1902.

Riis, Jacob. "A Blast of Cheer." In *Proceedings of the 28th National Conference of Charities and Correction,* 18–23. Boston: George H. Ellis, 1901.

Riis, Jacob A. *The Children of the Poor.* New York: Charles Scribner's Sons, 1892.

Riis, Jacob. "The Clearing of Mulberry Bend." *Review of Reviews* 12 (1895): 172–78.

Riis, Jacob. "Has Reform Made Good?" *Outlook* 75 (1903): 18–23.

Riis, Jacob. "Homeless Waifs of the City." *Harper's Young People*, January 22, 1889, 204–5.

Riis, Jacob A. *How the Other Half Lives: Studies among the Tenements of New York.* New York: Charles Scribner's Sons, 1890.

Riis, Jacob A. *The Making of an American.* New York: Macmillan, 1901.

Riis, Jacob A. *The Old Town.* New York: Macmillan, 1909.

Riis, Jacob A. *The Peril and the Preservation of the Home.* Philadelphia: George W. Jacobs, 1903.

Riis, Jacob A. *The Ten Years' War: An Account of the Battle with the Slum in New York.* Boston: Houghton Mifflin, 1900.

Riis, Jacob A. *Theodore Roosevelt: The Citizen.* New York: Macmillan, 1912.

Riis, Jacob. "What Settlements Stand For." *Outlook* 89 (1908): 69–72.

Riordon, William L. *Plunkitt of Tammany Hall.* New York: McClure, Phillips, 1905.

Roberts, Frederick T. *Theory and Practice of Medicine.* Philadelphia: P. Blakiston, Son & Co., 1884.

Roberts, Samuel Kelton, Jr. *Infectious Fear: Politics, Disease, and the Health Effects of Segregation.* Chapel Hill: University of North Carolina Press, 2009.

Rodgers, Daniel T. *Atlantic Crossings: Social Politics in a Progressive Age.* Cambridge, MA: Harvard University Press, 1998.

Rode's New York City Directory, for 1852–53. New York: Charles R. Rode, 1852.

Roohan, James Edmund. *American Catholics and the Social Question, 1865–1900.* New York: Arno, 1976.

Roosevelt, Theodore. "Value of an Athletic Training." *Harper's Weekly,* December 23, 1893, 1236.

Rosenberg, Charles E. *The Cholera Years: The United States in 1832, 1859, and 1866.* Chicago: University of Chicago Press, 1962.

Rosenzweig, Roy, and Elizabeth Blackmar. *The Park and the People: A History of Central Park.* Ithaca, NY: Cornell University Press, 1992.

Rosner, David, ed. *Hives of Sickness: Public Health and Epidemics in New York City.* New Brunswick, NJ: Rutgers University Press, 1995.

Rosner, Henry J. "The RFC Subsidizes Fred F. French." *Nation,* April 19, 1933, 438–39.

Rothman, Sheila M. *Living in the Shadow of Death: Tuberculosis and the Social Experience of Illness in American History.* Baltimore, MD: Johns Hopkins University Press, 1994.

Rothman, Sheila M. *Woman's Proper Place: A History of Changing Ideals and Practices, 1870 to the Present.* New York: Basic Books, 1978.

Rothstein, William G. *American Physicians in the Nineteenth Century: From Sects to Science.* Baltimore, MD: Johns Hopkins University Press, 1972.

Rousmaniere, John P. "Cultural Hybrid in the Slums: The College Woman and the Settlement House, 1889–1894." *American Quarterly* 22, no. 1 (1970): 45–66.

Rybczynski, Witold. *A Clearing in the Distance: Frederick Law Olmsted and America in the Nineteenth Century.* New York: Scribner, 1999.

Sachs, Theodore B. "Tuberculosis in the Jewish District of Chicago." *Journal of the American Medical Association* 43, no. 6 (1904): 390–95.

Sampsell-Willmann, Kate. *Lewis Hine as Social Critic*. Jackson: University Press of Mississippi, 2009.

Sayre, Wallace S., and Herbert Kaufman. *Governing New York City: Politics in the Metropolis*. New York: Russell Sage Foundation, 1960.

Scobey, David M. *Empire City: The Making and Meaning of the New York City Landscape*. Philadelphia: Temple University Press, 2002.

Sedgwick, William T. "Modern Medicine and the Public Health." *Public Health Reports* 36, no. 4 (1921): 109–16.

Shah, Nayan. *Contagious Divides: Epidemics and Race in San Francisco's Chinatown*. Berkeley: University of California Press, 2001.

Shanaberger, Manuel S. "Jeff." "Edward McGlynn: A Missionary Priest and His Social Gospel." *U.S. Catholic Historian* 13, no. 3 (1995): 23–47.

Shannon, William V. *The American Irish: A Political and Social Portrait*. Amherst: University of Massachusetts Press, 1963.

Shattuck, F. C. "Specialism, the Laboratory, and Practical Medicine." *Boston Medical and Surgical Journal* 136 (1897): 613–17.

Shea, John Gilmary. *The Catholic Churches of New York City*. New York: Goulding, 1878.

Shelley, Thomas J. "Ubiquitously Useful: The Jesuit College of St. Francis Xavier, New York City, 1847–1912." *Catholic Historical Review* 101, no. 3 (2015): 463–87.

Shrady, George F. "The Health Board and Its Official Diagnosis." *Medical Record* 51 (1897): 270–71.

Slayton, Robert A. *Empire Statesman: The Rise and Redemption of Al Smith*. New York: Free Press, 2001.

Smith, Alfred E. *Up to Now: An Autobiography*. Garden City, NY: Garden City, 1929.

Smith, F. B. *The Retreat of Tuberculosis, 1850–1950*. London: Croom Helm, 1988.

Smith, John Talbot. "The Homes of the Poor." *Catholic World* 45 (1887): 510–12.

Smith, John Talbot. "The Mayor and the Tenements." *Harper's Weekly*, October 15, 1881, 699.

Smith, Stephen. "Riots and Their Prevention." *American Medical Times* 7 (1863): 41–42.

Soja, Edward W. *Postmodern Geographies: The Reassertion of Space in Critical Social Theory*. New York: Verso, 1989.

Solomon, Barbara Miller. *In the Company of Educated Women: A History of Women and Higher Education in America*. New Haven, CT: Yale University Press, 1985.

"The Sources of Tammany's Power." *Outlook*, February 21, 1903, 419–21.

Sproat, John G. *"The Best Men": Liberal Reformers in the Gilded Age*. New York: Oxford University Press, 1968.

Stansell, Christine. *City of Women: Sex and Class in New York, 1789–1860*. Urbana: University of Illinois Press, 1987.

Starr, Paul. *The Social Transformation of American Medicine*. New York: Basic Books, 1982.

Stead, William. "Mr. Croker and Greater New York." *Review of Reviews* 16 (1897): 341–55.

Steffens, Lincoln. "Jacob A. Riis, Reporter, Reformer, American Citizen." *McClure's*, August 1903, 419–25.

Steffens, Lincoln. "New York: Good Government in Danger." *McClure's*, November 1903, 84–92.

Stella, Antonio. "Tuberculosis and the Italians in the United States." *Charities* 12 (1904): 486–89.

Stott, Richard B. *Workers in the Metropolis: Class, Ethnicity, and Youth in Antebellum New York City*. Ithaca, NY: Cornell University Press, 1990.

Stover, Charles. "Playground Progress in Seward Park." *Charities* 6 (1901): 386–93.

Stover, Charles. "Seward Park Playground at Last a Reality." *Charities* 10 (1903): 127–33.

Strong, George Templeton. *The Diary of George Templeton Strong*. Edited by Allan Nevins and Milton Halsey Thomas. New York: Macmillan, 1952.

Swett, Steven. "Test of a Reformer: A Study of Seth Low, New York City Mayor 1902–1903." *New-York Historical Quarterly* 44 (1960): 5–42.

Taylor, Graham Romeyn. "Chicago and the Social Settlement Movement." *Chicago the Great Central Market: A Magazine of Business* 4, no. 3 (July, 1907): 72–80.

Taylor, S. B. "The Duty of a Physician to a Tubercular Patient and to the Public." *Columbus Medical Journal* 18 (1897): 18–22.

Teller, Michael E. *The Tuberculosis Movement: A Public Health Campaign in the Progressive Era*. New York: Greenwood, 1988.

Thacher, David. "Olmsted's Police." *Law and History Review* 33, no. 3 (2015): 577–620.

Tice, Karen W. *Tales of Wayward Girls and Immoral Women: Case Records and the Professionalization of Social Work*. Urbana: University of Illinois Press, 1998.

Tolman, William. "The Tenement House Curse: Evils of the System." *Arena* 9 (1894): 659–62.

Tomes, Nancy. *The Gospel of Germs: Men, Women, and the Microbe in American Life*. Cambridge, MA: Harvard University Press, 1998.

Trow's New York City Directory. New York: J. F. Trow, 1872.

Trow's New York City Directory. New York: J. F. Trow, 1889.

Trow's New York City Directory. New York: J. F. Trow, 1903.

Trow's New York City Directory, 1857–58. New York: J. F. Trow, 1858.

Tsanoff, Stoyan Basil. "Children's Playgrounds." *Municipal Affairs* 2 (1898): 294–99.

Valentine, D. T. *Manual of the Corporation of the City of New York for 1855*. New York: McSpedon and Baker, 1855.

Valentine, D. T. *Manual of the Corporation of the City of New York for 1860*. New York: McSpedon and Baker, 1860.

Van Kleeck, Mary. "A Census of College Women." *Journal of the Association of Collegiate Alumnae* 11 (1918): 557–91.

Vaughn, Gerald F. "Katharine Coman: America's First Woman Institutional Economist and a Champion of Education for Citizenship." *Journal of Economic Issues* 38, no. 4 (2004): 989–1002.

Veiller, Bayard. *The Fun I've Had*. New York: Reynal and Hitchcock, 1941.

Veiller, Lawrence. *Housing Reform*. New York: Russell Sage Foundation, 1910.

Veiller, Lawrence. "New York's New Building Code." *Charities Review* 9 (1899): 388–91.

Veiller, Lawrence. "A Recent Phase of Relief Work." *Century Illustrated Magazine* 48, no. 3 (July 1894): 474–77.

Veiller, Lawrence. "Tenement House Exhibit of 1899." *Charities Review* 9 (1900): 19–25.

Veiller, Lawrence. "Tenement House Exhibition." *Gunton's Magazine* 17 (1899): 321–22.

Veiller, Lawrence. "Tenement House Reform in New York, 1834–1900." New York: Evening Post Job, 1900.

Villard, Oswald Garrison. "The Low Administration." *Nation*, January 2, 1902, 5–6.

Vrooman, Walter. "Municipal Playgrounds." *Garden and Forest* 9 (1896): 501–2.

Vrooman, Walter. "Playgrounds for Children." *Arena* 10 (1894): 286.

Wald, Lillian D. *The House on Henry Street*. New York: Henry Holt, 1915.

Walsh, Joseph. "History of the Pennsylvania Society." In *Annual Report of the Pennsylvania Society for the Prevention of Tuberculosis*, 3–13. Philadelphia: Pennsylvania Society for the Prevention of Tuberculosis, 1906.

Ward, David. *Poverty, Ethnicity, and the American City, 1840–1925: Changing Conceptions of the Slum and the Ghetto*. New York: Cambridge University Press, 1989.

Ward, Frank. "A Study of the Deaths from Tuberculosis in the Fifth Ward (Philadelphia) during a Period of Forty-Seven Years." *American Journal of Public Health* 3 (1913): 24–33.

Wardman, Ervin. "Men and Issues of the New York City Campaign." *Review of Reviews* 28 (1903): 545–55.

Ware, Louise. *Jacob Riis: Police Reporter, Reformer, Useful Citizen*. New York: D. Appleton-Century, 1938.

Warner, Emily Smith. *The Happy Warrior: A Biography of My Father, Alfred E. Smith*. Garden City: Doubleday, 1956.

Waugh, Joan. "'Give This Man Work!': Josephine Shaw Lowell, the Charity Organization Society of the City of New York, and the Depression of 1893." *Social Science History* 25, no. 2 (2001): 217–46.

Weber, Robert David. "The Social Function of New York Municipal Parks, 1850–1900." Master's thesis, University of Wisconsin, 1965.

BIBLIOGRAPHY

"Whole World Wars with Tuberculosis." *Charities* 11, no. 9 (1903): 176–78.

Wiebe, Robert H. *The Search for Order, 1877–1920*. New York: Hill and Wang, 1967.

Williams, Alberta. "White Collar Neighbors." *New Yorker*, November 24, 1934, 68–79.

Wilson, Leonard G. "The Historical Decline of Tuberculosis in Europe and America: Its Causes and Significance." *Journal of the History of Medicine and Allied Sciences* 45, no. 3 (1990): 366–96.

Wingate, Charles F. "The Moral Side to the Tenement-House Problem." *Catholic World* 41 (1885): 160–64.

Winslow, C.-E. A. *The Life of Hermann M. Biggs, M.D., D.Sc., LL.D., Physician and Statesman of the Public Health*. Philadelphia: Lea & Febiger, 1929.

Wood, Edith Elmer. *The Housing of the Unskilled Wage Earner*. New York: Macmillan, 1919.

Woodcock, H. de Carle. *The Doctor and the People*. London: Methuen, 1912.

Yochelson, Bonnie, and Daniel Czitrom. *Rediscovering Jacob Riis: Exposure Journalism and Photography in Turn-of-the-Century New York*. New York: New Press, 2007.

INDEX

INDEX

Tenement House Committee (THC), 39–40, 48, 50, 56

Tenement House Department of the City of New York (THD), 48, 54, 174n9; and Lung Block park campaign, 98, 100–101, 120–21, 126, 195n1; and "Lung Block" renovations, 141–42, 207n2

Tenement House Exhibition, 40–44, 46, 169n106, 169n108, 170n112, 172n156; "Lung Block" featured in, 51; significance, 27, 49

Tenement House Law of 1901, 47–48, 54, 141, 174n9

tuberculosis, 84, 176n35; and germ theory, 16; and growth of public-health establishment, 9–10, 17, 24, 159n47, 161n70; and housing reform, 27, 46, 51–52; and poverty, 53–54, 113; as basis for class conflict, 5–6, 143, 156n9; changing etiology, 10–12, 18, 53, 142, 157n11, 159n45, 159n52; definition, 10, 159n44; mortality, 55, 64, 66–67, 175n13, 179n72, 179n74, 179nn78–79; prevention and treatment strategies, 53, 57–58, 157n12, 160n56, 162n87, 174n3, 176n30; surveillance methods, 10, 18–21, 25, 160n61, 160n65; transmission theories, 21–23, 57–58, 123, 160n60, 161n77, 162n80, 207n5. *See also* antispitting measures; disease maps; "house infection"

University Settlement, 28–29, 31, 39, 143, 172n156, 195n1; and muckraking, 55, 69, 72, 79–80, 181n96, 182n106, 184n144

Van Wyck, Robert, 94, 128, 204n114

Veiller, Bayard, 163n5, 164n6; 164n11

Veiller, Lawrence Turnure, 4, 49–51, 119, 152, 173n164, 173n166; approach to reform, 27, 39, 47, 145, 147, 172n152, 208n22; background and education, 27–28, 164n6, 164n11; and Department of Buildings, 39–40, 168n92, 168n100; historians' portrayals, 27, 163nn4–5, 173n159; and Jacob Riis, 83, 95, 109, 165n25, 172n157; and Lung Block park campaign, 51–52, 97, 106, 110, 120–21, 125, 127; personality attributes, 38–39, 44, 48, 51, 69, 163n5

Wald, Lillian, 56, 90, 95, 146, 182n111; and Lung Block park campaign, 120, 123, 142, 208n24

Welch, William T., 13, 157n28

Wellesley College, 59–60, 68, 79, 177n44, 177n46, 177nn53–54

Willcox, William R., 99–100, 107–8, 110, 121, 123

Wingate, Charles F., 34, 36

women in social professions, 54–55, 59–60, 63–64, 78–79, 177n49, 178n69, 184n139